Oral Health Care Access

Guest Editor

GARY A. COLANGELO, DDS, MGA

DENTAL CLINICS OF NORTH AMERICA

www.dental.theclinics.com

July 2009 • Volume 53 • Number 3

SAUNDERS an imprint of ELSEVIER, Inc.

W.B. SAUNDERS COMPANY
A Division of Elsevier Inc.

1600 John F. Kennedy Boulevard • Suite 1800 • Philadelphia, Pennsylvania 19103-2899

http://www.dental.theclinics.com

DENTAL CLINICS OF NORTH AMERICA Volume 53, Number 3
July 2009 ISSN 0011-8532, ISBN-13: 978-1-4377-1207-0, ISBN-10: 1-4377-1207-X

Editor: John Vassallo; j.vassallo@elsevier.com
Developmental Editor: Theresa Collier

Dental Clinics of North America (ISSN 0011-8532) is published quarterly by Elsevier Inc., 360 Park Avenue South, New York, NY 10010-1710. Months of issue are January, April, July, and October. Business and Editorial Offices: 1600 John F. Kennedy Boulevard, Suite 1800, Philadelphia, PA 19103-2899. Customer Service Office: 11830 Westline Industrial Drive, St. Louis, MO 63146. Periodicals postage paid at New York, NY and additional mailing offices. Subscription prices are $207.00 per year (domestic individuals), $347.00 per year (domestic institutions), $100.00 per year (domestic students/residents), $246.00 per year (Canadian individuals), $437.00 per year (Canadian institutions), $297.00 per year (international individuals), $437.00 per year (international institutions), and $150.00 per year (international and Canadian students/residents. International air speed delivery is included in all *Clinics* subscription prices. All prices are subject to change without notice. **POSTMASTER:** Send address changes to *Dental Clinics of North America*, 11830 Westline Industrial Drive, St. Louis, MO 63146. **Customer Service (orders, claims, online, change of address): Elsevier Periodicals Customer Service, 11830 Westline Industrial Drive, St. Louis, MO 63146. Tel: 1-800-654-2452 (U.S. and Canada). Fax: 314-523-5170. E-mail: journalscustomerservice-usa@elsevier.com (for print support); journalsonlinesupport-usa@elsevier.com (for online support).**

Reprints. For copies of 100 or more, of articles in this publication, please contact the Commercial Reprints Department, Elsevier Inc., 360 Park Avenue South, New York, NY 10010-1710. Tel.: 212-633-3812; Fax: 212-462-1935; E-mail: reprints@elsevier.com.

The *Dental Clinics of North America* is covered in *MEDLINE/PubMed (Index Medicus), Current Contents/Clinical Medicine, ISI/BIOMED* and *Clinahl.*

Printed and bound by CPI Group (UK) Ltd, Croydon, CR0 4YY
Transferred to Digital Print 2011

Contributors

GUEST EDITOR

GARY A. COLANGELO, DDS, MGA
Clinical Associate Professor, Baltimore College of Dental Surgery, Dental School, University of Maryland, Baltimore, Maryland

AUTHORS

OSCAR AREVALO, DDS, ScD, MBA, MS
Assistant Professor and Chief, Division of Dental Public Health, Department of Oral Health Science, University of Kentucky College of Dentistry, Lexington, Kentucky

RENE CHAPIN, BSJ
Director of Membership and Communications, National Association of Dental Plans, Dallas, Texas

HONG CHEN, DDS, MS
Adjunct Assistant Professor, School of Dentistry, University of North Carolina, Chapel Hill, North Carolina

LEONARD A. COHEN, DDS, MPH, MS
Professor, Department of Health Promotion and Policy, Division of Health Services Research, University of Maryland Dental School, Baltimore, Maryland

GARY A. COLANGELO, DDS, MGA
Clinical Associate Professor, Baltimore College of Dental Surgery, Dental School, University of Maryland, Baltimore, Maryland

COUNCIL ON ACCESS, PREVENTION AND INTERPROFESSIONAL RELATIONS
American Dental Association, Chicago, Illinois

COUNCIL ON DENTAL PRACTICE, AMERICAN DENTAL ASSOCIATION
American Dental Association, Chicago, Illinois

ELAINE DAVIS, PhD
Member, CARES Advisory Board; Associate Dean for Student Affairs, and Associate Professor, Department of Oral Diagnostic Sciences, University at Buffalo, School of Dental Medicine, Buffalo, New York

JOAN M. DORIS, DSW
Assistant Professor, Department of Pediatric and Community Dentistry, School of Dental Medicine; Assistant Professor, School of Social Work; Research Director, CARES Program, University at Buffalo, Buffalo, New York

CYNTHIA DU PONT, MSW
Director, CARES Program, University at Buffalo, School of Dental Medicine, Buffalo, New York

BURTON L. EDELSTEIN, DDS, MPH
Founding Chair, Children's Dental Health Project of Washington DC, Washington, District of Columbia; Professor of Dentistry, College of Dental Medicine; and Professor of Health Policy and Management, Mailman School of Public Health, Columbia University, New York, New York

JAMES FRICTON, DDS, MS
Professor, University of Minnesota School of Dentistry, Minneapolis, Minnesota

SHELLY GEHSHAN, MPP
Director, Advancing Children's Dental Health Initiative, The Pew Charitable Trusts, Washington, District of Columbia

FRANK J. GRAHAM, DMD, ABO
Diplomate, American Board of Orthodontists; Chair, Council on Dental Practice, American Dental Association, Chicago, Illinois

KRISTEN L. HATHAWAY, BS
Director of Government Relations, National Association of Dental Plans, Dallas, Texas

BRITT HOLDAWAY, MSW
Assistant Director, CARES Program, University at Buffalo, School of Dental Medicine, Buffalo, New York

RICHARD J. MANSKI, DDS, MBA, PhD
Division of Health Services Research, Department of Health Promotion and Policy, Dental School, University of Maryland, Baltimore, Maryland

DAVID A. NASH, DMD, MS, EdD
William R. Willard Professor of Dental Education, and Professor of Pediatric Dentistry, Department of Pediatric Dentistry, College of Dentistry, University of Kentucky, Lexington, Kentucky

LINDSEY A. ROBINSON, DDS
Chair, Council on Access, Prevention and Interprofessional Relations, American Dental Association, Chicago, Illinois

JAMES T. RULE, DDS, MS
Professor Emeritus, Department of Pediatric Dentistry, University of Maryland Dental School, Easton, Maryland

ANDREW SNYDER, MPA
Senior Associate, Advancing Children's Dental Health Initiative, The Pew Charitable Trusts, Washington, District of Columbia

ERIC S. SOLOMON, MA, DDS
Executive Director, Department of Institutional Research, The Texas A&M Health Science Center; Professor, Department of Public Health Sciences, Baylor College of Dentistry, The Texas A&M Health Science Center, Dallas, Texas

CLEMENCIA M. VARGAS, DDS, PhD
Associate Professor, Department of Health Promotion and Policy, University of Maryland, Dental School, Baltimore, Maryland

JOS V.M. WELIE, MA, MMedS, JD, PhD
Professor of Medical and Dental Ethics, Center for Health Policy and Ethics, Creighton University, Omaha, Nebraska

Contents

The disadvantaged suffer disproportionately from dental problems. These persons are more likely to have untreated oral health problems and associated pain, and also are more likely to forego dental treatment even when in pain. There has been increased emphasis on the potential role of physicians in alleviating oral health disparities, especially among children. In addition, many adults lacking access to traditional dental services seek care and consultation from hospital emergency departments, physicians, and pharmacists. The delivery of oral health care services by non-dental health professionals may assume increasing importance as the population continues to age and becomes more diverse. This is because, in general, the elderly and ethnic and racial minorities face significant economic barriers to accessing private dental services.

This article documents the disparities in oral health among children, identifies barriers to access to care for children, describes the use of dental therapists internationally to improve access to care for children, documents previous efforts in the United States to train individuals other than dentists to care for children's teeth, describes the current status of the use of dental therapists in Alaska, justifies limiting the care given by dental therapists to children, suggests potential economic advantages of using dental therapists, and concludes by describing how dental therapists could be trained and deployed in the United States to improve access to care for children and reduce disparities in oral health.

Disparities remain among the United States population with regard to who receives dental treatment. This article assesses current programs designed to provide dental insurance coverage. This assessment examines person-level use and expenditures as a function of preferences, price, and the use of third-party coverage.

Dental coverage provides a means to obtain oral care, which is an important component of overall health. This article discusses the common forms of dental health plans, the services usually covered, and their relative costs.

Dentists and the dental health care industry have a renewed interest in clinical risk assessment, because they offer the potential to identify a patient's clinical needs for oral health care more specifically, to maximize prevention by early intervention, and to educate patients to become more informed consumers of oral health care and direct resources where they are most needed and can produce the greatest value. To realize this potential, risk assessment must be applied appropriately, and its indirect ramifications for access to care should be considered. Several ideas for the appropriate application of risk assessment are discussed and the ramifications for access to care are explored.

Despite vast improvements in the oral health status of the United States population over the past 50 years, disparities in oral health status continue, with certain segments of the population carrying a disproportionate disease burden. This article attempts to describe the problem, discuss various frameworks for action, illustrate some solutions developed by the private sector, and present a vision for collaborative action to improve the health of the nation. No one sector of the health care system can resolve the problem. The private sector, the public sector, and the not-for-profit community must collaborate to improve the oral health of the nation.

Teledentistry is an exciting new area of dentistry that fuses electronic health records, telecommunications technology, digital imaging, and the Internet to link health providers in rural or remote communities. For the patient located in underserved or remote areas, teledentistry improves ready access to preventive dental care and teleconsultation with specialists. It allows the dentist in the nearby community to provide easier access to preventive care to a patient who, otherwise, probably will not seek care. It enables the specialist located many miles away to make a diagnosis and recommend treatment options and/or referral.

Social work programs in dental schools and dental clinics have been operated successfully since the 1940s, and have been documented as contributing to patients' access to care and to dental education. However, unlike medical social work, with which it has much in common, social work in dentistry has failed to become a standard feature of dental schools and clinics. Few of the social work initiatives that have been implemented in dental schools have survived after initial grant funding ran out, or the institutional supporters of the program moved on. The authors hope that the CARES program serves as a model for the successful development of other programs at the intersection of social work and dentistry to the benefit of both dental patients and providers.

THE CLINICS ARE NOW AVAILABLE ONLINE!

Access your subscription at:
www.theclinics.com

Foreword

Dental access is a multifaceted problem and this issue of *Dental Clinics of North America* is equally multifaceted. Its contributors consider a wide range of issues: from ethical conundrums to logistic considerations, from private financing to national health policy, to informatics technology, and to workforce dynamics. Dr. Gary Colangelo, the Guest Editor for this issue, has approached the topic with a net as wide as the questions involved, engaging contributors who represent an equally wide range of philosophical and pragmatic perspectives.

Therefore, before launching into this text, it may be particularly helpful to gain an orientation to the problem of dental access. Stepping back to gain perspective before, and recurrently, during your reading of this text may help you identify the "take home" messages that will help define your personal response to the "access problem."

Since at least the late 1990s, access to healthcare, including oral healthcare, has been approached by government, the press, the healing professions, and advocates as a "disparities issue." The goal of much healthcare policy, whether public or private, local or national, has been to attain "health equity." Yet this approach is inherently curious as all of us recognize and typically accept the plethora of other social disparities daily: disparities in access to sound housing, effective transportation, fresh and nutritious foods, quality education, and safe streets. Unlike concerns for healthcare disparities, these other important social disparities are less commonly approached as issues of equity. Rather, they are typically addressed more from the perspective of assuring "basic" services. Judging from observations about our attitudes, actions, and public policies, our social compact appears to call for the guarantee of minimal, basic, humane levels of social services that are decent, if not equitable. Social Security, fair housing laws, building codes, mandatory public education, COBRA insurance continuation, the Food Stamp Program, Medicaid and Medicare, the Federal Deposit Insurance Corporation, and many other public programs all seek to ensure that everyone has access to basic social assurances. None of these typically American programs, however, calls for equity.

Yet healthcare is regarded differently, treated as an equity issue as though fairness in healthcare was of a different quality or magnitude than fairness in other social needs. This distinction is compounded by the growing understanding that health status is more significantly influenced by social determinants than by healthcare, making housing, education, safety, and nutrition issues more important than healthcare in achieving and maintaining health. One key question for the reader of this issue to keep in mind is the "what question": what is the goal of addressing dental access?

If the answer is minimal basic levels that are decent, if not equitable, the answer may lie in universal access to core services that at least relieve pain and infection. Current public policy, however, does not support even this level of response, because Medicare provides no coverage for treatment of dental conditions, and Medicaid leaves it to each state to determine whether even emergency oral heath services are available to adults. Until the Children's Health Insurance Program was amended in February 2009, not even children were assured of dental services as an essential component of basic healthcare coverage.

Dent Clin N Am 53 (2009) xi–xiii
doi:10.1016/j.cden.2009.03.013

dental.theclinics.com

If the answer is that all should have access to more sophisticated dental services, for example, access to services that restore people to oral function or reasonable aesthetics, then the access problem and challenges to its solution are considerably more demanding. Thus, a second question to keep in mind as you consider the contributions to this issue is "Access to what oral healthcare?"

Even as healthcare equity is debated, the question of personal versus public responsibility comes into play, particularly with regard to those made vulnerable by very young or very old age, by complicating health conditions (including both defects of birth and acquired diseases), and by our nation's racial and ethnic cultural diversity. Our collective legacy and continued attribute as a nation of immigrants further complicates this question of responsibility. The next question to keep in mind is "Whose problem is it?" Are differentials in access to oral healthcare a problem of government, the professions, parents, individuals, or all of the above?

Assuming that the answer is "all of the above," who has responsibility for which aspect? Is it essential that government provide, at a minimum, oral healthcare coverage for all and that the professions then deal with how to translate that coverage into care? Or is assurance of access to care a shared social responsibility, therefore attributable to government, and it is then the responsibility of individuals to use that care? These questions beg additional contextual questions. For example, are professional responses to access like Donated Dental Services, Missions of Mercy, Remote Access Medical, local voluntary efforts, and Give Kids a Smile exemplary displays of professional responsibility or insufficient patches to a failed system of care?

Policymakers speak of the "iron triangle," which details the seemingly irrefutable tradeoffs between cost, quality, and quantity of healthcare services. If we ensure that more people have access to care, it will either result in higher costs or will come at the cost of quality. Controlling costs must be offset either by providing fewer services or reducing quality of care. Raising quality can be offset either by spending more or providing care to fewer people. Already, healthcare costs are the single greatest expenditure in state budgets, with only public education competing for first place. In the larger context, US healthcare expenditures, of which oral healthcare comprises only one-twentieth, are the highest per capita and largest as a percentage of gross domestic product among developed countries, but our health outcomes are lower on almost every measure.

In working our way out of this triangle, some people call for massive deflation of our collective healthcare budget by emulating other countries' far lower payments to everyone involved in delivering services or by instituting more efficient administrative systems, like a single payer approach. Some people call for massive increases in spending to solve the access problem by using the approaches now in place to extend care to more people. Other people look to health information technology to reduce healthcare costs significantly by promoting best practices that deliver the most favorable outcomes at the lowest costs as defined by comparative health services research. Volunteerism is championed by others who see the best solution to access disparities in the professional compact and ethical charge to oral healthcare providers. Some people advocate building a safety net (our constellation of Federally Qualified Health Centers and community and school-based dental clinics) but others criticize it as "two-tiered healthcare." Rationing of some sort, whether explicit or implicit (as is now effectively the case with the lowest 20% of US population [per income] receiving the benefits of only 5% of dental expenditures) is intrinsic to the access issue, yet anathema to many and rarely discussed openly. Others look to competitive enterprise and to American private sector capitalism to solve the problems of access to oral healthcare. Indeed, Medicaid-only privately owned clinics for children have stepped into the access breach, taking risk, seeking reward, and in turn generating controversy among mainstream providers and the public. A completely alternative approach is to focus intensely on health promotion and disease prevention. Advocates for this approach note that dental services are overwhelmingly surgical and reparative, and they focus little on bona fide disease management techniques that include anticipatory guidance, primary prevention, and pharmaco-behavioral therapies for disease suppression. Each competing approach raises questions about resource allocation, personal and professional responsibility, roles for government and public policies, and even personal and shared values.

Questions as challenging as these lead inevitably to the "so what" question. Why does access to oral healthcare matter at either the individual or collective level? At last, this question has a clear answer and may serve as the basis for best understanding the contributions to this issue. Poor oral health and the failure to attend to acute treatment needs is consequential to individuals and to society, because it creates eating, speaking, and sleeping dysfunctions, lost productivity, impaired attentiveness to learning, and even lesser military readiness. From this observation, all must conclude that the question of access to oral healthcare services is important, timely, urgent, and worthy of your thoughtful consideration.

Burton L. Edelstein, DDS, MPH
Children's Dental Health Project of Washington DC
Washington DC, USA

College of Dental Medicine
Mailman School of Public Health
Columbia University
601 West 168th Street, Suite 32
New York, NY 10032, USA
E-mail address:
ble22@columbia.edu (B.L. Edelstein)

Preface

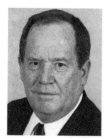

Gary A. Colangelo, DDS, MGA
Guest Editor

During the twentieth century, the dental profession gained remarkable technological advances that improved the oral health of many Americans. Systemic and topical fluoridation, the air rotor hand piece, and local anesthesia dramatically prevented disease and made surgical care efficient and painless. Despite these advances, access to optimal oral health care is limited or nonexistent for at least 40% of Americans. If the goal for Americans is to improve their oral health, the means to reach this goal is to improve access. Oral health care access includes more than receiving appropriate professional care. Access to disease prevention interventions and oral health knowledge also are essential to reach the goal of optimal oral health.

This issue of *Dental Clinics of North America* addresses the issue of oral health care access from multiple perspectives. Access is a complex issue with numerous variables and no absolute correct answers to improve access. This issue is an overview of oral health care access topics and not a comprehensive treatise. Health care professionals, policy makers, and advocates should find touch points of understanding and insight into potential solutions to improve access. The authors have provided extensive references for the reader to gain in-depth knowledge on a particular topic.

Through my 38 years of experiences as a dentist (formerly in private practice, a dental school faculty member, and most recently the director for a regional dental insurance plan), I have developed my own perspective of oral health care access issues. From my understanding of access and my work experiences, I am optimistic that we can improve the oral health of Americans by improving access. I am confident this will happen, because of the many dedicated and knowledgeable oral health and non-oral health professionals, policy makers, and advocates who continue to toil and innovate on improving access.

Twenty-two authors provided their thoughts and experiences for this issue. They have been a joy to work with, and I thank all authors for their time and effort. John Vassallo, Editor of the *Dental Clinics of North America*, has been patient, flexible, and understanding as the manuscripts were completed. I acknowledge the publisher,

Dent Clin N Am 53 (2009) xv–xvi
doi:10.1016/j.cden.2009.03.014
0011-8532/09/$ – see front matter **dental.theclinics.com**

Elsevier, for continuing to publish *Dental Clinics of North America*, a unique forum for sharing oral health knowledge.

Gary A. Colangelo, DDS, MGA
Baltimore College of Dental Surgery
Dental School
University of Maryland
39 Kenmare Way
Rehoboth Beach, DE 19971-1071, USA

E-mail address:
garycolangelo2@comcast.net (G.A. Colangelo)

How Dental Care Can Preserve and Improve Oral Health

Clemencia M. Vargas, DDS, PhD[a],*, Oscar Arevalo, DDS, ScD, MBA, MS[b]

KEYWORDS

- Oral health • Dental diseases • Dental care access
- Barriers to dental care • Prevention in oral health

RELEVANCE OF ORAL HEALTH
Connection With General Health

Oral health is important to an individual's well-being and overall health.[1] Therefore oral health must be considered in the context of the individual's environmental, behavioral, and socio-cultural factors. Poor oral health can have social, economic, behavioral, and quality-of-life effects.

Various studies have reported associations between oral health and systemic conditions. Studies assessing the link between coronary heart disease and periodontal diseases found that different presentations of periodontal diseases (gingivitis, tooth loss, periodontitis, and bone loss) were independent risk factors for coronary heart disease.[2] Moreover, it has been demonstrated that intensive treatment of periodontal disease resulted in improved endothelial function, which is a pathway to acute cardiovascular events.[3] The association between oral health and diabetes has been recognized for many years. This association goes both ways:[4] diabetes, particularly uncontrolled diabetes, is a risk factor for periodontal diseases. The presence of periodontal diseases among diabetics is so frequent that periodontal diseases have been considered the sixth highest ranked complication of diabetes.[5] On the other hand, there is strong evidence that periodontal diseases hinder diabetes control.[4] An association between chronic kidney disease and total tooth loss or edentulism also has been reported.[6] In this study, chronic kidney disease was more common among persons who had antibodies against the bacteria that cause periodontal diseases, but the investigators did not find any association between chronic kidney disease and clinical periodontal disease.[6] Studies have reported an association between

[a] Department of Health Promotion and Policy, University of Maryland, Dental School, 650 W. Baltimore St., Room 2217, Baltimore, MD 21201, USA
[b] Division of Dental Public Health, Department of Oral Health Science, University of Kentucky College of Dentistry, 800 Rose Street, M 129, Lexington, KY, 40536, USA
* Corresponding author.
E-mail address: cvargas@umaryland.edu (C.M. Vargas).

Dent Clin N Am 53 (2009) 399–420
doi:10.1016/j.cden.2009.03.011
0011-8532/09/$ – see front matter © 2009 Elsevier Inc. All rights reserved.

poor maternal oral health status, particularly periodontal diseases, and preterm and low birth weight babies.[7] It is not clear if this association is causal[7]; however, the association is sufficiently strong that recommending periodontal checkups before and during pregnancy is warranted.[8]

Among older adults, bacteria from the mouth can be aspirated during sleep and reach the lungs. Consequently, older persons who have poor oral health (caries lesions, periodontal diseases, and plaque) are more likely to present with pneumonia than older persons who have good oral health.[9] It also has been shown that respiratory diseases among older persons living in nursing homes and in ICUs can be prevented or limited with good oral hygiene.[9]

Quality of Life

Quality of life can be affected severely by conditions and diseases related to oral health. Poor oral health negatively affects a person's self-esteem, self-image, and overall well-being.[1] People who are embarrassed or self-conscious about their oral health frequently avoid showing their teeth, so that basic non-verbal expressions such as smiling, talking, and laughing are compromised; the absence of these non-verbal cues hampers social interactions.[1]

Functional problems of the oral cavity (eg, loss of teeth) also affect quality of life by causing difficulties eating. Masticatory efficiency is reduced as teeth are lost or replaced by total or partial dentures. Difficulties in chewing determine the frequency and types of food consumed.

Oral-facial pain also can affect quality of life. Acute pain associated with dental caries or periodontal diseases can be treated easily by a dentist. Most chronic pains related to the mouth are difficult to diagnose, however, and in many cases the cause cannot be identified or removed. In these cases, the treatment is limited to pain management.[1]

THE PROBLEM

The natural history of oral diseases is well understood. Most oral diseases are neither self-limiting nor self-repairing. For example, in the case of dental caries, the decaying process can continue until the destruction of the tooth and the compromise of adjacent tissues. The intervention of a dental professional at any stage of disease may help stop the disease and/or reduce its impact. With few exceptions, maintenance of oral health over a person's lifespan requires the participation of oral health professionals, and in many cases professional care is needed even before the disease process starts.[1] Prompt professional care is fundamental, given that oral diseases follow a downward spiral: incipient diseases requiring minimum dental care, if untreated, progress into diseases that require increasingly more complex and expensive treatments; increases in complexity and cost usually make the treatment even more out of reach for a large proportion of the population.[10]

Consequences of poor oral health carry over a lifespan.[11] Caries among children predict oral health problems among adults; current caries is the best predictor of future caries.[12] The United States population, however, does not receive the adequate dental care needed to preserve oral health. In 1958, Drs. Levell and Clark[13] reported, "despite the relative high number of well-qualified practicing dentists in this country and despite their highly developed means for restoring lost tooth structure, less than one-third of the dental needs of the country are given attention." Unfortunately, for the socially disadvantaged sectors of the population, the situation has not changed much since then.[1]

OVERVIEW OF THE MOST COMMON ORAL DISEASES

This section presents the most common oral diseases, their epidemiology, and their distribution and highlights potential interventions from the perspective of the levels of prevention. In 1953, Clark and Leavell[13] introduced the levels of prevention, and since then their model has been used widely. Although their model is illness oriented because it is based on the natural history of disease, it provides clear indication of the opportunities for prevention at each stage of disease. The model posits that treatment is one form of prevention that occurs after the disease process has started. Treatment is preventative in that it averts more serious damage.

Primary Prevention

Primary prevention seeks to thwart the start of the disease process. It includes measures that promote general health and more specific measures against the agents or circumstances associated with the disease in consideration. Primary prevention includes health promotion and specific protection.

Activities included in health promotion foster health in general and are applicable to any disease. They include health education, good nutrition, adequate housing, recreation, and agreeable working conditions. These activities for primary prevention have not changed significantly since Leavell and Clark[13] described them in their model of the levels of prevention. Currently, one would add an adequate environment free of pollutants and opportunities for physical exercise. All persons should have the opportunity to engage in adequate primary prevention activities. Leavell and Clark[13] indicated that the engaging in activities that promote health empower the individual to obtain the highest levels of health on his/her own.

Specific protection refers to measures that protect against specific disease agents, usually by establishing barriers against those agents. Therefore, specific protection intercepts the disease process before it starts. Community activities in oral health focus on specific protection.

Secondary Prevention

Secondary prevention takes place after the disease process has started, seeking to avoid the spread of diseases, to cure or arrest diseases, and to lessen disability. Secondary prevention includes early diagnosis, prompt treatment, and limiting disability. An individual's ability to act on this level of prevention depends on the availability and accessibility of dental care. Persons receiving limited or no dental care at this stage are destined to worse oral health outcomes and more expensive treatment.

Tertiary Prevention

The tertiary level of prevention refers to rehabilitation or the prevention of total disability after the disease has ran its course. If untreated, the most common oral health diseases (caries and periodontitis) are likely to result in tooth loss. Depending on the tooth or teeth that are lost, functionality and esthetics may be affected severely. Restoration of function and esthetics occurs with tooth replacement.

Caries

Caries is an infectious disease caused by bacteria that reside in the dental plaque. *Streptococcus mutans* is the most cariogenic bacteria because of its ability to produce acid. If early caries prevention measures, such as plaque removal, fluoride, and sealants, are not in place, the acid demineralizes the tooth surface, appearing initially as white spots. At this early stage, the caries process can be reversed by remineralizing the enamel with fluoride varnish. Otherwise, the white spots may progress until they result in a cavity, which if untreated may extend to other tooth structures such as the dentin or the tooth's pulp.

Dental caries is a highly prevalent disease. Among children in the United States, caries is five times more frequent than asthma, and 95% of adults have had dental decay in their permanent teeth.[1,14] Dental caries are more common among the socially disadvantaged: the poor and racial ethnic minorities (**Figs. 1** and **2**).[15]

Primary prevention

General promotion A good diet is particularly important for the prevention of caries. Fermentable carbohydrates, which include sugars and cooked starches, are the most cariogenic foods.[16] Caries develops more easily when these sugars and starches are consumed between meals.[16,17] For example, feeding infants juice between meals has been associated with dental caries.[18] The consumption of milk, on the other hand, has been found not to be associated with caries.[19] A visit to the dentist during a baby's first year will give the opportunity for caregivers to discuss and learn about health, diet, and behaviors conducive to good oral health.

Specific protection Effective preventive agents are available to prevent caries. Community water fluoridation is arguably the most cost-effective of all measures. Water fluoridation provides fluoride to all persons residing in the water system catchment area, regardless of socioeconomic condition, at a very low cost.[8] Fluoride in toothpaste is another effective mechanism to prevent caries. In fact, fluoridated toothpaste has been considered responsible for the global decline in caries in the late twentieth century.[20] Dental sealants also provide significant caries prevention. Sealants are plastic coats that are applied by dental professionals to the surface of teeth that have pits and fissures. Sealants isolate the tooth surface from the bacteria that colonizes the dental plaque and the acids produced by the bacteria, so that caries cannot develop.

Oral hygiene is considered a part of expected personal grooming and is fundamental to prevent periodontal diseases. For caries prevention, the most important effect of oral hygiene is the exposure of dental surfaces to fluoride from toothpaste.[8] Plaque control by tooth brushing or flossing prevents caries by reducing the amount of cariogenic bacteria in the mouth.[21] The well-accepted recommendation is to brush the

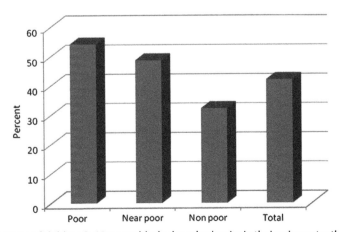

Fig. 1. Percentage of children 2–11 years old who have had caries in their primary teeth, by poverty status. (*Data from* Dye BA, Tan S, Smith V, et al. Trends in oral health status: United States, 1988–1994 and 1999–2004. National Center for Health Statistics Vital Health Stat 2007;11(248):20.)

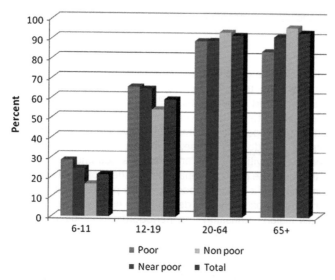

Fig. 2. Percentage of persons who have had caries in their permanent teeth, by age group and poverty status. (*Data from* Dye BA, Tan S, Smith V, et al. Trends in oral health status: United States, 1988–1994 and 1999–2004. National Center for Health Statistics Vital Health Stat 2007;11(248):23, 31, 43, 69.)

teeth regularly with fluoridated toothpaste. Children under 2 years of age who are at high risk for caries should be brushed with a "smear" of fluoridated toothpaste; children 2 to 4 years of age should be brushed with a "small pea size" of toothpaste.[22] Older children and adults should use an mount of toothpaste equal to the size of a pea.[22]

Secondary prevention

Early diagnosis Early diagnosis of caries by a dental professional can limit the spread of the disease. Considering the downward spiral model of disease, early diagnosis results in shorter and easier treatments for the patient at a lower cost. Caries also can be diagnosed and reversed before cavitation occurs, when there is only a white spot.

Prompt treatment Dental caries lesions should be treated as soon as they are diagnosed to minimize the loss of tooth structure and the complexity of treatment. White spot lesions can be reversed with fluoride varnish, which can be applied by dental or medical professionals. Once the white spot lesion becomes a cavity, a dentist's intervention is necessary. Neglecting small lesions is likely to result in large cavities that require more involved and more expensive treatment.

Limiting disability Dental cavities result in loss of tooth structure and, in many cases, pain. To restore the teeth to their full functional capacity, the dentist must remove all the decayed tissue, apply materials to replace the lost structure, and reproduce its original shape. If unrestored, teeth will continue to erode, resulting in lost structure and potential pulp involvement. Once the pulp has been affected, more complex or radical treatment such as endodontic or surgical treatment will be required.

Tertiary prevention

Teeth with extensive dental caries usually must be extracted surgically. After surgery, the next opportunity for prevention is rehabilitation to avoid the consequences of impaired function and affected esthetics. Rehabilitation consists of tooth replacement with bridges anchored on remnant neighboring teeth, with implants, or with removable partial or full dentures.

Periodontal Diseases

"Periodontal disease" is a generic term describing diseases affecting the gums and tissues that support the teeth.[8] The two main diseases included in periodontal diseases are gingivitis and periodontitis.[23–25] Although both diseases are infections of bacterial origin linked to dental plaque and calculus, the severity of periodontitis is determined strongly by genetic factors and by any form of tobacco use.[26] Gingivitis, the mildest form of periodontal disease, is an inflammation of the gums around the teeth. In untreated gingivitis, plaque and calculus accumulate between the gums and the teeth and force the gums to separate from the tooth root (loss of attachment). This separation results in a space or pocket where plaque accumulates, resulting in inflammation that develops freely and destroys the nearby bone. The opinion that all or most gingivitis lesions transition into periodontitis has been revised; it is clear now that only few patients will develop periodontitis subsequent to gingivitis.[8] Timely dental care will prevent the disease from progressing to advanced stages. In the absence of dental intervention, treatment becomes more complex and expensive. In some instances, untreated periodontitis can remain as a chronic disease for years with the possibility of causing the loss of the affected teeth. Moreover, untreated periodontal diseases have the potential of affecting the general health of the individual because of its association with cardiovascular diseases, preterm and low birth weight pregnancy outcomes, diabetes, and kidney disease.[3,4,6,7]

The symptoms of periodontal diseases may include red, swollen, or tender gums; bleeding while brushing, flossing, or eating hard food; tooth sensitivity; receding gums; loose or separated teeth, pus between gums and teeth; persistent bad breath; or a change in either how the teeth fit together or in the fit of partial dentures.[1]

Gingivitis has decreased considerably in the United States. It is more common in children and adolescents than in adults,[8,27] but severe gingivitis is uncommon in children.[27] Periodontitis is more likely to be present among low-income persons and African Americans.[14] Among adults 20 to 64 years of age, moderate or severe periodontitis has decreased from 9.63% in the period from1988 to 1994 to 5.08% (SE 0.34) in the period from 1999 to 2004 (**Fig. 3**).[14]

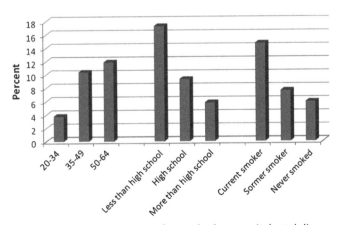

Fig. 3. Percentage of adults 20 to 64 years of age who have periodontal disease. (*Data from* Dye BA, Tan S, Smith V, et al. Trends in oral health status: United States, 1988–1994 and 1999–2004. National Center for Health Statistics Vital Health Stat 2007;11(248):63.)

Primary prevention

General promotion It is likely that periodontal diseases are the oral diseases that can benefit the most from health promotion activities. Avoidance of tobacco products is a first step to prevent periodontal diseases. Smokers are four times more likely than non-smokers to have periodontitis.[28] Uncontrolled diabetes is strongly associated with periodontal diseases. Therefore, diabetes control is another general health promotion activity that will help prevent periodontal diseases.

Specific protection Tooth brushing is the main intervention to prevent and treat gingivitis.[1] Prevention of gingivitis will prevent the incidence of periodontitis. It is believed that inclusion of tooth brushing as part of the routine personal grooming has helped in the reduction of gingivitis in the United States and other countries.[8] Daily regular dental flossing also helps prevent gingivitis and periodontitis by reducing the amount of bacteria between the teeth.[21] Brushing and flossing should be performed despite bleeding gums. Although oral home care is the cornerstone in preventing periodontal diseases, it might not be sufficient for persons who have a strong genetic predisposition to periodontal diseases.[29]

The role of the dental team is essential in preventing periodontal diseases. Plaque that deposits above the gums can be removed with tooth brushing and flossing. When the plaque accumulates below the gum line, a professional dental cleaning is necessary.[8] Moreover, the guidance of a dental professional usually is necessary to achieve effective oral home care.

Secondary prevention

Early diagnosis Early intervention of a dentist is fundamental in determining the presence of periodontal diseases, which can have a slow, silent start. Although resolution of inflammation in a timely matter can prevent or reduce damage to the tissues of support, failure to bring the gums to their natural state results in chronic inflammation and destruction of tissues.[30]

Prompt treatment With new techniques and medications, periodontal treatment is not particularly painful and does not involve days of recovery.[29] The treatment guidelines from the American Academy of Periodontology emphasize that the treatment of periodontal diseases should be the least invasive possible. The dentist should start with nonsurgical treatment to clean the plaque and calculus (tartar) from the roots of the teeth and make them smooth so that plaque will be less likely to adhere again. In many cases, this cleaning might be sufficient to treat periodontal diseases; in other cases periodontal surgery is necessary to reinstate tissues' anatomy and to facilitate oral hygiene.[30]

Limiting disability In some instances, surgical treatment is necessary to maintain or recover the functionality of the teeth and to reconstruct the damaged tissue. For example, when the gums have receded and the teeth roots are exposed, a soft tissue graft can be used to cover those exposed roots, avoiding additional recession and subsequent bone loss. In these cases, the graft surgery results in esthetic improvement, reduction of sensitivity to hot or cold liquids, and a decrease in the risk of developing root caries.

Tertiary prevention

Once periodontal diseases have destroyed the supporting bone, the teeth become mobile and are at high risk of being lost. Dentists can rehabilitate teeth severely affected by periodontitis with surgical procedures to regenerate some of the lost bone. A very extensive loss of support tissue requires extraction of the tooth. Teeth lost because of periodontal disease can be replaced with bridges, dental implants, or partial/full dentures.

Oral Cancer

Oral cancer includes cancer of the lip, tongue, buccal mucosa, salivary glands, and pharynx. Most oral cancers (80%) are squamous cell carcinomas, which are located most commonly on the tongue, lips, and the floor of the mouth.[1] The strongest risk factors for oral cancer are tobacco use (smoking or chewing) and alcohol consumption.[1]

The most frequent symptoms of oral cancer are small wounds that bleed easily and do not heal and constant pain in the mouth. Other possible symptoms include a lump or thickening in the cheek; a white or red patch inside the mouth; a sore throat or a feeling of something stuck in the throat; and difficulties chewing, swallowing, or moving the tongue or jaw.[31]

It is estimated that in 2008 there were 35,310 new cases and 7590 deaths from oral cancer in the United States.[31] Oral cancer is twice as common in men as in women and is particularly common among African American men,[8] possibly because men are more likely to use tobacco and alcohol over long periods of time.[31]

Primary prevention

General promotion Legislation such cigarette taxes discourage smoking and thereby reduce the risks associated with smoking. Because the strongest risk factors for oral cancer are alcohol and tobacco use, the general health recommendations about avoiding smoking and smokeless tobacco (not starting or quitting) and limiting alcohol ingestion probably will protect individuals against oral cancer. Tobacco cessation as part of routine treatment provided by dentists and dental hygienists will help patients overcome their addiction to tobacco.

Specific protection Lip cancer has been linked to high sun exposure. Therefore, the use of sun blocker lip balm and hats with a wide brim will provide protection against lip cancer.

Secondary prevention

Early diagnosis is of the utmost importance in oral cancer and truly can make the difference between life and death. The devastating consequences of oral cancer treatment also are lessened by early diagnosis.

Early diagnosis and prompt treatment As with most cancers, oral cancer usually is treatable in its earlier stages, and the sooner the cancer is detected, the more conservative the treatment can be. Dentists and physicians should provide oral cancer examinations as part of routine examinations. Patients also should request them from their health care providers.

Limiting disability Cancer treatment usually involves removal of the affected tissue by surgery coupled with radiation therapy. Because of the multifunctionality of the oral cavity, cancer treatment is likely to have devastating consequences on the individual's quality of life.

Tertiary prevention

Treatment of advanced cancers usually results in serious disabilities. Rehabilitation usually involves other health professionals to address plastic surgery reconstructions, speech limitations, swallowing difficulties, and other issues.

FACTORS THAT DETERMINE AVAILABILITY AND ACCESS TO ORAL HEALTH CARE

Access to oral health care figures prominently among the health care problems facing the United States population. According to *Oral Health in America: A Report of the Surgeon General,* one third of Americans are without access to oral health care.[1] Barriers to oral health care are multifactorial and include issues related to the work-force, structural and patient issues, behavioral, and socio-cultural issues. The following sections describe these factors and their impact on different subpopulations.

Workforce

Shortage and maldistribution of providers

An adequate number of dentists is necessary to address the oral health needs of Americans. The dentist-to-population ratio in the United States has been declining since 1995 and is expected to continue decreasing.[32] The number of dentists per 100,000 United States inhabitants in 2002 was 59 and is expected to decrease to 54.3 in 2022. According to the American Dental Association, a projected increase in dentists' clinical productivity will offset the demands of population growth.[33] Unfortunately, dentists are not distributed evenly around the country; studies have documented that the geographic distribution of dentists is related significantly to population size and per capita income.[34,35] Accordingly, the number of Dental Health Professional Shortage Areas (D-HPSA), a federal designation for areas with a deficit in the number of dentists (population-to-dentist ratio higher than 5000:1), has increased from 805 in 1991 to 3951 in 2008.[36] A full 47 million people live in these dental shortage areas. The reality is that, for individuals residing in rural and low-income inner city areas and for some groups such as the Medicaid population, a shortage of dental providers exists.

A number of factors contribute to the shortage of dentists in economically deprived areas, including the high level of educational debt carried by recent dental school graduates and the limited availability of loan repayment and scholarship programs. According to the American Dental Education Association (ADEA), the average reported educational debt upon graduation from dental school in 2006 was $145,465.[37] The average educational debt upon graduation increased 93.5% between 1992 and 2002, a rate that significantly exceeded the inflation rate.[38] This impending debt pressures recent dental school graduates to choose practices in more financially lucrative areas rather than in inner-city and rural locations.[39] The National Health Service Corps (NHSC), a federally supported loan repayment program, was established to increase the availability of health care by placing professionals in urban and rural communities that lack ready access to a range of health services. Unfortunately, this program has been affected by continuously low numbers of participating health care professionals, low retention rates, and underfunding.[40,41] In 2006, 415 dentists were part of the NHSC, a far cry from the 9321 dentists required to meet the dental needs of populations in D-HPSA.[42,43]

Limited scope of practice for auxiliary personnel

An important factor in the disparity of access to oral health care in the United States may be that allied dental personnel are not being used to provide all the health services for which they easily could be trained. According to the Bureau of Labor Services, in 2006 there were 167,000 dental hygienists and 280,000 dental assistants in the United States.[44] Their scope of practice is limited, however, and requirements that auxiliary personnel work under the supervision of a dentist suggest that the declining number of dentists will restrict the capacity of the dental care delivery system.[45] From an economic standpoint, restrictions in the scope of practice lead to decreased productivity and higher profits for the dentists.[46] Changes in dental practice acts have the potential to increase capacity and, as a result, access to care.

Racial/ethnic homogeneity of the dental workforce

Persons from racial/ethnic minority groups are more likely to seek a health care provider who belongs to their racial/ethnic group. For instance, African Americans and Hispanics seek care from physicians of their own groups because of personal preference and language, not solely because of geographic accessibility.[47] This preference also could be related to patients seeking culturally competent care. Surveys of practice show among dentists that dentists who belong to racial/ethnic minority groups treat significantly higher proportions of urban, less formally educated, and lower-income patients than do their non-minority colleagues.[48] Similarly, African American dentists are more likely than their non-African American colleagues to practice in areas that have a higher residential African American population.[49] African American patients are more likely to receive care from an African American dentist. Effectively, 62% of black patients are seen by black dentists, and only 10.5% of black patients receive their care from white dentists.[49,50]

Despite changes in the racial and ethnic mix of the country, the representation of racial and ethnic minorities in the dental profession lags behind their representation in the general population.[51] African Americans and Latinos represent 27% of the total population of the United States but only 11% of the students entering dental schools.[52,53] This lack of racial/ethnic diversity in the dental work force is recognized as a major concern for the profession and the public[54,55] because it hampers the profession's ability to provide adequate care to racial/ethnic minority groups.

Curricular and training deficiencies

The curricula of dental education have been characterized as overcrowded.[56] A packed 4-year curriculum does not allow comprehensive exposure to certain population groups, limiting the graduates' ability to deal with the particular needs of these groups. Certain groups, such as the frail elderly, patients who have special needs or who are medically compromised, and young children face considerable barriers in accessing dental care. It is possible that the dental workforce is not trained appropriately to address the oral health needs of these populations. This problem is exacerbated by the perception of many dentists that these individuals are more difficult to treat and that the reimbursement is inadequate to cover operational expenses.[57] A survey conducted among dental schools in 2003 showed that during the past 20 years the didactic teaching of geriatric dentistry had increased significantly, but the clinical experience had not kept pace.[58] As a result, in 2002 dental school seniors reported that they were not well prepared to provide care for older individuals.[38] The ADEA survey of graduating dentists in 2000 showed less satisfaction with the time devoted to pediatric dentistry education than in previous years.[59] A shrinking number of faculty members and a limited number of patients seem to affect the ability of dental institutions to train general dentists appropriately in the management of the pediatric patient.[60–62]

Structural Issues

Financing of dental care, dental insurance, and use of services

In 2006, $91.1 billion was spent on dental care; $86 billion was paid by private sources, and only $5.5 billion was paid by the federal and state governments,[43] Although in 1990 expenditures for dental services represented 11.1% of total health expenditures, in 2005 that figure had decreased to 6.3%.[43] The resources allocated for oral health determine the scope and magnitude of programs targeting disadvantaged populations. Reduced state and federal budgets for oral health programs have led to increased numbers of uninsured and underinsured individuals and to an overburdened safety net.

The availability of dental insurance is important because the cost of dental care is a barrier to receiving regular care and maintaining good oral health. A review of the literature on the effects of dental insurance on the demand for dental care found that insured individuals are more likely than their uninsured counterparts to seek dental care.[63] Although 47 million Americans lack health insurance, 108 million lack dental insurance;[64] in 2004, 35% of the United States population was uninsured for dental care for the whole year.[65] The elderly, racial/ethnic minorities, and low-income persons are recognized as having the most critical need for dental care. Unfortunately, they are the least likely to have the financial resources or dental insurance to pay for dental care. Among older Americans, the ability to pay for dental care deceases with retirement because of the decrease in income and the loss of employer-based insurance coverage.[66–68] According to the 2004 Medical Expenditure Panel Survey (MEPS), poor and low-income families were more than likely high-income families to be uninsured (41% and 47% versus 25%).[65] Likewise, African Americans and Hispanics were more likely than non-Hispanic whites to have public dental insurance coverage. Lamentably, even when the financial barrier is removed, use seems to vary by insurance group. According to the same study, 57% of the population with private insurance had a dental visit, but only 32% of the population with public dental insurance visited the dentist.[65]

Inadequate federal and state programs

Publicly subsidized programs such as Medicaid and the State Children's Health Insurance Program (SCHIP) provide coverage for dental care for low-income individuals. These programs, however, have limitations that hamper their effectiveness in increasing access to dental services at the community level.

Even though Medicaid provides dental benefits for selected adults in some states, both the Medicaid and SCHIP programs target mainly low-income children. Very low participation from dentists in the Medicaid and SCHIP program is a chronic problem. Approximately only 25% of all dentists reported seeing Medicaid patients in their offices.[40,69] Providers often cite inadequate reimbursement as the reason for their low rate of participation. Other issues include administrative problems, such as complicated paperwork, slow reimbursement, and claims denials, and patient-related issues, including poor compliance in keeping appointments and following treatment recommendations.[70–72] A review of the literature concluded that higher reimbursement rates were necessary but not sufficient to increase provider participation in Medicaid. To improve their programs, Medicaid agencies must revamp administrative practices and build partnerships with dental societies.[73]

The SCHIP program was designed to provide access to care for children in working poor families, that is, families with incomes above the threshold of eligibility for Medicaid (up to 200% of the federal poverty level). A few studies have documented the effect of SCHIP on dental use and inferred limited positive impact.[74–76]

Dental coverage for adults is elective, and benefits vary greatly by state. In many instances coverage is limited to emergency care, and the extent of benefits fluctuates according to state budgets. Expanding dental coverage for adults might decrease access barriers.

Limited dental public health infrastructure

The infrastructure for dental public health is the foundation on which public dental programs and activities are planned, implemented, and evaluated. Unfortunately, the dental public health workforce is underappreciated and has a low priority in the United States society in general, with limited resources to address the great unmet needs of the country.[42] An assessment of the dental public health infrastructure concluded that the workforce is small, most state programs have limited funding, the discipline has minimal presence in academia, and its role in the regulation of dentistry and dental hygiene is small.[77] The number of public health dentists is limited: in the United States, 2032 dentists and only 155 active board-certified specialists work in public health.[42]

Federally qualified health centers and rural health centers often serve as safety net providers for dental care. Currently, around 1200 health centers deliver care through more than 6600 service delivery sites serving 18 million Americans nationwide.[78] In 2003, 65% of the federally funded community health care centers and 85% of the migrant health care centers provided some type of dental care.[77] A study that examined the capacity of the dental safety net to meet the needs of the underserved population concluded that the current system had the capacity to care for about 7 to 8 million people annually with the potential of increasing this figure to 10 million.[79] A comparison of this limited capacity with the high number of uninsured and low-income individuals led to the conclusion that any substantial strategy to address the unmet dental needs of Americans will require the participation of private practitioners.

Population Issues

Patient behavioral and socio-cultural issues

Removing structural and financial barriers is an important step toward eliminating disparities in access, but it is not sufficient, because there are other important determinants. Care for patients, especially those from vulnerable groups, is a complex issue.[80] A major factor leading to underutilization of dental care is the educational and cultural gap between patients and dentists.[80–83] Patient characteristics such as race, education level, cultural values associated with oral health, level of perceived disease burden, and disease severity have an influence on treatment.[84,85] Negative experiences when trying to access dental care services, such as difficulty finding a provider, scheduling convenient appointments, transportation, long waiting times, taking time off work, and discriminatory treatment, may affect the willingness of patients to seek dental care.[81,86–88]

Another important barrier to dental care is the choice socially disadvantaged populations must make between fulfilling basic needs and seeking and paying for dental care. In this situation, dental care becomes a luxury that is relegated to a second place after basic needs are fulfilled.[89] Lack of awareness about the benefits of regular dental visits, as opposed to episodic visits, also affects the use of dental care. It is particularly important that caregivers of low-income children be aware of the need for measures for preserving oral health, because such awareness is a strong predictor of children's use of dental care.[90,91]

Similarly, dentists' characteristics, including practice specialty, practice style, and attitudes or bias about patients' ethnicity and social background, may influence the type and quality of services rendered.[84,85,92] As the dental profession deals with an increasingly diverse population, the lack of cultural and linguistic competence among providers represents an additional barrier to care.[93]

POPULATIONS WITH LIMITED DENTAL CARE USE

The factors described in the previous section affect certain populations more than others. The following sections describe their particular impact on a selection of dentally underserved populations.

Low-Income Individuals

An individual's socioeconomic status and disposable income is the strongest determinant of dental care use and expenditures. Consequently, low-income persons who cannot afford to pay for dental services become a severely underserved group. Data from the MEPS 2004 showed that 58% of individuals from high-income families had at least one dental visit during the past year, compared with 30% of individuals from low-income families.[65] Low-income adults, in particular, are peril, because most dental insurance is provided as a work-related benefit. Low-paying jobs and federal programs such as Medicaid provide few dental benefits, and the Medicare program does not cover dental care unless it is related to the treatment of a medical condition.

Racial/Ethnic Minorities

The oral health of racial/ethnic minorities is relatively poor. These populations have the highest levels of oral diseases and at the same time have limited access to oral health care.[1] Racial/ethnic minorities are more likely than non-Hispanic whites to have low family income that makes dental care inaccessible. Low-income populations reside in economically depressed areas where the availability of dental care is limited. Access to health care for racial/ethnic minority groups also is hindered by a shortage of culturally competent practitioners. The lack of a diverse workforce may foster linguistic and cultural barriers, bias, and clinical uncertainty within the patient–provider relationship.[94,95] On the other hand, diversity in the workforce has been associated with increased satisfaction with care received and with improved patient–provider communication.[94,96,97]

Rural Residents

Adult and children living in rural areas are more likely than urban residents to report poor oral health and to have more unmet dental needs. Adults in rural areas are more likely than their urban or suburban counterparts to have lost all of their teeth.[98,99] They also are less likely to report having a dental visit during the past year. This finding is not a surprise; residents of rural areas face a unique challenge that limits access to dental services: an acute shortage of dental professionals relative to the rest of the country. Dentists are significantly underrepresented within rural counties, especially in smaller and more isolated locations.[100,101] In urban areas of the United States, there are 61 dentists per 100,000 people, but rural areas have only 29 dentists per 100,000 people.[102]

Pregnant Women

Dental care is of great importance during pregnancy, because normal changes in the woman's body may increase the possibility of oral health problems. For example, the gingival tissues can be irritated easily, resulting in gingivitis, and nausea and vomiting predispose the pregnant woman to dental erosion.[103–105] Dental care should be started as early in pregnancy as possible, and involved procedures should be scheduled early in the second trimester; however, women should be encouraged to attain their optimal oral health level before becoming pregnant.[103,106] Although dentists agree that dental care should be provided during pregnancy,[107] dental care usually is delayed until after delivery[105] for fear of harming the fetus. It has been shown, however, that dental care during pregnancy is safe for the fetus.[104] Because of this overly cautious behavior by dentists, pregnant women are an underserved population for dental care.

Prisoners

The National Commission on Correctional Health Care has established standards for prisons and jails, including standards for oral health care.[108] According to the Bureau of Justice statistics, on June 30, 2007, 2.3 million individuals were held in federal or state prisons or in local jails.[109] The few publications that have addressed oral health among inmates agree that their oral health status is generally poor.[110–112] Federal facilities generally are equipped with dental clinics staffed by dentists from the US Public Health Service; state correctional facilities may lack these resources.[111] Limited financial resources and difficulties in recruiting dentists to work in the correctional system are major barriers to providing dental care to inmates.[113,114]

Elderly Population

Although children's oral health has received a great deal of national attention in the last few years, public policy efforts to provide dental benefits for the growing elderly population have been limited. Data from the 2004 MEPS showed that approximately 70% of older adults did not have any dental insurance coverage. Lacking financial assistance to cover dental expenses through retirement benefits or Medicare, the elderly often avoid or delay seeking care.[65] Medicare, the public insurance program for the elderly, does not provide dental benefits unless dental services are part of specific disease-related medical treatments or in preparation for certain kinds of radiation treatment.

Moreover, because geriatric dentistry is not recognized as a specialty of the American Dental Association, there is scarcity of dentists formally trained to address the needs of elderly patients, specifically those who are medically compromised and/or cognitively impaired.[115] A report from *Oral Health America* noted that older Americans suffer disproportionately from oral conditions and that the problem is particularly serious for individuals living in long-term care facilities.[116] As a result of age-related changes that result in lower sensitivity to oral pain, many older adults are unaware of oral disease until the disease has advanced and extensive services are required to manage it.[117]

Victims of Natural Disasters

Dental services, along with the communities they serve, are affected by natural or human disasters. Because dental services require stable sources of electricity and water, even small disasters limit dentists' ability to provide care. Relief efforts are not likely to include dental services, and when these services are included they must be provided with considerable limitations. One of the few times when the emergency response included dental care was after Hurricane Katrina. Dentists then had to provide care in mobile vans using portable equipment installed in a tent, knowing that there was no follow-up for their patients.[118]

Provision of dental care is of utmost importance in large-scale disasters because chronic problems become acute in emergency situations, and previous needs become current needs.[119] The most common needs for dental care are extractions because of toothaches, denture adjustment or replacement, and temporary fillings.[118–120] After the emergency situation is addressed, local dentists must spend significant resources and time setting up their dental offices again. In the mean time, the community is without available dental care.

Recent Immigrants

Immigrant populations face particular challenges when accessing dental care: lack of knowledge of the health care system, limited knowledge of English, fear associated with their legal status,[121] and cultural beliefs.[122] To add to these difficulties, in most states recent immigrant children, who usually come from families with limited economic resources, are not eligible for Medicaid coverage.

Special Needs Populations

People who have special needs are defined as individuals who face difficulty accessing health care services because of complicated physical, medical, social, or psychological conditions.[123] In 2002, 51.2 million Americans had some sort of developmental, physical, and/or intellectual disability.[124] Several publications have documented that people who have special needs have more dental disease and more difficulty obtaining access to dental care than other members of the general population.[40,125–128] As a result, they face increased medical care costs, diminished quality of life, and unnecessary suffering.[129] These problems particularly affect those living in rural areas.[130,131] Factors leading to disparities in access for people who have special needs include a trend toward deinstitutionalization, relying on a dental delivery system not suited to provide care for this population, the limited availability of dental services for special needs adults because few states provide dental benefits as part of Medicaid, low reimbursement rates for providers, and limited exposure to and training in managing the special needs patient during dental education.[1,128,132,133] People who have special needs are more likely than non-disabled individuals to be unemployed and to live in poverty,[134] conditions that augment their difficulties in accessing dental care.

SUMMARY

Oral health is associated with overall health, and lack of access to dental care has consequences that go far beyond esthetics. Most oral diseases are preventable and are relatively easy and inexpensive to address at early stages, but multiple barriers make dental care unreachable for a sizable portion of the United States population, who consequently have higher incidence and prevalence of disease. Achieving meaningful improvements in oral health status among these groups will require a revamping of the dental infrastructure, augmenting the productivity and skills of the dental workforce, and increasing the population's oral health literacy.

ACKNOWLEDGMENTS

The authors thank Daniel Saman for his research and editorial assistance.

REFERENCES

1. U.S. Department of Health and Human Services. Oral health in America: a report of the Surgeon General. Rockville (MD): National Institutes of Health, National Institute of Dental and Craniofacial Research; 2000.
2. Humphrey LL, Fu R, Buckley DI, et al. Periodontal disease and coronary health disease incidence: a systematic review and meta-analysis. J Gen Intern Med 2008;23(12):2079–86.

3. Tonetti MS, D'Aiuto F, Nibali L, et al. Treatment of periodontitis and endothelial function. N Engl J Med 2007;356(9):911–20.
4. Taylor GW. Bidirectional interrelationships between diabetes and periodontal diseases: an epidemiological perspective. Ann Periodontol 2001;6(1):99–112.
5. Loe H. Periodontal disease: the sixth complication of diabetes mellitus. Diabetes Care 1993;16(1):329–34.
6. Fisher MA, Taylor GW, Papanou PN, et al. Clinical and serologic markers of periodontal infection and chronic kidney disease. J Periodontol 2008;79(9): 1670–8.
7. Scannapieco FA, Bush RB, Paju S. Periodontal diseases as a risk factor for adverse pregnancy outcomes. A systematic review. Ann Periodontol 2003; 8(1):70–8.
8. Burt BA, Eklund SA. Dentistry, dental practice, and the community. 6th edition. St. Louis (MO): Elsevier Saunders; 2005.
9. Azarpazhooh A, Leake JL. Systematic review of the association between respiratory diseases and oral health. J Periodontol 2006;77:1465–82.
10. Vargas CM, Ronzio CR. Relationship between dental needs and dental care utilization. U.S. 1988–94. Am J Public Health 2002;92(11):1816–21.
11. Thomson WM, Poulton R, Milne BJ, et al. Socioeconomic inequalities in oral health in childhood and adulthood in a birth cohort. Community Dent Oral Epidemiol 2004;32(5):345–53.
12. O'Sullivan DM, Tinanoff N. The association of early dental caries patterns with caries incidence in preschool children. J Public Health Dent 1996;56(2):81–3.
13. Leavell HR, Clark EG. Preventive medicine for the doctor in his community. An epidemiologic approach. 3rd edition. New York: McGraw-Hill Book Company; 1965.
14. Dye BA, Tan S, Smith V, et al. Trends in oral health status: United States, 1988–1994 and 1999–2004. National Center for Health Statistics Vital Health Stat 11 2007;(248):1–92.
15. Vargas CM, Crall JJ, Schneider DA. Sociodemographic distribution of pediatric dental caries: NHANES III, 1988–1994. J Am Dent Assoc 1998;129:1229–41.
16. McDonald RE, Avery DR, Stookey GK. Dental caries in the child and adolescent. In: McDonald RE, Avery DR, editors. Dentistry for the child and adolescent. 6th edition. St. Louis (MO): Mosby, Inc.; 2000. p. 209–46.
17. Marshall TA, Broffitt B, Eichenberger-Gilmore J, et al. The roles of meal, snack, and daily total food and beverage exposures on caries experience in young children. J Public Health Dent 2005;65(3):166–73.
18. Marshall TA, Levy SM, Broffitt B, et al. Dental caries and beverage consumption in young children. Pediatrics 2003;112(3 Pt 1):e184–91.
19. Bowen WH, Lawrence RA. Comparison of the cariogenicity of cola, honey, cow milk, human milk, and sucrose. Pediatrics 2005;116(4):921–6.
20. Bratthall D, Hansel-Petersson G, Sundberg H. Reasons for the caries decline: what do the experts believe? Eur J Oral Sci 1996;104:416–22.
21. Corby PMA, Biesbrock A, Bartizek R, et al. Treatment outcomes of dental flossing in twins: molecular analysis of the interproximal microflora. J Periodontol 2008;79(8):1426–33.
22. Maternal Child Health Bureau. Topical fluoride recommendations for high-risk children. Recommendations from MCHB Expert Panel, Oct. 22–23, 2007. Available at: http://mohealthysmiles.typepad.com/Topical%20fl% 20recommendations%20for%20hi%20risk%20children.pdf. Accessed April 10, 2009.

23. Page RC, Schroeder HE. Pathogenesis of inflammatory periodontal disease. A summary of current work. Lab Invest 1976;33:235–49.
24. Lindhe J, Okamoto H, Yoneyama T, et al. Longitudinal changes in periodontal disease in untreated subjects. J Clin Periodontol 1989;16:662–70.
25. Machtei EE, Hausman E, Dunford R, et al. Longitudinal study of predictive factors for periodontal disease and tooth loss. J Clin Periodontol 1999;26:374–80.
26. Kornman KS, Crane A, Wang HY, et al. The interleukin-1 genotype as a severity factor in adult periodontal disease. J Clin Periodontol 1997;24:72–7.
27. McDonald RE, Avery DR, Weddell JA. Gingivitis and periodontal disease. In: McDonald RE, Avery DR, editors. Dentistry for the child and adolescent. 6th edition. St. Louis (MO): Mosby, Inc.; 2000. p. 440–84.
28. Tomar SL, Asma S. Smoking-attributable periodontitis in the United States: findings from NHANES III. National Health and Nutrition Examination Survey. J Periodontol 2000;71(5):743–51.
29. Genco RJ. Clinical innovations in managing inflammation and periodontal diseases: the Workshop on Inflammation and Periodontal Diseases. J Periodontol 2008;(Suppl):1609–11.
30. American Academy of Periodontology. Periodontal procedures. Available at: http://www.perio.org/consumer/procedures.htm. Accessed November 25, 2008.
31. American Cancer Society. Oral cancer. Available at: http://www.cancer.org/downloads/PRO/OralCancer.pdf. Revised March 2008. Accessed September 23, 2008.
32. Brown LJ. Dental work force strategies during a period of change and uncertainty. J Dent Educ 2001;65:1404–16.
33. Brown LJ. Regional issues in dental education and workforce distribution. In: Brown LI, Meskin LH, editors. The economics of dental education. Chicago: American Dental Association, Health Policy Resources Center; 2004.
34. Beazoglou TJ, Crakes GM, Doherty NJ, et al. Determinants of dentists' geographic distribution. J Dent Educ 1992;56:735–40.
35. Bailit HL, Beazoglou TJ. State financing of dental education: impact on supply of dentists. J Dent Educ 2003;67:1278–85.
36. U.S. Department of Health and Human Services. Health Resources and Services Administration. Shortage designation: HPSAs, MUAs & MUPs. Available at: http://bhpr.hrsa.gov/shortage/index.htm. Updated July 30, 2008. Accessed September 29, 2008.
37. Chmar JE, Harlow AH, Weaver RG, et al. Annual ADEA survey of dental school seniors, 2006 graduating class. J Dent Educ 2007;71(9):1228–53.
38. Weaver RG, Haden NK, Valachovic RW. Annual ADEA survey of dental school seniors: 2002 graduating class. J Dent Educ 2002;66(12):1388–404.
39. Gordy A. The impact of declining dentist-to-population ratios. Community Health Forum 2001;2:6;28–31.
40. U.S. General Accounting Office. Oral health: dental disease is a chronic problem among low-income populations. Washington, DC: US General Accounting Office; 2000. Pub No GAO/HEHS-00-149.
41. Marwick C. National Health Service Corps faces reauthorization during a risky time. JAMA 2000;283:2461–2.
42. Allukian M, Adekugbe O. The practice and infrastructure of dental public health in the United States. Dent Clin North Am 2008;52(2):259–80, v.
43. U.S. Department of Health and Human Services. Center for Medicare and Medicaid Services. National health expenditures aggregate amounts and average annual percent change, by type of expenditure: selected calendar years

1960–2005. Available at: http://www.cms.hhs.gov/NationalHealthExpendData/downloads/tables.pdf. Accessed October 10, 2008.

44. U.S. Department of Labor. Occupational employment statistics. Available at: www.bls.gov. Accessed on October 9, 2008.

45. Jones K, Tomar SL. Estimated impact of competing policy recommendations for age of first dental visit. Pediatrician 2005;115(4):906–14.

46. Getzen TE. Health economics: fundamentals and flow of funds. 2nd edition. New York: John Wiley & Sons, Inc.; 2003.

47. Saha S, Taggart SH, Komaromy M, et al. Do patients choose physicians of their own race? Health Aff 2000;19(4):76–83.

48. Brown LJ, Wagner KS, Johns B. Racial/ethnic variations of practicing dentists. J Am Dent Assoc 2000;131(12):1750–4.

49. Solomon E, Williams C, Sinkford J. Practice location characteristics of black dentists in Texas. J Dent Educ 2001;65(6):571–8.

50. Sullivan Commission. Missing persons: minorities in the health professions 2004; Washington, DC. Available at: http://www.kaisernetwork.org/health_cast/uploaded_files/092004_sullivan_diversity.pdf. Accessed April 10, 2009.

51. Neumann LM. Trends in dental and allied dental education. J Am Dent Assoc 2004;135:1253–9.

52. American Dental Association. In: 2002–03 survey of predoctoral education: academic programs, enrollment and graduates, Vol. 1. Chicago: American Dental Association; 2004.

53. Weaver RG, Valachovic RW, Haden NK. Applicant analysis: 2000 entering class. J Dent Educ 2002;66:430–48.

54. Haden NK, Catalanotto FA, Alexander CJ, et al. Improving the oral health status of all Americans: roles and responsibilities of academic dental institutions: the report of the ADEA President's Commission. J Dent Educ 2003;67:563–83.

55. Casamassimo PS, Harms KA, Parrish JL, et al. Future of dentistry: the dental work force. J Am Dent Assoc 2002;133:1226–35.

56. ADEA Commission on Change and Innovation in Dental Education. The case for change in dental education. J Dent Educ 2006;70(9):921–4.

57. Kuthy RA, McQuistan MR, Riniker KJ, et al. Students' comfort level in treating vulnerable populations and future willingness to treat: results prior to extramural participation. J Dent Educ 2005;69(12):1307–14.

58. Mohammad AR, Preshaw PM, Ettinger RL. Current status of predoctoral geriatric education in US dental schools. J Dent Educ 2003;67(5):509–14.

59. Weaver RG, Haden NK, Valachovic RW. Annual ADEA survey of dental seniors—2000 Graduating Class. J Dent Educ 2001;65(8):788–802.

60. Feigal RJ. Producing the next generation of professional educators in pediatric dentistry. Pediatr Dent 1997;19(3):189–92.

61. Davis MJ. Pediatric dentistry workforce issues: a task force white paper. American Academy of Pediatric Dentistry Task Force on Work Force Issues. Pediatr Dent 2000;22(4):331–5.

62. Seale NS, Casamassimo PS. Access to dental care for children in the United States: a survey of general practitioners. J Am Dent Assoc 2003;vol.134(12):1630–40.

63. Bendall D, Asubonteng P. The effect of dental insurance on the demand for dental services in the USA: a review. J Manag Med 1995;9(6):55–68.

64. DeNavas-Walt C, Proctor BD, Smith JC. U.S. Census Bureau, current population reports, P60-235, income, poverty, and health insurance coverage in the United States: 2007. Washington, DC: U.S. Government Printing Office; 2008.

65. Manski RJ, Brown E. Dental use, expenses, private dental coverage, and changes, 1996 and 2004. MEPS Chartbook No.17. Rockville (MD): Agency for Healthcare Research and Quality; 2007. Available at: http://www.meps.ahrq.gov/mepsweb/data_files/publications/cb17/cb17.pdf. Accessed October 13, 2008.

66. Manski RJ, Goodman HS, Reid BC, et al. Dental insurance visits and expenditures among older adults. Am J Public Health 2004;94(5):759–64.

67. Niessen LC. Extending dental insurance through retirement. Spec Care Dentist 1984;4:84–6.

68. Jones JA, Adelson RA, Niessen LC, et al. Issues in financing dental care for the elderly. J Public Health Dent 1990;50:268–75.

69. American Dental Association, Survey Center. 2000 survey of current issues in dentistry: Dentists' participation in Medicaid programs. Vol. 1. Chicago; American Dental Association; 2001–2002.

70. Damiano PC, Momany ET, Willard JC, et al. Factors affecting dentist participation in a state medicaid program. J Dent Educ 1990;54:638–43.

71. Lang WP, Weintraub JA. Comparison of Medicaid and non-Medicaid dental providers. J Public Health Dent 1996;46:207–11.

72. Venezie RD, Vann WF Jr, Cashion SW, et al. Pediatric and general dentists' participation in the North Carolina Medicaid program: trends from 1986 to 1992. Pediatr Dent 1997;19(2):114–7.

73. National Academy for State Health Policy. Increasing access to dental care in Medicaid: does raising provider rates work? Available at: www.chcf.org/documents/policy/IncreasingAccessToDentalCareInMedicaidIB.pdf. Accessed October 17, 2008.

74. Lave JR, Keane CR, Lin CJ, et al. The impact of dental benefits on the utilization of dental services by low-income children in western Pennsylvania. Pediatr Dent 2002;24(3):234–40.

75. Damiano PC, Willard JC, Momany ET, et al. The impact of the Iowa S-SCHIP program on access, health status, and the family environment. Ambul Pediatr 2003;3(5):263–9.

76. Hughes RJ, Damiano PC, Kanellis MJ, et al. Dentists' participation and children's use of services in the Indiana dental Medicaid program and SCHIP: assessing the impact of increased fees and administrative changes. J Am Dent Assoc 2005;136(4):517–23.

77. Tomar SL. An assessment of the dental public health infrastructure in the United States. J Public Health Dent 2006;66(1):5–16.

78. National Association of Community Health Centers. America's Health Centers fact sheet. Available at: www.nachc.org/client/documents/America%27s_Health_Centers_updated_8.13.08.pdf. Accessed October 15, 2008.

79. Bailit H, Beazoglou T, Demby N, et al. Dental safety net: current capacity and potential for expansion. J Am Dent Assoc 2006;137(6):807–15.

80. Patrick DL, Lee RS, Nucci M, et al. Reducing oral health disparities: a focus on social and cultural determinants. BMC Oral Health 2006;6(Suppl 1):1–17.

81. Frazier PJ, Jenny J, Bagramain RA, et al. Provider expectations and consumer perceptions of the importance and value of dental care. Am J Public Health 1977;67(1):37–43.

82. Bailit HL, Newhouse J, Brook R, et al. Dental insurance and the oral health of preschool children. J Am Dent Assoc 1986;113(5):773–6.

83. Tetuan TM, McGlasson D, Meyer I. Oral health screening using a caries detection device. J Sch Nurs 2005;21:299–306.

84. Milgrom P, Weinstein P. Early childhood caries: a team approach to prevention and treatment. Seattle (WA): University of Washington in Seattle; 1998.

85. Borrell LN, Taylor GW, Borgnakke WS, et al. Perception of general and oral health in white and African American adults: assessing the effect of neighborhood socioeconomic conditions. Community Dent Oral Epidemiol 2004;32:363–73.

86. Gift HC. Utilization of professional dental services. In: Cohen LK, Bryant PS, editors. Social sciences and dentistry: a critical bibliography, Vol. 2. London: Quintessence Publishing Company Ltd; 1984. p. 202–67.

87. Mofidi M, Rozier RG, King RS. Problems with access to dental care for Medicaid-insured children: what caregivers think. Am J Public Health 2002;92:53–8.

88. Tickle M, Milsom KM, Humphries GM, et al. Parental attitudes to the care of the carious primary dentition. Br Dent J 2003;195:451–5.

89. Maslow AH. A theory of human motivation psychological review. Psychol Rev 1943;50:370–96.

90. Kim YO. Reducing disparities in dental care for low-income Hispanic children. J Health Care Poor Underserved 2005;16(3):431–43.

91. Sohn W, Ismail A, Amaya A, et al. Determinants of dental care visits among low-income African-American children. J Am Dent Assoc 2007;138(3):309–18.

92. Lam M, Riedy C, Milgrom P. Improving access for Medicaid-insured children: focus on front-office personnel. J Am Dent Assoc 1999;130:365–73.

93. Garcia RI, Cadoret CA, Henshaw M. Multicultural issues in oral health. Dent Clin North Am 2008;52(2):319–32.

94. Institute of Medicine Committee on Understanding and Eliminating Racial and Ethnic Disparities in Health Care. Unequal treatment: confronting racial and ethnic disparities in health care. Washington, DC: National Academy Press; 2002.

95. Formicola AJ, Stavisky J, Lewy R. Cultural competency: dentistry and medicine learning from one another. J Dent Educ 2003;67:869–75.

96. Institute of Medicine of the National Academies. In the nation's compelling interest: ensuring diversity in the health care workforce. Washington, DC: National Academies Press; 2004.

97. Terrell C, Beaudreau J. 3000 by 2000 and beyond: next steps for promoting diversity in the health professions. J Dent Educ 2003;67:1048–52.

98. Vargas CM, Dye BA, Hayes KL. Oral health status of rural adults in the United States. J Am Dent Assoc 2002;133:1672–81.

99. Vargas CM, Ronzio CR, Hayes KL. Oral health status of children and adolescents by rural residence, United States. J Rural Health 2003;19(3):260–8.

100. Larson EH, Johnson KE, Norris TE, et al. State of the health workforce in rural America: profiles and comparisons. Seattle (WA): University of Washington, WWAMI Rural Health Research Center; 2003.

101. Knapp KK, Hardwick K. The availability and distribution of dentists in rural zip codes and primary care health professional shortage areas (PC-HPSA) zip codes: comparison with primary care providers. J Public Health Dent 2000;60:43–8.

102. Eberhardt MS. Health, United States, 2001. Urban and rural health chartbook. Hyattsville (MD): U.S. Dept. of Health and Human Services, Centers for Disease Control and Prevention, National Center for Health Statistics; 2001. DHHS (Public Health Service) 01-1232-1.

103. Task Force on Periodontal Treatment of Pregnant Women, American Academy of Periodontology. American Academy of Periodontology statement regarding periodontal management of the pregnant patient. J Periodontol 2004;75(3):495.

104. Michalowicz BS, DiAngelis AJ, Novack MJ, et al. Examining the safety of dental treatment in pregnant women. J Am Dent Assoc 2008;139(6):685–95.

105. Silk H, Douglass AB, Douglass JM, et al. Oral health during pregnancy. Am Fam Physician 2008;77(8):1139–44.
106. Hilgers KK, Douglass J, Mathieu GP. Adolescent pregnancy: a review of dental treatment guidelines. Pediatr Dent 2003;25:459–67.
107. Hueber C.E. Milgrom P. Lee R, et al. Dental care for pregnant women. Abstract #1908. International Association of Dental Research 2008. Toronto.
108. National Commission on Correctional Health Care. Available at: www.ncchc.org/resources/standards.html. Accessed November 7, 2008.
109. US Department of Justice. Office of Justice Programs. Bureau of Justice Statistics. Available at: www.ojp.usdoj.gov/bjs/. Accessed November 4, 2008.
110. Salive ME, Carolla JM, Brewer TF. Dental health of male inmates in a state prison system. J Public Health Dent 1989;49:83–6.
111. Mixson J, Eplee H, Feil P, et al. Oral health status of a federal prison population. J Public Health Dent 1990;50:257–61.
112. Clare JH. Survey, comparison, and analysis of caries, periodontal pocket depth, and urgent treatment needs in a sample of adult felon admissions, 1996. Journal of Correctional Health Care 1998;5:89–101.
113. Treadwell HM, Formicola AJ. Improving the oral health of prisoners to improve overall health and well-being. Am J Public Health 2005;98(9 Suppl):S171–2.
114. Makrides J, Schulman J. Dental health care of prison populations. J Correctional Health Care 2002;9:291–303.
115. Lamster IB. Oral health care services for older adults: a looming crisis. Am J Public Health 2004;94(5):699–702.
116. A state of decay: the oral health of older Americans. Available at: http://www.csg.org/pubs/Documents/sn0610StateofDecay.pdf. Accessed April 10, 2009.
117. Locker D, Jokovic A. Using subjective oral health status indicators to screen for dental care needs in older adults. Community Dent Oral Epidemiol 1996;24(6):398–402.
118. Mosca NG, Finn E, Joskow R. Dental care as a vital service response for disaster victims. J Health Care Poor Underserved 2007;18:262–70.
119. Bhalla N. Relief after the wave. Special article. Br Dent J 2006;200(2):116–8.
120. Kanehira T, Honda O, Kawakami S, et al. Dental care for refugees at shelters after the eruption of Mt. Usu. J Dent Health 2003;53(2):145–9.
121. Marcus M, Maida CA, Guzman-Becerra N, et al. Policy implications of access to dental care for immigrant communities. California Policy Research Center, University of California, California Program on Access to Care; 2001. Available at: http://www.ucop.edu/cpac/documents/dentalaccess.pdf. Last accessed November 4, 2008.
122. Obeng C. Culture and dental health among African immigrants school-aged children in the United States. Health Educ 2007;107(4):343–50.
123. Glassman P, Anderson M, Jacobsen P, et al. Practical protocols for the prevention of dental disease in community settings for people with special needs: the protocols. Spec Care Dentist 2003;23(5):86–90.
124. Seinmetz E. Americans with disabilities: 2002. US Census Bureau, current population reports 2006; P70–07 Available at: http://www.census.gov/prod/2006pubs/p70-107.pdf. Accessed December 3, 2008.
125. Feldman CA, Giniger M, Sanders M, et al. Special Olympics, special smiles: assessing the feasibility of epidemiologic data collection. J Am Dent Assoc 1997;128:1687–96.
126. Waldman HB, Perlman SP, Swerdloff M. Use of pediatric dental services in the 1990s: some continuing difficulties. J Dent Child 2000;67:59–63.

127. Oral Health America. Oral health report card. 2001. Available at: www. oralhealthamerica.org/pdf/2001-2002ReportCard.pdf. Accessed November 15, 2008.
128. Glassman P, Subar P. Improving and maintaining oral health for people with special needs. Dent Clin North Am 2008;52(2):447–61.
129. Glassman P, Folse G. Financing oral health services for people with special needs: projecting national expenditures. J Calif Dent Assoc 2005;33(9): 731–40.
130. Wilson KI. Treatment accessibility for physically and mentally handicapped people—a review of the literature. Community Dent Health 1992;9:187–92.
131. Skinner AC, Slifkin RT, Mayer ML. The effect of rural residence on dental unmet need for children with special health care needs. J Rural Health 2006;22(1): 36–42.
132. Schriver T. Testimony before a Special Hearing of a Subcommittee of the Committee on Appropriations of the United States Senate. One Hundred Seventh Congress, First Session. Anchorage (AK). March 5, 2001.
133. Dao LP, Zwetchkenbaum S, Inglehart MR. General dentists and special needs patients: does dental education matter? J Dent Educ 2005;69(10):1107–15.
134. U.S. Census Bureau. Census 2000 brief; disability status 2000, March 2003. Available at: http://www.census.gov/prod/2003pubs/c2kbr-17.pdf. Accessed April 10, 2009.

The Dilemma of Access to Care: Symptom of a Systemic Condition

James T. Rule, DDS, MS[a],*, Jos V.M. Welie, MA, MMedS, JD, PhD[b]

KEYWORDS

• Dental ethics • Professionalism • Access to care • Disparities
• Disconnectedness • Public trust • Social engagement

The standard ethical arguments that prescribe dentistry's involvement in improving access to oral health care are based on two related ideas. The first is that the ethics of social justice compels dentistry to make the distribution of its services more equitable, with special attention to the most vulnerable in the population.[1] The other is that, because disparities in oral health are, by their nature, unfair, then dentistry, with its eminently strategic position in oral health care, is obligated to do something about the disparities.[2]

The authors agree with these positions, but they also acknowledge that there is a wide gap between the theoretical ideals of justice and their application to actual practice. Overcoming this gap often is difficult. An egalitarian's delight may be a libertarian's nightmare. When it comes to getting things done, the principle of justice often invites a stalemate, not a solution.

In this article the authors present the view that ethical principles will fail to have an impact unless they are supported by a robust sense of professionalism. This theme is elaborated in the context of two broad goals.[1] The authors first show that the issue of access is a symptom of a broader problem in dentistry, namely the lack of connectedness that dentists feel between themselves and their profession, their community, and society at large. They argue that this pattern of disconnectedness (or isolation) also contributes to other urgent challenges to the profession.[2] The authors then show how the introduction of "connectedness" can facilitate the resolution of these problems. The authors believe that their proposal to "get connected" actually harkens back to the very roots of the dental profession, to the early 1830s at a time of crisis both for the country and its early dental practitioners, when visionary dental leaders managed to establish the foundation of public trust on which the fledgling profession

[a] Department of Pediatric Dentistry, University of Maryland Dental School, 8842 High Banks Drive, Easton, MD 21601, USA
[b] Center for Health Policy and Ethics, Creighton University, 2500 California Plaza, Omaha, NE 68178, USA
* Corresponding author.
E-mail address: jrule0807@verizon.net (J.T. Rule).

Dent Clin N Am 53 (2009) 421–433
doi:10.1016/j.cden.2009.03.008
0011-8532/09/$ – see front matter © 2009 Published by Elsevier Inc.

dental.theclinics.com

was accepted and grew. The authors argue that a more robust connectedness between dentists, their patients, their profession, their community, and society at large will facilitate the resolution of many of the systemic problems that dentistry currently faces, including the issue of access to care.

ACCESS TO CARE AS A SYMPTOM OF DENTISTRY'S DISCONNECTEDNESS

The United States Surgeon General's report, *Oral Health Care in America*, brought to public attention the extent and seriousness of oral disease in this country's most vulnerable people, that is, "poor children, the elderly, and many members of racial and ethnic minority groups."[3] Disparities in oral health have many different causes, some of which are far beyond the scope of the profession, as is true of most of the systemic challenges faced by dentistry today, and indeed by all professions. Individual dentists and the dental profession at large are also part of the problem, however, and do share in the responsibility for correcting it.

The authors submit that the root cause for dentistry's relative ineffectiveness in reducing disparities in oral health (relative, that is, to other health professions) lies in its longstanding pattern of disconnectedness, or isolationism. As the American Dental Education Association (ADEA) has pointed out: "Reduced access to oral health care is one of the prices of professional isolation that has too often characterized dentistry."[4]

The tendency of dentists to focus on their own privacy negatively affects their inclinations and attempts to deal with broader issues, including the staggering disparities in oral health. Many dentists consequently point outside dentistry—to state and local government, to insurance companies, to patients themselves—for solutions to oral health disparities. Even the American Dental Association (ADA) in its Code of Ethics (under the section devoted to justice) lists only one tangible duty vis-à-vis the problem of access: "[T]his principle expresses the concept that the dental profession should actively seek allies throughout society on specific activities that will help improve access to care for all."

Dentistry has a long history of disconnectedness. Throughout its existence, it has been practiced largely in separation from other branches of medicine. Whereas the traditional medical disciplines of internal medicine, surgery, and obstetrics gradually merged, dentistry remained a separate discipline. Before the very recent emergence of podiatry and optometry, the teeth were the only part of the body that always retained its own group of healers; all the other body parts, organs, and organ systems were treated by medically trained healers.

This isolation of the oral cavity from the rest of the body has had far-reaching consequences. Dental education is largely separate from medical education. Dentists and physicians have separate licensing boards and regulations. Dental and medical insurance plans are organized separately, and in many countries dental care is not part of publicly supported health care financing systems. For example, the US Medicare program, which makes health care available to the elderly, does not cover dental care. Moreover, as the ADEA points out, dentistry's disconnectedness "gives the impression to other health professionals, policymakers, and the public that oral health is not as important as general health."[4] It may even be that many dentists themselves are less appreciative of the importance of oral health compared with medical care and perhaps consider themselves as less important than physicians.

Structural forces at work in dentistry foster these patterns of isolation. Most physicians, even those with private outpatient practices, tend to work closely with other physicians in clinics and hospitals. They cooperate with a diverse cadre of other professionals such as nurses, physical therapists, clinical psychologists, and social workers. Dentists, on the other hand, generally work in relatively small practices that include a few hygienists and dental assistants. They clearly like that way of practicing, as evidenced by the persistence of this practice model. Dentists like to be their own bosses, run their own offices, and practice dentistry their way. They tend to be suspicious of protocols and use reviews, practice standards, professional regulations, and governmental control.

At the same time, many citizens in the United States suffer unnecessarily from treatable and even preventable oral conditions. In turn, this lack of care leads to significant economic losses because of missed days of work, and, in the case of children, far too many missed days at school. More serious still are delays in the diagnosis of oral cancer, leading in extreme cases to premature death. The problem of disparities in oral health is exacerbated further by the unevenness of their distribution. Everyone in the path of an earthquake or tsunami is subject to devastation, but the unmet needs for oral health care are distributed disproportionately because of poverty, race, or co-morbidity.

Other Symptoms of Disconnectedness

The authors submit that dentistry's relative failure to tackle the problem of oral health disparities head-on is only one symptom among many. They also see dentistry's isolationism reflected problematically, for example in dentistry's reluctance to engage in and submit to constructive peer review. Internal regulation is a hallmark of any profession. Dentistry has been less forthcoming than most professions in developing effective peer review programs.

Another example of dentistry's disconnectedness from society concerns the aforementioned widespread aversion to policies and treatment protocols. The individual dentist, however, is no longer able to stay abreast of rapid scientific and technological advances, and there is the grave risk that a failure to do so will undermine the public's trust in the profession of dentistry. A case in point is the 1997 *Reader's Digest* article, "How Honest Are Dentists?"[5] The article described the experiences of a journalist-patient who visited 50 different dentists to receive examinations and treatment plans. The results showed that the treatment plans varied greatly, as did the costs, which ranged from $500 to $30,000. The article—and even more so the magazine's cover title, "How Dentists Rip Us Off"—certainly outraged dentists, but it also was unsettling to patients.

There are other signs that dentistry's high ranking by the public as a trusted profession is faltering. A 2001 monthly column by Gordon Christensen[6] in the *Journal of the American Dental Association* noted the weakening of public trust and attributed it to the public's perception that dentists are preoccupied with making money and with their own interests. Also of concern is the recent flurry of very serious cheating scandals involving many United States dental students.

Finally, the authors believe that the ever-increasing practice of commercial competition between dentists, as evidenced by advertising, in-office product sales, and an ever-greater emphasis on elective treatments, is driven at least in part by dentistry's tendency toward disconnectedness. Some observers within the profession believe that what is at stake in this most onerous demonstration of isolationism is nothing less than the transformation of dentistry from a profession to a business.

Dentistry cannot have its cake and eat it too. Dentists cannot claim professional status but operate primarily according to a business model. The public will not accept such ambiguity. Indeed, in the late 1970s, the ADA's right to professional self-regulation was curbed dramatically when the Federal Trade Commission and the US Supreme Court found that the ADA (and likewise the American Medical Association and American Bar Association) was a trade organization, primarily aimed at the business interests of its members, and therefore could not prohibit advertising.

More recently, despite vigorous opposition by the dental profession, state legislatures passed various laws on the credentialing of foreign dentists and dental auxiliaries in an attempt to increase access to oral health care services. Some states now are preparing regulations for a whole new cadre of oral health practitioners. In 2006, the ADA failed to block an access-to-care plan operated by the Alaska Native Tribal Health Consortium. Furthermore, there now are published (although challenged) reports about the acceptable quality of care in the Alaska program.

The points in the previous paragraph illustrate that the profession and the public are at odds about a very important issue, and the profession's view is not prevailing. Arguably, dentists either must respond more effectively to the needs of the public or pay the price of decreased public esteem and trust. The next section shows how to deal with these problems in a way that capitalizes on the profession's thoughtful evaluation of itself.

ESTABLISHING CONNECTEDNESS

If disconnectedness is the problem—or at least a significant part of the problem—the obvious solution is to foster its opposite. What is needed, in the words of Hershey,[7] is "a willingness to be *connected*—a willingness to go beyond the isolation of narrowly interpreting one's professional role to be connected to the concerns of other individuals and to the overall well-being of society." The literature is replete with terms that capture this sense of "connectedness"; among them are "belonging," "civil engagement," "community spirit," "community mindedness," "public conscience," "social responsibility," and even "cultural competence." The authors submit that if dentists acquire a more robust sense of connectedness, it will be an important first step in the reduction of oral health disparities and other social problems of the profession. In addition it will render dentists more inclined, comfortable, and capable, as stated by DePaolo and Slavkin,[8] "of meeting the nation's need for oral health professionals engaged in the practice of clinical oral health care, public health practice, biomedical and health services research, education, and administration and who can contribute to the fields of ethics, law, public policy, government, business, and journalism."

Four Realms of Connectedness

Even if organized dentistry has a long history of contributing to the isolation of its members, and even if individual dentists willingly seek some degree of isolation, most dentists increasingly are cognizant that good oral health care demands connectedness. The days in which the dentist paternalistically could decide what patients need without involving them in the decision are long gone. Patients must inform their dentists honestly about their needs, symptoms, habits, fears, and expectations and in turn must be fully informed by their dentists about their diagnoses and treatment options. Dentists must diligently foster their patients' trust by maintaining confidentiality, allowing them full access to their records, and abstaining from any behaviors that could jeopardize patient trust. Just as patients must respect the professional autonomy of dentists, realizing that they cannot demand treatment, so dentists must respect their patients' autonomy and always obtain consent before initiating treatment.

These examples all underscore the importance of connectedness between dentist and patient. There is widespread acknowledgment today that a strong fiduciary relationship, in which the patient is a full partner in the therapeutic process, is essential for successful outcomes. This understanding of connectedness, however, is limited to the sphere of dentists and their particular patients. The kind of connectedness that Hershey[7] and DePaolo[8] advocate goes beyond the dental office. Besides a commitment to their patients, connectedness can be broken down into three additional realms: (1) the profession that dentists choose to be part of; (2) the community in which they practice; and (3) the society at large with which the profession has an implicit contract.

Nothing in this analysis is radical or even new. These three additional realms of connectedness already are acknowledged, even if not as explicitly and robustly as they should be. Consider, for example, the issue of professional commitment. The very definition of a "profession" is intrinsically a social concept:

> Many individual expert service providers are committed to serve others and may have even promised to do so publicly. But the social phenomenon of a profession always refers to a collective. It does not make sense for anyone to claim the status of a professional if there is no profession to which one belongs. Indeed, society's trust in professionals is not vested in the individual service providers but in the profession at large.[9]

Furthermore, many dentists already assume leadership roles in their communities and apply their specific expertise and skills for the betterment of those communities. Their engagement ranges from health education projects in schools to the provision of oral health care for the homeless, and from lobbying for water fluoridation to serving in elective office.

Many dentists likewise exhibit deep concern for the well-being of society at large and understand the importance of cooperating with other players in society. Public health dentistry is an acknowledged specialty today and indeed is a concern of every dentist. The ADA's code of ethics specifically states, "[T]he dentist's primary obligation is service to the patient and the public-at-large" (Section 3). More recently, environmental protection has come to the foreground. As Mandel[10] points out, "[D]ental practice today involves a growing list of safety concerns that are important areas for discussion—as well as oral health research—and include infection control, radiation safety, mercury hygiene, amalgam and silver halide disposal, waterline biofilms, and nitrous oxide leakage and its reproductive effects." Access to oral health care is yet another issue of concern.

If dentistry is to overcome its historical tendency toward isolationism, and if one grants that dentists must develop a more robust sense of connectedness not only to their own patients but also to the profession of which they have chosen to be part, to the community in which they will be practicing, and to society at large, then practitioners themselves must take the first step.

Practitioners as Agents of Change

The history of how professions, dentistry included, are formed is a story of grassroots leadership by dedicated practitioners over long periods of time that results in society's recognition of their particular expertise as being worthy of public trust.[11] It begins with the practitioners of a given occupation coming together to form associations. Working within that framework, the early practitioners recognize that their survival depends on their credibility. The recognition of their credibility by the public is accomplished over time through the requirement of formalized training and ultimately by the granting of licensure. Gradually the professional associations become powerful enough to acquire legislative recognition by the government. This recognition gives the aspiring profession competitive advantages in the marketplace, permitting its membership to function effectively as a monopoly.

The evolution from occupation to profession comes about only if practitioners can gain the public's trust, and that trust is given only if (and as long as) services are provided with dedication and a sense of integrity.[11] Ultimately, professional status is not a right but a privilege awarded by society. In a similar vein, the ADEA[4] in its 2003 report, "Improving the Oral Health Status of All Americans: Roles and Responsibilities of Academic Dental Institutions," reminds dentists that "knowledge about oral health is not the property of any individual or organization; rather, society grants individuals the opportunity to learn at academic dental institutions with an assumed contract that this knowledge will benefit the society that granted the opportunity to obtain it."

How did the early profession of dentistry gain this trust? Much of dentistry's crucial history occurred nearly 200 years ago, in the 1830s, a time of great instability in the national experience. Financial speculation was rampant. Banks failed, and bankruptcies were common. Unemployment was rampant.[1,2] At that time American dentistry existed without any well-established system for either education or oversight, even though many dentists were quite competent as a result of the limited apprenticeship training that was available in various places. Because of the absence of standards for entrance to the practice of dentistry, however, anyone who chose to do so could engage in dental practice. In the 1830s, as a result of widespread unemployment, many out-of-work persons viewed dentistry as a golden opportunity to make money in a very short time. By arranging individual agreements with dental practitioners, farmers or shop men could move from the farm or the factory to the dental chair within a few months, often within a few weeks.[12] As a result, the ethical practices and overall competence of dental practitioners took a tailspin, and public concerns about the quality of care rose accordingly.[11]

A potentially disastrous situation for both the public and for dentistry was averted because leaders came forward from the ranks of practitioners and worked diligently in the public interest against their unscrupulous colleagues who were practicing unorthodox remedies and who had no compunction about using aggressive advertising to promote them.

This leadership culminated in three key developments: the publication of the first dental journal in the United States, the creation of the Baltimore College of Dental Surgery in 1840 (the world's first dental school), and the formation of the American Society of Dental Surgeons (the first national dental society), also in 1840.

Each of these events was a necessary milestone in the recognition of dentistry as a profession. Without the creative leadership of dedicated practitioners in the early decades of the 1800s, dentistry's movement toward recognition as a profession almost certainly would not have occurred for many more decades to come, and its development might well have been far less auspicious than it has been.

At present, the country is once again in deep financial distress. Unlike the 1830s, the profession of dentistry seems to be thriving. There are, however, cracks in the profession's foundation that represent serious challenges to its future. The next section details a plan for meeting these challenges that, like dentistry's actions in the 1830s, should be led by the practitioners themselves.

The Scope of Planning

The plan presented here offers practical suggestions for developing connectedness in the professional lives of dentists. The authors believe this sense of connectedness can be achieved through a continuous process of critical self-definition. They encourage each individual practitioner and the organizations to which they belong to define for themselves the kind of professional person they and their colleagues should be, by responding to a series of questions designed to reevaluate professional values (see Appendix 1). The answers to these questions will differ for different groups, reflecting differences in community experiences both for the profession and the public, regional oral health needs, and regional cultural influences. This is a period of changing values, both for society at large and for dentistry. As traditional values are challenged, dentists must be aware of the historical and cultural influences that surround them.

The authors take their prototype for reorientation from that used by the Bon Secours Health System, Inc. (BSHSI) of Marriotsville, Maryland.[13] The BSHSI developed its format decades ago as a way to revitalize its organization and present itself more favorably in a competitive marketplace. Its current *Ethics Quality Plan 2005* is "intended to take BSHSI to a higher level of ethical awareness, expertise and behavior." Its goals include ensuring (1) that "excellence in ethics" is a BSHSI hallmark, serving both clinical and organizational needs; (2) that BSHSI "is capable of meeting the challenges of [the] future; and (3) that both "leadership and co-workers develop a suitable understanding of ethical issues and consistent habits of acting ethically."

The BSHSI plan differs from many other such institutional statements about ethics and values in its implementation into everyday activities. BSHSI takes the process seriously. It uses the process to guide the routine function of its health care system (James DeBoy, Vice President, Mission, BSHSHI, personal communication, June 6, 2005). All its institutions post their mission and values statements in conspicuous places. Each new employee is familiarized with its values, and each year the values are reinforced during staff meetings. In fact, the values are so much a part of the institution that they permeate all its decision-making processes, from clinical care to the making of budgets.

The authors present this plan with no illusions. Re-evaluation of life's directions never is easy, but dentistry's professionalism and its value system area at stake. If the profession wants to see changes in access to care and other serious issues, it must re-evaluate what dentists and dentistry ought to stand for and to judge how close they are to meeting those standards. The process, however difficult, will be interesting and certainly rewarding.

Leadership and Key Players

As with the grassroots activities in the 1830s, leadership must come from practitioners working through their various dental associations. Presumably, the primary organizations with which to collaborate are the state dental associations because of their broad representation of the profession. Other organizations to consider include the American College of Dentists, which has ethics and professionalism as a primary focus, and the Academy of General Dentistry, which also has a history of concern for ethics. Similarly, the various state boards of dental examiners have a vested interest in the ethical direction of the profession, as do specialty organizations.

Ideally, the process described here would take place in multiple communities all across the nation. Depending on the geographic context, the locus of such action may be as large as a whole state or as small as a city. Groups of two or three concerned dentists could work to persuade their organization to undertake the project. To maximize success, a broad base of key contacts should include the president, members of the board, and members of key committees or councils that pertain to issues germane to this project. These committees might include those dealing with charitable activities, peer review, governmental relations, and ethics and professionalism, among others.

If the organization is interested in participating, there should be opportunities for discussion in general forums such as the annual meeting of the association. The goal of these discussions is to inform the membership about the project and to generate support for it.

The actual work would be done by a committee composed of 18 to 20 individuals. Committee membership would consist, in part, of officers of the organization, members of pertinent committees, and representatives from the general membership. In addition, because such a project has implications that go beyond the profession, other groups should be represented as well. Examples include a member of the board of dental examiners, the state department of dental health, non-dentist members of the dental team, physicians, and representatives from the general community. In addition, if there is a nearby dental school, one might consider including representatives from the student body and dental faculty.

The entire committee would meet initially for the purpose of general orientation. It then would be divided to function as two small groups during the data collection phase, which consists of discussions of challenging questions about the committee members' views concerning the ideals, values, scope, and obligations of the dental profession.

Questions for Discussion: The Heart of the Process

The questions to be raised are by far the most important component in this process. The small-group discussions are led best by someone with experience and skill in working with diverse groups. In the discussions, it is essential to nurture a climate in which everyone feels comfortable in expressing their views, including views that are unpopular, without the risk of disapproval. Discussion leaders should try to summarize the views expressed on each question. When disagreement occurs, the discussion leaders should determine the point at which disagreement occurs.

Collectively, the questions should help the organization define its vision of how dentists should function as professionals as they interact with their patients, their profession, their community, and society in general. From the responses to these questions, value statements, as described in the next section, can be established that reflect the beliefs of the committee about what constitutes professionalism. At this point, the two separate committees combine in an attempt to prepare a final document. Ultimately, the agreed-upon value statements are presented to the membership at large for ratification.

Suggested questions for discussion appear in the Appendix at the end of this article. The questions are adaptations from papers by the present authors on the role of dental schools in the development of professional values,[14,15] but each organization is encouraged to edit these questions freely and to create new ones according to its needs.

Using the Information

Guiding value statements should be developed based on the information collected during discussion of the questions by the small groups. Each completed value statement should include three components: (1) a characterization of the essence of the statement in a single word or a phrase that serves as a lead-in to a full statement; (2) a definition of the value; and (3) an illustration(s) that includes a descriptive interpretation of its practical applicability. For example, if a particular organization decides that the altruism is part of its identity, altruism could be defined as "placing the interest of the other above one's own interest." The descriptive interpretation could be "Dentists as professionals recognize their own interests but strive to keep them in perspective as they recognize the vulnerability of their patients. They especially recognize the interests of those who need care and, with their colleagues, look for appropriate ways to contribute to those persons' well being."

Once the data have been collected and processed, the value statements need to be ratified by the organization. The organization then needs to put the values it has endorsed into action. The authors offer the following suggestions for helping the organization act most effectively:

- Establish a committee that will both monitor and promote the program
- Inform all existing and new members of the organization about the program and the organization's commitment to it. Effective mechanisms of communicative may include the organization's Web sites and print media
- Compile a list of examples for members to act upon, beginning with the examples that are presented in the descriptive interpretations of the value statements
- Catalog the activities of the membership in professional, interprofessional, or community activities for appropriate use within the organization or for public relations
- Formulate policies that foster participation in collaborative efforts with medical or other health disciplines
- Encourage collaboration with nearby dental schools in projects of mutual interest, such as participation in the teaching of ethics or in community-oriented projects designed to reduce oral health disparities
- Support initiatives that affect general societal welfare, including public health initiatives and other societal measures of merit, such as those involving public nutrition, environment, ecology, or racial discrimination
- Encourage members' participation in non-dental community outreach groups, such as Big Brother or Big Sister organizations or those that focus on HIV, juvenile diabetes, church outreach, or soil conservation.
- Celebrate the leadership of the organization's members, both individually and collectively, in worthy causes

To initiate and carry out the process described is a challenging endeavor. It should not be undertaken, however, without considering how to assess its impact—an even more difficult challenge. A recently published article by Patthoff[16] proposes an interesting self-assessment system that members of professional organizations might wish to consider. In fact, this program already is in the process of being developed. Its goal is to help practitioners build ethically sound practices. It is patterned after the Baldrige Awards, which were created by Congress in 1987 to recognize outstanding quality and performance in the business world.[17] The basic idea of the Baldrige process is to use voluntary self-assessment in seven categories of business activity, ranging from leadership to customer and market focus. Adapting the Baldrige process to the needs of dentistry requires a significant reorientation. As Patthoff[16] points out, its "purpose would be to advance professional ethics rather than gaining a 'competitive edge.'" Thus, in dentistry issues such as fiduciary relationships would be considered, along with collegial cooperation, community interaction, and social engagement.

SUMMARY

The authors have argued that the challenge of reducing disparities in oral health is tied directly to the challenge of developing a more robust sense of professionalism by strengthening dentists' connectedness to their patients, profession, community, and society at large. Leadership must come from the ranks of individual practitioners, working through their various dental associations, just as occurred in the 1830s when American dentistry was emerging as a profession. The authors recognize that dentistry's tendency toward isolation has centuries-old roots and has remained a forceful and indeed much cherished characteristic of modern dentistry. Hence, making changes such as those proposed here is a most difficult task. Treating the challenge of oral health disparities not as a separate "illness" but rather as an indication of a more systemic problem, and tackling it at its very roots, has the added benefit that other symptoms of the same condition will improve also. Even if the problem of disparities in oral health often may seem to many individual practitioners to be a non-dental problem, few will argue that the sustenance of the professionalism of the dental profession can or should be left to non-dentists. It is up to dentists to tackle this challenge.

ACKNOWLEDGMENT

The authors thank Dr. Gary Colangelo for his helpful perspectives at the outset of writing this article.

APPENDIX 1: QUESTIONS FOR DISCUSSION

The questions are organized according to the four levels of connectedness described in the body of this article: (1) between dentists and their patients; (2) between dentists and their profession; (3) between dentists and their communities; and (4) between dentists and society at large with which the profession has an implicit contract.

Connectedness Between Dentists and their Patients

What is the nature of the relationship between dentist and patient? Is it (still?) a fiduciary relationship and, if so, what does that mean? What are the rights and responsibilities of either party in this relationship? What does it mean to consider the patient as a full partner in the fiduciary relationship? Give some examples of failure to be a full partner.

Are the days of paternalism in the dental office really long gone? What is the difference between being paternalistic and making recommendations based on the patient's clinical needs? Are a patient's clinical needs synonymous with a patient's best interests? Is it possible for a professional to know the best interests of the patient, and if so, how?

If a dentist sells electric toothbrushes for profit in his or her office, is it an acceptable business practice? Does its acceptability depend upon the degree of marketing? Does its acceptability depend upon the dentist's disclosure of profit? Is this practice consistent with a fiduciary relationship?

Are you satisfied with your informed consent process? How do you view it? Is it an important risk management procedure? Is it the demonstration of your relationship with your patient? How do your patients view your informed consent process?

How important is confidentiality in dental practice as compared with medical practice?

Think about your answers for each of the questions in terms of the values they represent.

Connectedness Between Dentists and their Profession

Is the optional membership and voluntary leadership that currently characterizes most professional dental organizations sufficient to sustain the profession of dentistry? Do dentists have a responsibility to participate in the education of future dentists and the advancement of the science of dentistry? What strategies can motivate individual dentists to take a more active role in professional organizations, dental education, and dental research?

Most professional peer review committees function to resolve disputes between patients and their dentists. Is the peer review process suited to fulfill an expanded role, for example, one that includes patient safety and error prevention programs? Should peer review committees perform monitoring functions related to patient care? What can be done to motivate dentists to engage in and submit to constructive collegial multi-disciplinary peer review activities?

With respect to colleagues who are incompetent, how should dentists interact with them upon learning of a problem? Are the considerations the same with impaired colleagues? What about dishonest colleagues or those who engage in legally dubious behaviors? Under what circumstances, if any, should dentists act as whistleblowers against incompetent, impaired, or dishonest colleagues? What should be the role, if any, of state boards in these issues?

It is clear that professionals may advertise legally. Many dentists, however, believe that advertising is unprofessional. What are the boundaries between acceptable and unacceptable advertising? How can the profession assure that advertisements by its members foster the public's trust in the profession?

Regarding the issue of the encroachment of commercialism on the profession, what are the examples of concern, if any? Are any or all of the examples a threat to the public? To the profession?

What kinds of professional activities give you the most satisfaction? Why?

Think about your answers for each of the questions in terms of the values they represent.

Connectedness Between Dentists and their Communities

Should dentists and professional dental organizations be involved in oral health programs that exceed the scope of the individual dentist's typical practice parameters, such as oral health disparities, geriatric care in nursing homes, or fabrication of mouth guards? If so, in what way? Financial support? Through actions in their offices? Community clinics? Medicaid?

Should individual dentists and professional dental organizations be involved in general health issues such as heart disease, breast cancer, smoking cessation? If so, in what way? Financial support? Volunteer activities? Involvement in community clinics? Collaboration with medical organizations?

Should dentists consider their arena of interest or responsibility to include being involved in non–health-related community activities, such as town or city government, charity drives, bank directorships, homeless shelters? If so, with what motivation?

If dentists choose to participate in any or all of these activities, is it important for the public to recognize their involvement with these issues? Why or why not?

Think about your answers for each of the questions in terms of the values they represent.

Connectedness Between Dentists and Society at Large

At the general societal level, how should dentists view their responsibilities to become involved in socially based oral health problems such as access to care? Is there any duty at all to participate at some level? If so, what is the extent of a dentist's duty to do so? Is the dentist's obligation equal to or more than that of the average citizen?

The same question can be asked with respect to societal concerns of a general health nature.

Are dentists obligated to be engaged in public causes, such as gender or racial discrimination, environmental issues, or global projects in developing countries?

If dentists were to be involved in politics, given their membership in a helping profession, is their influence best placed in certain categories of activity?

Think about your answers for each of the questions in terms of the values they represent.

REFERENCES

1. Winslow GR. Just dentistry and the margins of society. In: Welie JV, editor. Justice in oral health care. Ethical and educational perspectives. Milwaukee (WI): Marquette University Press; 2006. p. 7–16.
2. Welie JVM. Are oral health disparities merely unfortunate or also unfair? In: Welie JVM, editor. Justice in oral health care. Ethical and educational perspectives. Milwaukee (WI): Marquette University Press; 2006. p. 97–125.
3. US Dept of Health and Human Services. Oral health in America: a report of the Surgeon General. MD. Rockville (IN): USDHHS, NIDCR, NIH; 2000.
4. Haden NK, Bailit H, Buchanan J, et al. Improving the oral health status of all Americans: roles and responsibilities of academic dental institutions. Report of the ADEA President's Commission. Washington, DC: American Dental Education Association; 2003.
5. Ecenbarger W. How honest are dentists? Read Dig 1997;50–6.
6. Christensen GJ. The credibility of dentists. J Am Dent Assoc 2001;132:1163–5.
7. Hershey GH. Profession and professionals: higher education's role in developing ethical dentists. J Am Coll Dent 1994;61(2):29–33.
8. DePaolo DP, Slavkin HC. Reforming dental health professions education: a white paper. J Dent Educ 2004;68(11):1139–50.
9. Welie JV. Is dentistry a profession? Part I: professionalism defined. J Can Dent Assoc 2004;70(8):529–32.
10. Mandel ID. Oral health research and social justice: the role and responsibility of the university and dental school. J Public Health Dent 1997;57(3):133–5.
11. Rule JT, Veatch RM. The structure of professions and the responsibilities of professionals. In: Rule JT, Veatch RM, editors. Ethical questions in dentistry. 2nd edition. Chicago (IL): Quintessence; 2004. p. 19–40.
12. Asbell MB. The professionalization of dentistry. Part 1. Compendium 1993;14(8):992, 994, 996.
13. BSHSI – Bon Secours Health System, Inc. Bon Secours Ethics Quality Plan. Marriotsville (MD): BSHSI; 2005. Available at: http://www.bshsi.com/strategic-direction/lead-in-catholic/ethics-purpose.htm. Accessed October 31, 2005.
14. Welie JV, Rule JT. Overcoming isolationism. Moral competencies, virtues and the importance of connectedness. In: Welie JV, editor. Justice in oral health care. Ethical and educational perspectives. Milwaukee (WI): Marquette University Press; 2006. p. 97–125.

15. Rule JT, Welie JV. Justice, moral competencies, and the role of dental schools. In: Welie JV, editor. Justice in oral health care. Ethical and educational perspectives. Milwaukee (WI): Marquette University Press; 2006. p. 233–50.
16. Patthoff DE. The future of dental ethics: promises needed. J Am Coll Dent 2008; 75(3):21–7.
17. Baldrige National Quality Program. National Institute of Standards and Technology, 2008. Available at: http://www.quality.nist.gov/Criteria.htm. Accessed April 3, 2008.

Dental Workforce

Eric S. Solomon, MA, DDS[a,b,*]

KEYWORDS

- Workforce • Dental economic trends
- Dental education trends • Future of dentistry

Dental workforce refers to the number, distribution, and characteristics of dentists, dental auxiliaries, and other support staff involved in the provision of oral health care. During the past half century, the perception of the dental workforce has fluctuated from fears of a shortage to warnings of an oversupply. Consequently, it is pertinent to view the factors that can affect changes in the supply of the dental workforce as well as the attitudes regarding the adequacy of that supply. The dental workforce supply is influenced by a variety of factors; prominent among them are demographics, dental disease rates, economics, and consumer habits. Changes in these factors in turn influence the manner in which dentistry is practiced. Patterns of dental practice can affect the supply and distribution of the dental workforce. Thus, examining these data will enhance the understanding of the changes in the dental workforce and help anticipate future trends.

Since 1950, the population of the United States has almost doubled, from 152,271,417 to an estimated 301,621,157 in 2007.[1] Moreover, the population today can be subdivided into a variety of demographic cohorts based on their year of birth. **Fig. 1** shows the distribution of population and identifies some of the most common cohorts. Individuals born before the end of World War II (1945) are referred to as the "World War II generation." There were approximately 68 million of these individuals in the United States in 2005. The Baby Boomers were born between 1946 and 1964, and there were approximately 80 million of them in 2005. Members of Generation X were born between 1965 and 1979. This cohort is smaller, with approximately 50 million individuals. Generation Y sometimes is referred to as the "Baby Boom echo." They were born between 1980 and 2001, and there are 75 million of them. In 2005, almost 46% of the population of the United States was comprised of the World War II and Baby Boomer generations.

By 2020, as these population cohorts age, their relative contribution to the total population will change. The number of members of the World War II generation will drop to just under 23 million, and the number of Boomers will decrease to about 74.5 million.

[a] Department of Institutional Research, The Texas A&M Health Science Center, Dallas, TX, USA
[b] Department of Public Health Sciences, Baylor College of Dentistry, The Texas A&M Health Science Center, Dallas, TX, USA
* Corresponding author. Department of Institutional Research, The Texas A&M Health Science Center, Baylor College of Dentistry, 3302 Gaston Avenue, Dallas, TX 75246.
E-mail address: esolomon@bcd.tamhsc.edu

Dent Clin N Am 53 (2009) 435–449
doi:10.1016/j.cden.2009.03.012
0011-8532/09/$ – see front matter © 2009 Elsevier Inc. All rights reserved.

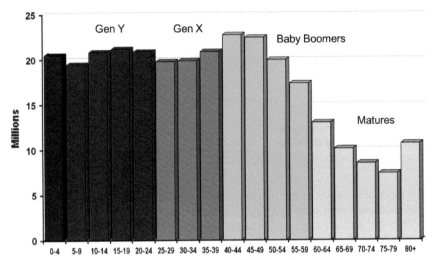

Fig. 1. United States population by age groups, 2005. (*Data from* U.S. Census Bureau. Population pyramids. Available at: http://www.census.gov/ipc/www/idb/pyramids.html. Accessed August 13, 2008.)

Together these two cohorts will represent only about 29% of the total population. The size of the various cohorts impacts changes in dental disease.

Dental caries is the most prevalent disease of the oral cavity. Since the early 1970s, caries rates generally have declined in children.[2] In 1971, children between the ages of 5 and 17 years had an average of 7.1 decayed, missing, and filled tooth surfaces (DMFS) in their permanent dentition. By 1991, the average of DMFS in children of that age had dropped to 2.5, a 64.8% decrease. Recent data suggest that the decline in DMFS in the permanent teeth of children has continued but at a slower rate. These recent data also show a slight, but not statistically significant, increase in caries in primary teeth.[3]

Increased exposure to fluoride has been widely recognized as a significant cause for this decline in caries.[4] In 1967, only 40% of the population lived in communities that had fluoridated water. By 2006, 69.2% of communities had fluoridated water.[5] Fluoride also is found in most toothpaste and in many mouthwashes. Greater awareness of the need to maintain good oral hygiene through improved home care also contributes to decreasing caries rates. **Fig. 2** charts the decline in dental caries, the increased percentage of community fluoridation, and how the decrease in dental caries has affected the generational cohorts. The Baby Boomer generation was at the very beginning of the caries decline. Generation X experienced the largest decline in caries rates, dropping from an average of 5.95 DMFS to 2.62. Generation Y and those generations that follow will reap the benefits of lower caries rates.

Expenditures for dental services increased from just under $2.0 billion in 1960 to $91.5 billion in 2006, an increase of more than 45-fold. The U.S. Centers for Medicare and Medicaid Services (formerly the Health Care Financing Administration) have projected the level of expenditures to the year 2017.[6] These projections show expenditures for dental services increasing annually to $169.6 billion by the end of the projection period—an additional increase of $78.1 billion in total annual expenditures for dental services over the next 11 years. These expenditure data were divided by the total population of the United States to arrive at per capita expenditures for dental services. Per capita expenditures for dental services increased from $10.86 in 1960 to $305.20 in 2006, an increase of more than 28-fold or an average annual increase

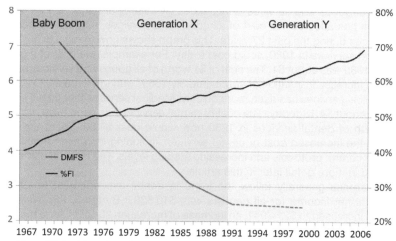

Fig. 2. Incidence of DMFS in children age 5 to 17 years and percentage of communities with water fluoridation. (*Data from* Refs.[2–4])

of 7.4% per year. Per capita expenditures are projected to increase to $517.50 by 2017, or an average annual increase of 4.9% per year. The total expenditures for dental services divided by the number of active dentists provides a rough estimate of the gross income per dentist. Expenditures per dentist increased from $21,787 in 1960 to $586,781 in 2007, an increase of more than 26-fold or an average annual increase of 7.3%. If the projections hold true, expenditures per dentist should rise to $1,150,583 by 2017, an average annual increase of 6.3%.

The mix of payment methods for dental services also has undergone major shifts. In 1960, out-of-pocket expenditures accounted for more 97% of dental payments. Insurance as a source of dental payments increased rapidly through the decades of the 1970s, 1980s, and early 1990s, peaking at 52.3% of dental expenditures in 1996. Since then, insurance as a source of payment has decreased slowly to 49.6% in 2006.[6] Government sources of dental payments were virtually nonexistent in 1960, accounting for less than 1% of all expenditures. Government funding has risen slowly since then to 6.0% in 2006. Consequently, the profile of expenditures for dental services in 2006 was 49.6% from insurance, 44.4% from out-of-pocket payments by patients, and 6.0% from government sources. In contrast, government sources accounted for 34.2% of expenditures for physician and clinical services in 2006. The U.S. Centers for Medicare and Medicaid Services predicts insurance, as a source of expenditures for dental services, will decline only slightly, to 49.5%, in 2017. They also estimate out-of-pocket expenditures will decline slightly, to 43.5% of expenditures, and that government sources will increase to 7.0% of all dental expenditures by 2017. This projection estimates that government expenditures for dental services will double by 2017 to approximately $11.8 billion. Historically, government expenditures for dental services have not increased at this rate.

Long-term economic trends are heavily influenced by changes in the inflation rate. By adjusting actual data (real dollars) using the Bureau of Labor Statistic's Consumer Price Index (CPI),[7] one can compensate for inflationary effects and view these economic trends in constant dollars. Therefore, the income and expenditure data presented here are adjusted by the CPI to reflect constant dollars. In this way, one can better ascertain real rather than inflation-induced growth.

The cost of goods and services is influenced by inflationary factors. **Fig. 3** shows how inflation has affected the cost of all goods and services, medical services, and dental services during the past 27 years. This graph shows how much a dollar's worth of goods and services in 1980 would cost today. For example, the cost of a gallon of gasoline in 1980 was about $1. The cost of $1 worth of all goods and services has risen to $2.56, an increase in inflation of approximately 156% during the past 27 years. The cost of medical services has risen more quickly. Medical services that cost $1 in 1980 would cost about $4.18 today. The cost of dental services has risen even more. That dollar's worth of dental services in 1980 now would cost $4.60. There are several reasons for the increased cost of dental services, including increased requirements for infection control protocols and increasing staffing levels. The issue of staffing level is discussed in more detail later in this article.

Dental incomes generally follow the trend in dental expenditures. In 1952, the average total net income for all dentists was $10,539.[8] By 2005, the average net income had increased to $214,941, an increase of more than 20-fold.[9] As in the expenditure data, these income figures are influenced by inflationary trends. To see whether dentists' incomes really have improved, the income data were adjusted by the CPI. Real dental incomes (in 1950 dollars) have not always increased. Between 1972 and 1983, the average real income per dentist fell by 26.3%, but it increased by 21.8% in the next decade (1982–1991), and from 1992 to 2005 the real average income increased by 41.1%.

As these data suggest, periods of high inflation have a negative impact on dental incomes. Real dental incomes fell between 1973 and 1983 as the CPI increased by a whopping 124% (an average inflation rate of 8.2% per year). As incomes rose steeply from 1992 to 2005, the average annual increase in inflation was only 2.6%. During periods of double-digit inflation, dentists generally are not able to increase their fees to keep pace with inflationary pressures; consequently, real incomes tend to fall during these times.

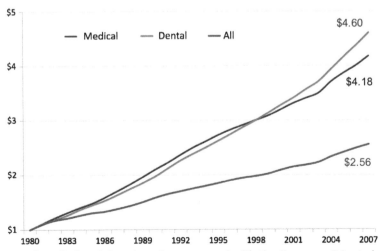

Fig. 3. Cost of medical and dental services compared with the Consumer Price Index, 1980 to 2007. (*Data from* U.S. Department of Labor. Bureau of Labor Statistics consumer price index. Available at: http://data.bls.gov/PDQ/outside.jsp?survey=cu. Accessed September 17, 2008.)

An important economic measure is the percentage of the population who visit the dentist on a regular basis.[10] During the past half-century, Americans have established a tradition of visiting the dentist on a regular basis. In 1950, less than one third of the total population and less than 15% of the population aged over 64 years had at least one dental visit during that year (**Fig. 4**). By 1998, almost two thirds of the total population (66.2%) and more than 56% of the population aged over 64 years had an annual dental visit. Since 1998, however, these percentages have been rather flat. In 2005, 65.8% of the total population and 57.7% of the population over 64 years of age had a dental visit. A greater awareness of the benefits of regular, monitored oral health care probably is responsible for the increase in annual patient visits in the overall population, and decreasing levels of edentulism is the likely principal cause for the higher visitation rates among older population groups.

The mix of services provided in the dental office also has changed appreciably during the past 40 years (**Fig. 5**). In 1958, 42% of all services in the dental office were examinations and prophylaxis. Amalgams accounted for an additional 41% of all services.[11] Extractions made up an additional 13% of services. Thus the typical visit to the dentist in the 1950s comprised an examination, a cleaning, amalgams, and the occasional extraction. By 1999, this profile of services for the general practitioner had changed considerably.[12] In 1999 Examinations and prophylaxis represented 76% of all dental services in the office. Restorations comprised 13% of the procedures, and there were more plastic restorations than amalgams. The remaining 11% of procedures comprised prosthodontic, endodontic, periodontal, and other specialty-type procedures. Only 3% of all procedures were extractions. Data from the American Dental Association's (ADA) electronic claims database suggest these trends are continuing. In 1983, 86% of the claims were from either diagnostic or preventative procedures, and restorative procedures accounted for only 6% of the claims. Obviously, the distribution of fees for these procedures was quite different. Nevertheless,

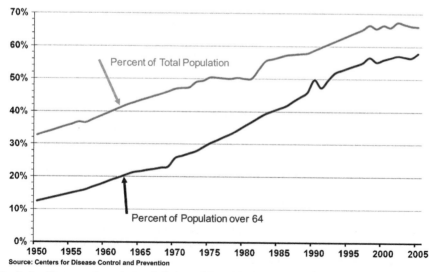

Source: Centers for Disease Control and Prevention

Fig. 4. Percentage of total population and percentage of population over 64 years of age that visited the dentist, 1950 to 2005. (*Data from* National Center for Health Statistics. National health interview surveys. Available at: http://www.cdc.gov/nchs/nhis.htm. Accessed October 9, 2008.)

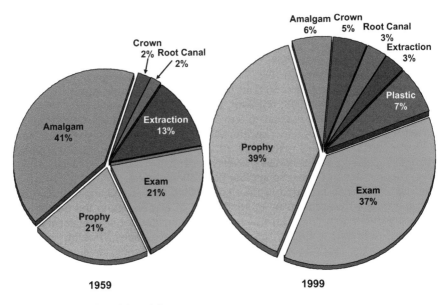

Source: American Dental Association

Fig. 5. Distribution of patient services, 1959 and 1999. (*Data from* American Dental Association. The 1959 survey of dental practice. Chicago (IL): American Dental Association; 1960. p. 64; and American Dental Association. Future of dentistry. Chicago (IL): American Dental Association; 2002. p. 56.)

the diagnostic and preventative procedures accounted for more than half the fees (54%), and the restorative procedures accounted for 22% of the fees.

The shift in the types of services provided has prompted a change in the mix of personnel involved in the provision of these dental services. Since 1955, there has been a significant increase in the auxiliary personnel involved in the dental office, with the exception of dental laboratory technicians, which has not changed appreciably.[13] The percentage of dentists who employ at least one dental assistant has increased from about 70% in 1955 to nearly 100% of all dentists today. The most dramatic change, however, has been in the employment of dental hygienists. In 1955, only about 10% of dentists employed a dental hygienist. In 2000, about 74% of general dentists employed a dental hygienist. This increase in the use of dental hygienists follows the shift toward more preventive services, a higher percentage of the population receiving routine dental care, and a general decline in the caries rate.

The increased use of dental auxiliaries strongly indicates that the number of dental office personnel has expanded, and that is certainly the case. The average size of a dental office staff has increased by about 450% during the past half century. The average number of staff members in the dental office in 1950 was less than one—a significant number of dentists still worked alone. Today's dental office is far more complex, with multiple assistants, dental hygienists, and front desk personnel. There was an average of 4.5 staff members in the dental office in 2000, and the trend for increasing staff size is likely to increase.

Another way of looking at this trend is to view the total number of dental personnel in the labor force (**Fig. 6**). In 1950, there were approximately 155,000 dental office personnel, including dentists, dental hygienists, dental assistants, and other staff; slightly more than 50% of these individuals were dentists.[14] By 2006, the number of

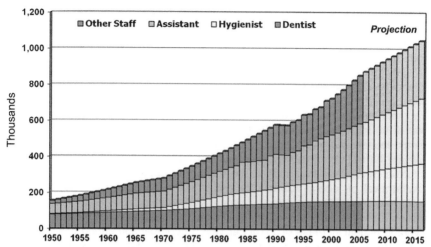

Fig. 6. Dental personnel in the labor force. (*Data from* Sixth report to the President and Congress on the status of health personnel in the United States. Chapter 5. Washington, DC: Department of Health and Human Services; 1988. p. 5–24, 5-35–5-37; and Bureau of Labor Statistics. Occupational outlook handbook, 2008–09 edition. Available at: http://www.bls.gov/oco/. Accessed October 21, 2008.)

dental office personnel had risen by more than fivefold, to more than 875,000, but less than 20% of these individuals were dentists. The Bureau of Labor Statistics predicts a continuing increase in the employment of dental hygienists, assistants, and other dental office personnel.[15] By 2016, the number of dental hygienists is predicted to increase from 160,122 in 2006 to 209,019 (30.5%); the number of dental assistants is predicted to increase from 280,000 in 2006 to 362,000 (29.3%); and other dental office personnel are predicted to increase from 277,441 in 2006 to 319,401 (15.1%). Based on these projections, more than 1 million persons will be employed in dental offices in 2014, and dentists will represent about 15% of these personnel.

These changes have a profound impact on the dental workforce levels, the state of the profession, and people's attitudes toward the profession of dentistry. For young adults, it may influence their perception of the viability of dentistry as a potential career. This perception, along with the perception of the viability of competing careers, has a profound influence on the size and character of the applicant pool for dental schools.

ENROLLMENT

During the past half-century, dramatic changes have occurred in the number of applicants to dental school, demonstrating these changing attitudes.[16,17] Wide swings in the number of applicants can influence dental schools to increase or decrease enrollment, open new schools, or close existing schools. Between 1963 and 1975, the number of applicants to dental schools increased by almost 10,000 from 5770 to 15,734. In the late 1970s and throughout the 1980s there was a growing perception that there were too many dentists and that the decreases in dental caries levels would dramatically reduce the need for dentists in the future. As a result, the number of applicants decreased as rapidly as it had risen, falling to 4996 in 1989. Since then, the number of applicants to dental school has increased again, to 10,731 in 2005—the largest applicant pool since 1978. The percentage of women applicants generally has increased as well. Between 2002 and 2005, the percentage of women applicants hovered around 44%.

Since 1950, first-year dental school enrollments have gone through four distinctly different periods (**Fig. 7**).[18] Between 1950 and 1965, first-year enrollment increased slowly from 3226 to 3808 (18.0%), an increase of about 1.2% per year. During this period, new dental schools were being established, increasing from 42 to 49 (16.7%) by 1965, in part, because of an influx of federal support. The period between 1965 and 1978, when the Baby Boomer generation went to dental school, is marked by rapid growth in first-year enrollment, increasing from 3808 to 6301 (65.6%); an average annual increase of 5.0%. New dental schools continued to open, reaching a total of 60 in 1978. Between 1978 and 1989, the rapid rise in enrollment in the previous decade was matched by an equally dramatic decline. By 1989, first-year enrollment had fallen to 3979, a decrease of 2322 students (36.9%). The decline was fueled by a precipitous drop in the number of applicants to dental school and the withdrawal of federal support for enrollment expansion. By 1989, five dental schools had closed or were in the process of closing. First-year enrollment has increased slowly since 1989, rising to 4770 in 2007 (an increase of 791 students), an average annual increase of 1.0% per year. In comparison during this period, the United States population increased by 1.2% per year. During this time, one additional dental school closed, and five new schools opened.

The pattern of dental school graduates obviously follows that of first-year enrollment (**Fig. 8**). Slightly more than 90% of entering dental students complete the program. There are two noteworthy periods. During the 10-year period from 1975 to 1984, the number of dental school graduates exceeded 5000 per year, peaking at 5756 in 1982. Between 1990 and 1996, however, there were fewer than 4000 graduates per year. In the United States, the number of dental school graduates generally has increased each year since then, rising to 4714 in 2007. The number of dental school graduates is expected to continue to increase slowly over the next 14 years, exceeding 5000 by 2016. There are several reasons for this estimate. Several new dental schools have opened in the past few years, and it is likely that a few more schools may open during the next decade. All the schools that have opened recently

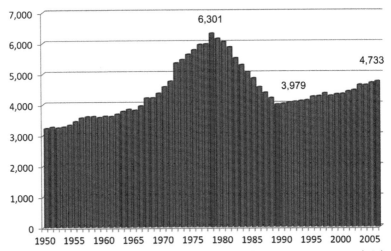

Fig. 7. First-year enrollment in dental school. (*Data from* American Dental Education Association. Applicant analysis. Washington, DC: American Dental Education Association; 1963–2005.)

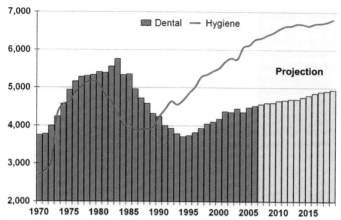

Fig. 8. Numbers of graduates from dental school and from dental hygiene programs. (*Data from* American Dental Association. Survey of dental education, Vol. 1. Chicago (IL): American Dental Association; 1950–2006.)

are located in areas of high population growth, and three are in states that previously did not have a dental school. In contrast, existing dental schools are unlikely to increase their enrollment. Today, dental schools generally are in a restricted fiscal condition because of cutbacks in state funding and the need to control tuition increases. Enrollment expansion is a costly proposition, generally involving the renovation or replacement of existing facilities. In addition, many schools are focused on a more pressing problem—recruiting and retaining a quality faculty. As long as the dental school is the primary site for providing clinical education, the number of graduates is likely to increase only moderately.

The trend in dental hygiene graduates mirrors that in dental graduates up to 1990 (**Fig. 8**). After that, the number of hygiene graduates increases at a significantly greater rate. Between 1986 and 2006, the number of hygiene graduates increased from 3880 to 6273 (61.7%). This trend should continue for at least the next decade, because the demand for dental hygiene services remains high. In addition, the cost of educating a dental hygienist has decreased because of a change in the educational setting for training dental hygienists. In 1967, almost 40% of dental hygiene programs were located in dental schools. In 2006, fewer than 9% of the dental hygiene programs were located in dental schools, and 83.2% of the programs were located in 2-year institutions such as community colleges and technical schools. If this enrollment trend continues, 44% more hygienists than dentists would graduate in 2020.

Fig. 9 shows the projected number of dental school graduates and the projected number of retiring dentists.[19] Until now, the number of dental school graduates has exceeded the number of retiring dentists. Around 2010, however, as the Baby Boomer dentists begin to retire, the number of dental retirees could surpass the number of dental school graduates. Between 2010 and 2020 the total number of active dentists in the United States actually might decline. The graph clearly shows how the enrollment bulge of the 1970s and early 1980s is mirrored in the retirement bulge that will take place during the next 10 to 15 years. Economic conditions will affect the accuracy of these predictions. Favorable economic conditions could result in a higher number of retirees at an earlier time. On the other hand, poor economic conditions could reduce significantly the retirement rate of dentists over the next decade. In addition, the retirement projections assume similar retirement ages as in the past.

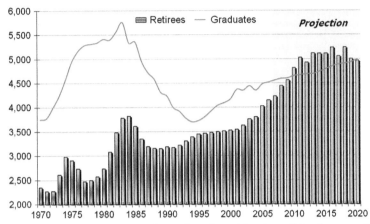

Fig. 9. Number of dentists entering practice and number of dentists retiring from practice. (*Data from* American Dental Association. Survey of dental education, Vol. 1. Chicago (IL): American Dental Association; 1950–2006; and Beazoglou T, Bailit H, Brown LJ. Selling your practice at retirement. Are there problems ahead? J Am Dent Assoc 2000;131(12):1694.)

WORKFORCE PROJECTIONS

The rate of dental retirements versus dental school graduates obviously will affect the projection of the number of dentists. If the number of retirees exceeds the number of dental school graduates, the number of active dentists in the United States will decline. The age distribution of dentists clearly shows the effect of the Baby Boomer bulge in dental enrollment and shows why the number of dental retirees may exceed that of dental school graduates. According to the ADA, 40.4% of independent dentists will be 55 years old or older by 2020.[20] Should historical patterns prevail, most of these dentists will retire or significantly cut back on their practice time during the next decade. In contrast, only 13.1% of dentists are under 40 years of age.

Since 1900, the number of dentists in the United States generally has increased (**Fig. 10**). The one exception was during the Great Depression of the 1930s when the total number of dentists actually fell. Currently, however, the number of active dentists in the United States is approaching a peak. As the anticipated number of dentists retiring potentially rises above the number of dental school graduates, the total number of dentists in the United States could begin to decline slowly around 2016. Dentistry could become the only major health profession with decreasing numbers. Because of relatively slow growth in the number of dental school graduates, the total number of active dentists in the United States could continue to decrease slowly until 2026.

Fig. 11 shows the total number of active dentists by gender. In 1980, fewer than 3% of all dentists were women. There has obviously been a rapid increase, with women currently representing an estimated 19% of dentists. Dental enrollment trends indicate that in 2020 approximately 30% of dentists will be women. As women become a larger segment of the total number of dentists, the number of male dentists necessarily declines. These data indicate that the number of male dentists probably began to decline around 2000.

Not all dentists work full-time. **Fig. 12** shows the number of dentists by full-time or part-time work status. Full-time dentists are defined as those working at least 30 hours per week. Historical data indicate that most dentists worked full-time during the first

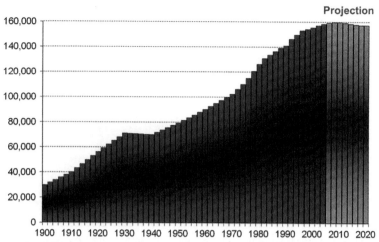

Fig. 10. Number of dentists in the United States. (*Data from* Sixth report to the President and Congress on the status of health personnel in the United States. Chapter 5. Washington, DC: Department of Health and Human Services; 1988. p. 5–24, 5-35–5-37.)

half of the twentieth century.[18] In 1975, fewer than 10% of the active dentists worked part-time. The number of dentists working part-time has increased during the past quarter century. Currently, an estimated 20% of all active dentists work part-time. If current trends persist, one in four dentists (25%) might work part-time by 2020. This change could have a significant effect on the effective workforce supply.

Recent data suggest a relationship between gender and work status.[21] In 1999, female dentists who were younger than 40 years old were more than five times more likely than their male counterparts to work part-time (5.6% versus 31.3%). Female dentists between the ages of 40 and 59 years were more than three times

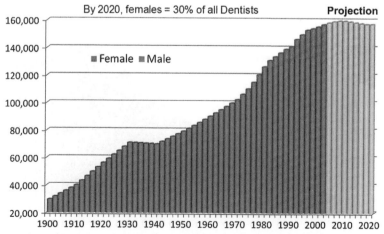

Fig. 11. Number of dentists in the United States by gender. (*Data from* Sixth report to the President and Congress on the status of health personnel in the United States. Chapter 5. Washington, DC: Department of Health and Human Services; 1988. p. 5–24, 5-35–5-37.)

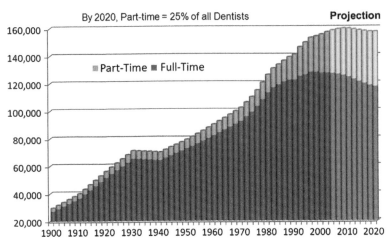

Fig. 12. Number of dentists working full time and part time. (*Data from* Sixth report to the President and Congress on the status of health personnel in the United States. Chapter 5. Washington, DC: Department of Health and Human Services; 1988. p. 5–24, 5-35–5-37.)

more likely to work part-time (8.7% versus 28.6%). Most dentists who are at least 60 years old are male, and about half of these dentists (46.2%) work part-time. As the number of female dentists increases, their impact on the dental workforce will be significant if gender differences in work status persist.

Another relatively recent phenomenon is the growth in the proportion of dentists who are dental specialists (**Fig. 13**). Most of this growth has occurred during the past 30 years. In 1970, fewer than 10% of all active dentists were specialists. Currently, about 22% of dentists are specialists. This percentage should increase slowly to about 27% by 2020. The number of both dental school graduates and specialty graduates has stabilized; therefore, it is unlikely that the proportion of

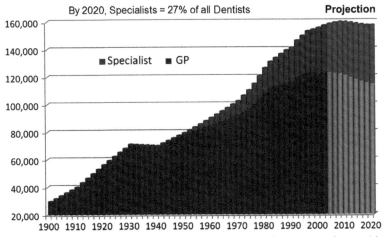

Fig. 13. Number of dentists by specialty status. (*Data from* Sixth report to the President and Congress on the status of health personnel in the United States. Chapter 5. Washington, DC: Department of Health and Human Services; 1988. p. 5–24, 5-35–5-37.)

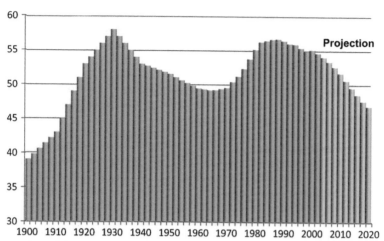

Fig. 14. Number of dentists per 100,000 population. (*Data from* Sixth report to the President and Congress on the status of health personnel in the United States. Chapter 5. Washington, DC: Department of Health and Human Services; 1988. p. 5–24, 5-35–5-37.)

dentists that are specialists will increase beyond 2020. The converse of the higher proportion of specialists is that there are fewer general dentists. In fact, the number of general dentists in the United States probably started declining at the very end of the twentieth century and probably will continue to decline throughout the projection period. This trend probably will affect the supply of dentists, particularly in non-urban areas. The overwhelming majority of specialists are located in urban areas. A decreasing number of general dentists could have a negative impact on the supply of dentists in rural areas.

Another way of looking at the supply of dentists is to compare the number of dentists with the population. The ratio of dentists to the population (dentists per 10,000 people) is dramatically different than the distribution of dentists (**Fig. 14**). The dentist-to-population ratio peaked twice during the twentieth century, once before the Great Depression and again in the late 1980s. Since the late 1980s, the dentist-to-population ratio generally has fallen. The rate of decline thus far has been relatively slow, but if the actual number of dentists begins to decline, this rate of decline will increase. By 2020, the dentist-to-population ratio could be similar to the ratios experienced almost a century earlier.

SUMMARY

The practice of dentistry underwent a fundamental change during the second half of the twentieth century. From a profession meeting a demand that was largely episodic and disease-driven, dentistry now is centered on prevention, maintenance, function, and esthetics. Changes in the workforce have followed the changes in practice; however, these changes largely involved increases in the number of auxiliaries and support staff. In 1950, the average dental office had one support person; now the average is close to six.

Three major trends converge in the first decade of the twenty-first century: a decrease in the supply of dentists relative to the population, an increase in the proportion of older groups in the population, and an increased recognition that dentistry must serve a larger segment of the population. Oral health now is recognized more widely as an integral element in overall health. Accordingly, organized dentistry and governmental agencies are trying to develop strategies that would increase the proportion of the population that has access to oral health care. The most difficult aspect of this issue is providing oral health care to the traditionally underserved segments of society.

Thus, the major workforce issue for the early decades of the twenty-first century is centered on the strategies used to provide dental services to two different population groups: the traditional population that routinely seeks dental care and the nontraditional population, many of which are referred to as the "dentally underserved" population. The current fee-for-service model of dental practice should have sufficient workforce to accommodate the traditional patient population. Increases in staffing levels and technical advances will continue to improve the efficiency of the traditional dental office. These increases in efficiency should be more than adequate to accommodate increases in demand for restorative care from older population groups that are retaining their teeth and will require routine maintenance.

Roughly 100 million Americans do not seek dental care on a routine basis. Some of these individuals can afford oral health care but do not choose to do so. Many others, however, are identified as the dentally underserved population. They do not seek dental care for a variety reasons, including inadequate financial resources, cultural barriers, and geographic isolation. Attempts to expand oral health care services to the underserved population will stimulate changes in the number and characteristics of dental health personnel. The ADA has proposed the creation of two new members of the dental workforce: the oral preventive assistant and the community dental health coordinator. These new categories of oral health care providers were designed expressly to help solve issues regarding access to the oral health care. Programs currently are being developed to educate these individuals. The Minnesota House of Representatives has approved the creation of an Advanced Dental Hygiene Practitioner. The specific duties of this new class of oral health care worker currently are under discussion, but the concept is that the duties of this individual will fall somewhere between those of a general dentist and a dental hygienist. This new provider is being developed expressly to address the oral health care needs of individuals in rural areas and the underserved population within the state.

Expanding oral health care services to the underserved will require more than simply defining new categories of oral health care providers. To address these issues successfully, adequate and reliable sources of funding must be secured. In addition, programs must be developed that also address the non-financial barriers to access to care. If these steps are taken, these new oral health care providers could play a meaningful role in the expansion of oral health care to the underserved population. In any event, attempts to address access to care issues will continue to stimulate changes in the mix and characteristics of the oral health care team.

REFERENCES

1. U.S. Census Bureau. Population pyramids. Available at: http://www.census.gov/ipc/www/idb/pyramids.html. Updated: March 27, 2008. Accessed August 13, 2008.
2. U.S. Department of Health and Human Services. Oral health in America: a report of the Surgeon General. Rockville, MD: National Institute of Dental and Craniofacial Research, National Institutes of Health; 2000. p. 2.
3. Centers for Disease Control and Prevention. National Center for Chronic Disease Prevention and Health Promotion. Available at: http://www.cdc.gov/mmwr/

preview/mmwrhtml/ss5403a1.htm#tab5. Published: August 26, 2005. Accessed August 11, 2008.

4. Centers for Disease Control and Prevention. National Center for Chronic Disease Prevention and Health Promotion. Available at: http://www.cdc.gov/nccdphp/publications/factsheets/Prevention/oh.htm. Updated: November 25, 2005. Accessed August 11, 2008.

5. Centers for Disease Control and Prevention. National Center for Chronic Disease Prevention and Health Promotion. Available at: http://www.cdc.gov/fluoridation/statistics/cwf_status.htm. Updated: October 8, 2008. Accessed October 14, 2008.

6. U.S. Centers for Medicare and Medicaid Services. National health expenditure data. Available at: http://www.cms.hhs.gov/NationalHealthExpendData/02_NationalHealthAccountsHistorical.asp#TopOfPage. Updated: July 7, 2008. Accessed September 17, 2008.

7. U.S. Department of Labor. Bureau of Labor Statistics consumer price index. Available at: http://data.bls.gov/PDQ/outside.jsp?survey=cu. Updated: August 27, 2008. Accessed September 17, 2008.

8. American Dental Association. The 1953 survey of dental practice. Chicago, IL: American Dental Association; 1954. p. 12.

9. American Dental Association. The 2006 survey of dental practice, income from the private practice of dentistry. Chicago, IL: American Dental Association; 2006. p. 4.

10. National Center for Health Statistics. National health interview surveys. Available at: http://www.cdc.gov/nchs/nhis.htm. Updated: October 15, 2008. Accessed October 9, 2008.

11. American Dental Association. The 1959 survey of dental practice. Chicago, IL: American Dental Association; 1960. p. 63–4.

12. American Dental Association. Future of dentistry. Chicago, IL: American Dental Association; 2002. p. 56.

13. American Dental Association. The 2006 survey of dental practice, Employment of dental practice personnel. Chicago, IL: American Dental Association; 2006. p. 6.

14. Sixth report to the President and Congress on the status of health personnel in the United States. Chapter 5. Washington, DC: Department of Health and Human Services; 1988. p. 5–24, 5-35–5-37.

15. Bureau of Labor Statistics. Occupational outlook handbook, 2008–09 edition. Available at: http://www.bls.gov/oco/. Accessed October 21, 2008.

16. American Dental Education Association. Applicant analysis. Washington, DC: American Dental Education Association;1963–2005.

17. Okwuje I, Anderson E, Siaya L, et al. U.S. dental school applicants and enrollees, 2006 and 2007 entering classes. Journal of Dental Education 2008;72(11):1350–91.

18. American Dental Association. Survey of dental education, Vol. 1. Chicago, IL: American Dental Association; 1950–2006.

19. Beazoglou T, Bailit H, Brown LJ. Selling your practice at retirement. Are there problems ahead? J Am Dent Assoc 2000;131(12):1693–8. p. 1694.

20. American Dental Association Health Policy Resource Center 2006. American Dental Association dental workforce model: 2004–2005. Chicago (IL): American Dental Association, Health Policy Resource Center; 2006. p. 10.

21. American Dental Association, Future of Dentistry. Chicago, IL: American Dental Association; 2002. p. 36.

The Role of Non-Dental Health Professionals in Providing Access to Dental Care for Low-Income and Minority Patients

Leonard A. Cohen, DDS, MPH, MS

KEYWORDS

- Dental problems • Hospital emergency departments
- Physician offices • Pharmacists

In the United States, poor oral health represents a significant public health problem. The 1989 National Health Interview Survey (NHIS) reported that approximately 39 million adults had suffered from some type of orofacial pain more than once during the preceding 6-month period.[1] Orofacial pain and other dental problems contribute to reduced quality of life, physical disabilities, emotional distress, and impaired functioning across a variety of life domains. In addition to causing pain and suffering, dental problems also affect economic productivity. Data from the 1996 NHIS revealed that adults missed approximately 2,442,000 days of work because of acute dental conditions,[2] and it has been estimated that children who have oral health problems lose 52 million hours from school[3] and poor children suffer from approximately 12 times as many days of restricted activity caused by dental problems as children from families with higher incomes.[4] These data probably understate the scope of the problem because orofacial pain and associated dental problems contribute to reduced productivity and a diminished learning environment even when individuals do not miss work or school. Additionally, low-income individuals report the greatest number of days of restricted activity and of lost work hours because of poor oral health,[3] suggesting that the poor are most vulnerable to the deleterious effects of orofacial pain and other dental problems.

Individuals without a usual source of medical care are less likely to gain access to needed health services.[5–7] Similarly, many individuals who lack access to dentists may be forced to use hospital emergency departments (EDs), physician offices, or

Department of Health Promotion and Policy, Division of Health Services Research, University of Maryland Dental School, 650 West Baltimore Street, Baltimore, MD 21201, USA
E-mail address: lacohen@umaryland.edu

Dent Clin N Am 53 (2009) 451–468
doi:10.1016/j.cden.2009.03.001
0011-8532/09/$ – see front matter © 2009 Elsevier Inc. All rights reserved.

dental.theclinics.com

other nontraditional settings and providers to deal with their dental problems. The poor and minorities are more likely than other segments of the population both to experience dental emergencies and to see non-dentists for the treatment of these problems because they experience greater levels of oral disease[8–14] and frequently face cost and other barriers in gaining access to dentists.[15,16]

Children residing in low-income communities are five times as likely to have untreated cavities, but only 36% of poor children had a dental visit during the preceding year compared with 70% of children from families with high income.[17] The use of dental services has been linked consistently to economic status.[18] Furthermore, individuals with dental insurance are more likely to use dental services.[19] Not surprisingly, the poor, Hispanics, and African Americans are less likely to have dental insurance.[20] Among children overall, medical insurance is approximately three times as prevalent as dental coverage.[21] Even with dental insurance, African Americans and Hispanics continue to make fewer dental visits than whites and are less likely to have visited the dentist in the previous year.[20,22] Most states limit or exclude dental benefits for adults.[23] The State Children's Health Insurance Program, passed in 1997, directed increased resources for improving children's access to needed oral health services, but use rates for adult Medicaid recipients continue to deteriorate as many states facing financial difficulties tighten eligibility criteria and restrict and/or entirely eliminate adult dental benefits.[23]

For adults, in particular, opportunities to receive free care at public clinics are extremely limited. Delay in obtaining needed dental services often results in additional pain and treatment that is more expensive and less conservative than would have been required initially. Although some poor individuals lacking coverage or facing loss of coverage because of Medicaid cutbacks may choose to pay for treatment out of pocket at a dental office, others may consult EDs, physicians, or pharmacists for pain relief. The following sections explore the role of these non-dentist health professionals in the provision of oral health care services.

USE OF EMERGENCY DEPARTMENTS FOR DENTAL PROBLEMS

Although data on the use of EDs for the treatment of dental problems are limited, African Americans and the poor have been found to be more likely than other groups to use EDs for medical care.[8] The inappropriate use of EDs for non-urgent primary medical care services has received wide attention. Similarly, many of the patients seeking care for dental-related problems could be managed by dentists in their offices.[24] Numerous reports have examined dental treatment provided in the hospital setting. Studies have involved care provided to both children[25–27] and adults,[28–30] and often have focused on oral trauma.[31,32] Most studies have focused generally on hospitals with dedicated departments of dentistry and have described services provided by dentists in dental clinical facilities. Only a few studies have described the actual services provided in EDs or patient satisfaction with the care received.[33,34]

Overall, visits to EDs increased approximately 14% during the period from 1992 to 1999.[33] Nationally, from 1997 to 2000 there was an average of 738,000 visits annually to EDs for complaints of tooth pain or tooth injury.[34] Overall, diseases of the teeth and supporting structures accounted for 0.7% of all visits to EDs. Individuals visiting EDs for dental rather than medical problems were significantly more likely to indicate Medicaid or self-pay as the payer, rather than private insurance. Only approximately 10% of dental-related visits had an associated procedure, as compared with 42% of ED visits for other problems. More than 80% of the visits resulted in prescriptions, most frequently for pain medications and antibiotics. This study raised the important issue of whether patients ever received definitive care for their dental problem. The authors concluded that EDs were an important source of care for dental-related problems, particularly for individuals lacking private dental insurance, but that ED services needed to be enhanced to provide better triage, diagnosis, and basic treatment.[34]

More recently, diseases of the teeth and supporting structures were reported to account for 0.9% of all visits to EDs.[35] National data from the 2001 Medical Expenditure Panel Survey (MEPS) revealed that 2.7% of all individuals who sought care for a dental problem outside of dental offices received care in an ED.[36] Whites and middle- and high-income individuals were more likely to receive prescriptions for their dental problems than were African Americans and low-income individuals. Given the higher levels of dental needs among African Americans and those with lower incomes, it was assumed that these groups would be more likely to receive prescriptions. It was not possible to assess whether these demographic-linked differences were based on clinical findings or were influenced by practitioner knowledge, attitudes, or culturally based biases. The role of cultural issues in the delivery of oral health care services is receiving increased attention.[37,38]

Several reports have examined changes in ED use at the University of Maryland Medical System following the elimination in 1993 of Medicaid reimbursement to dentists for the treatment of adult dental emergencies.[39,40] Visits to the ED by Medicaid patients increased by 22% following the elimination of dentist reimbursement. ED use for dental conditions, unlike medical conditions, was most common on weekends. This finding suggested an inability to access dental offices on weekends.[40] This hospital-specific project led to a statewide study covering all adult Medicaid-eligible persons treated in all Maryland hospitals and by office-based physicians.[41] The rate of ED claims was 12% higher after dentist reimbursement was eliminated. The most frequent diagnosis codes cited were "unspecified disorder of the teeth and supporting structures" (34%), "periapical abscess" (24%), and "dental caries" (22%). During the 4-year study period, 85 hospital admissions resulted from ED Medicaid dental-related visits. The average cost for claims associated with hospital admissions was $5793.[42] Although the objective of the original policy change eliminating dentist reimbursement from Medicaid achieved the goal of reducing overall dentist–related Medicaid expenditures from approximately $7.5 million for the 2-year period before the change to zero after the policy change, the policy change also resulted in poorer health outcomes and a diminution of access to care.[43]

More recently, a Maryland telephone study examined the characteristics of low-income minority adults who had sought relief from toothache pain during the previous 12 months at EDs and physician offices as compared with those who sought care from dentists.[44] In addition, it assessed patient satisfaction with the services received. A majority of the respondents suffering from toothache pain (58.6%) sought relief from dentists; only 8.7% and 20.1% contacted EDs or physician offices, respectively. ED contacts were least likely to be reported by the elderly, Hispanics, and higher-income respondents and were most likely to be reported by African Americans and the poor. The overwhelming majority of respondents who contacted an ED (80.5%) subsequently contacted a dentist for relief. Irrespective of demographic characteristics and consistent with other reports,[34,45] ED use was positively associated with the severity of the pain experience. More than three fourths of the respondents (78.6%) reported that pain was the most important reason for contacting the ED. The only reason given by Hispanics for contacting EDs, however, was lack of knowledge of any dentists to contact. This finding highlights the importance of addressing access problems of Hispanics if disparities in oral health are to be reduced.[46] The majority of all respondents (71.4%) reported that they were told to see a dentist; approximately

35% were given a prescription. No one received definitive treatment for the pain. Nevertheless, most respondents reported that the treatment or advice provided helped "a lot" (65.9%). Paradoxically, this high level of perceived effectiveness may reflect a high concordance of expectations with the actual care received.[47]

Thus, it seems that many individuals lacking access to traditional dental services may use EDs for temporary pain relief. Unfortunately, most EDs lack readily available dental services and therefore generally do not provide definitive treatment.[48] Nevertheless, costs are incurred when patients are assessed standard charges for ED visits (facility and physician charges). The magnitude of this problem is unknown. ED services would be enhanced by the addition of dental staff or ED physicians who have received specialized training in the delivery of emergency dental services.

PROVISION OF ORAL HEALTH CARE SERVICES BY PHYSICIANS
Services for Children

There has been increased emphasis on the potential role of physicians in alleviating disparities in oral health, especially among children.[46,49–51] Even though the availability of Medicaid services for children has improved, there is evidence that this step alone will not guarantee access to needed services.[52] Concurrently, there has been a growing awareness of the need for better integration between medicine and dentistry if oral health disparities among children are to be addressed adequately.[53] This need was reflected in the 1995 report by the Institute of Medicine, "Dental Education at the Crossroads," which called for closer integration of medicine and dentistry at the levels of research, education, and patient care.[54] In 2006 a major initiative of the American Dental Education Association and the Association of American Medical Colleges published a report highlighting the need for changes in professional curricula to foster a greater integration of medicine and dentistry.[55] Numerous reports, conferences, and government agencies have recognized the need to address oral health disparities among children and have issued recommendations and promoted strategies to do so, including, notably, an increasing role for pediatricians and family physicians.[21,53,56,57]

There is a strong rationale for using primary care physicians for delivering preventive services to children. Interventions are needed early in life, and well-child visits to pediatricians begin early and occur frequently. Poor children have better access to medical care than to dental care: 90% of poor children have a usual source of medical care.[58] Furthermore, most general dentists will not treat young children, and in many areas of the country the number of pediatric dentists is very limited. There are, however, approximately 88,000 family physicians and 40,000 pediatricians, and 50% of all primary care office visits are provided by family physicians.[59] It has been suggested that children who are found to be at risk for the development of dental caries or who possess recognized risks should be encouraged to establish a dental home 6 months after the eruption of the first tooth or by age 1 year, whichever occurs first.[60] Pediatricians and family physicians are well placed to make this determination and subsequent dental referral.

Professional organizations have taken the lead in recognizing and advancing the role of physicians in providing needed oral health care services to children. For example, the American Academy of Family Physicians has published a practical guide on infant oral health,[61] as has the Society of Teachers of Family Medicine Group on Oral Health.[62] Furthermore, the American Academy of Pediatrics has established a policy describing the role of pediatricians in the oral health risk assessment of children and emphasizing the need for pediatric health care professionals to develop the knowledge to provide assessments on all patients beginning at the age of 6 months.[60]

Unfortunately, there is evidence of only very limited involvement of medical schools, residency programs, and continuing medical education programs with oral health content. In general, the overall level of training in oral health of pediatricians at all levels is inadequate to provide the competencies needed to provide quality oral health care to children.[63] Several studies have questioned physicians about the amount of oral health training they received while in medical school. A survey of pediatricians and family practitioners in Alabama found that 59% of the respondents reported receiving no preventive oral health information during their medical school training,[64] and a national study of pediatricians reported that half of the respondents received no training in dental health issues during their medical school or residency experiences.[51] Similarly, a survey of 3000 pediatricians revealed that 76% considered that participatory experiences and learning opportunities during their pediatric residency in the area of dentistry were insufficient.[65] Unfortunately, recent reports indicate that there has been little improvement. A 2006 survey of graduating pediatric residents found that during their training, 32% received no oral health care training; among those who received training, 75% received less than 3 hours, and only 14% spent clinical time with a dentist. On a positive note, more than 85% of respondents believed pediatricians should perform oral screenings and counsel patients about correct brushing techniques.[66]

Thus, although the need for further training is evident, physicians have indicated that they recognize the importance of and are interested in providing oral health care services to children. Nationally, more than 90% of the responding pediatricians agreed that they had an important role in identifying oral health problems in children and in providing counseling on caries prevention. Furthermore, 74% indicated that they were willing to provide fluoride varnish.[51] Although physicians have expressed a willingness to provide preventive services to young children, the effectiveness of physician interventions aimed at preventing and managing dental caries in preschool children has not been established.[67] The U.S. Preventive Services Task Force reviewed the effectiveness of five possible physician interventions: screening and risk assessment, referral, provision of dietary supplemental fluoride, application of fluoride varnish, and counseling. The Task Force concluded that there was not sufficient evidence to support the effectiveness of screening, referral, and counseling to prevent dental caries in preschool children. There was fair evidence of the effectiveness of fluoride supplementation and varnish. Unfortunately, there also was fair evidence that the physicians' consideration of fluoride exposure was inadequate and therefore contributed to an increased risk of fluorosis among children receiving supplements.

In a related area, the characteristics of medical providers that influence their decision to refer children at risk for dental problems have been examined. The study population included 69 pediatric practices and 49 family medicine practices and focused on the referrals among Medicaid-eligible children in North Carolina.[68] Overall, approximately 78% of all primary care clinicians reported that they probably would refer children who had signs of early dental caries or were at high risk. The most common method of referral was to provide the caregiver with a dentist's name (96%); less frequently, calls were made from the physician's office to a dental office to make an appointment for the referred child (54%). Practitioners who had a high degree of confidence in their screening abilities and low referral difficulty were most likely to make referrals. Another study used national data from the 2003 Medical Panel Expenditure Survey to examine the role of non-dentist health care providers in providing advice to children and adolescents on obtaining a dental checkup.[69] Approximately 45% of children age 2 to 17 years were advised by a non-dentist health care provider to seek a dental checkup. Although no differences in likelihood of referral were found based on patient income, children from higher-income families were more likely to seek dental care. Similarly, the potential role of Early Head Start programs in providing referrals to primary care providers for the delivery of preventive dental care has been examined.[70] Staffs were questioned about their opinions on the ability of physicians and nurses to screen children for dental problems and to provide preventive dental services during medical visits. The opinions generally were favorable, but education was deemed necessary for staff lacking familiarity with this approach to care delivery.

A number of studies have begun to explore the role of physicians in providing preventive dental services to children. A statewide project in North Carolina focused on the involvement of medical practices in the prevention of early childhood caries in low-income children.[71] That program, "Into the Mouths of Babes," targeted low-income children from birth until 35 months of age. Pediatricians, family physicians, and providers in community health centers received Medicaid reimbursement for providing preventive dental services including risk assessments, screening, referral, fluoride varnish applications, and counseling. Providers received lectures and interactive sessions, practice guidelines for the interventions, case-based problems, implementation strategies, resource materials, and follow-up training. Preliminary evaluations demonstrated that non-dental personnel were able to integrate preventive dental services into their practices.

The effectiveness of preventive services provided by physicians depends in part on the frequency of well-child visits. Therefore, another study attempted to assess the number of follow-up preventive dental visits in medical offices and their determinants among children who had received dental screenings, fluoride varnish, and counseling.[72] Children were found to have received approximately 66% of the recommended number of remaining well-child visits. The authors concluded that efforts to increase the frequency of preventive dental visits may need to be linked to efforts directed at increasing well-child visits for medical care.

In another program, dental, medical, and educational faculty from the University of Washington Academic Health Center worked together to provide evidence-based, culturally appropriate pediatric oral health training to family medicine residents in five community-based programs.[73] The educational program was directed at children from birth to 5 years of age and included dental development, the caries process, dental emergencies, and special needs topics. Preliminary evaluations of knowledge gained, attitudes and self-efficacy, and behavioral changes were encouraging. In another study directed at pediatric and family practice residents, residents received 1- or 2-hour training sessions in infant oral health.[74] At a 1-year follow-up, the participants' behaviors had improved, with 73% reporting referrals to dentists at age 1 year (compared with 28% at baseline); however, fluoride-prescribing practices showed little improvement.

Questions addressing the effectiveness of physician interventions are beginning to be addressed. Another North Carolina study was conducted at a private pediatric group practice to determine the accuracy of the care provider's screening and referral for early childhood caries.[75] Independent, blinded oral screening results and referral recommendations made by the pediatricians were compared with those of a pediatric dentist. The pediatricians received 2 hours of training in infant oral health that included clinical slides illustrating dental caries, instructions on how to recognize cavitated lesions, and information about determining the need for a dental referral. Providers were told to refer any child who had one or more cavitated carious lesions, soft tissue pathology, or oral trauma. Results indicated that with limited training, the pediatric primary care providers attained an adequate level of accuracy in identifying children needing referral. Only 70% of the children needing referral actually were referred, however. The authors concluded that it would be easy to incorporate dental screenings into a busy pediatric practice.

It seems likely that programs aimed at increasing the preventive oral health services provided by primary care providers will increase. For example, the Health Foundation of South Florida recently announced a new educational program directed at 700 pediatricians and family practice physicians in several Florida counties.[76] The program will train providers who accept Medicaid to provide dental screenings, preventive procedures, and counseling to children. North Carolina continues to expand its "Into the Mouths of Babes" program.[77] Presently more than 425 private practices and local health departments and 3000 providers have received training, resulting in more than 100,000 preventive visits per year. Similarly, the Washington Dental Services Foundation is working to increase primary care providers' involvement in oral health by training family medicine residents and by developing and distributing continuing education materials.[59] Recently, Baltimore became the first city in the country to provide fluoride vanishes to children in medical clinics.[78] Plans are underway to expand the program statewide by July 2009.

Despite these positive steps, roadblocks to greater participation by primary care providers must be addressed. Experiences related to oral health must be increased for primary care residents, and continuing education opportunities must be made available for current practitioners.[63] At the same time, the efficacy of physician interventions must be established. In addition, the ease of obtaining referrals to pediatric and general dentists must be enhanced if primary care providers are not to become frustrated, because only approximately 5000 pediatric dentists and few general dentists see children under the age of 3 years.[79] Finally, time constraints imposed on busy practitioners[63] as well as limited reimbursement for preventive services other than fluoride varnish probably will pose further impediments.[80]

Services for Adults

Several authors have discussed the role of medical practitioners in addressing dental pain,[81-83] providing treatment for temporomandibular disorders,[84] and in the early detection of oral cancer.[85,86] Compared with the increased emphasis on the role of physicians in providing needed oral screening and preventive services for children, however, studies examining the role of physicians in providing services to adults for the treatment of dental emergencies or other dental problems are limited. "Oral Health in America: A Report of the Surgeon General" commented on the lack of data on physician-based services for oral and craniofacial conditions.[21] Several overseas studies have documented the use of medical practitioners for the treatment of adult dental problems.[87,88] In the United States, the role of non-dental professionals in providing adult pain relief has been recognized also,[89] and several studies, although limited in scope, have established that patients suffering from toothache pain have sought relief from non-dentist professionals.[90,91] For example, among older Florida adults reporting toothache pain during the prior 12 months, approximately 11% reported seeing a physician. More generally, although in 1995 there were approximately 700 million total patient visits to physician offices in the United States, only 0.2% of these visits had a principal diagnosis relating to diseases of the teeth and supporting structures.[92] From 1999 to 2000, visits for dental-related problems accounted for approximately 0.3% of all physician office visits.[35] In 2002, there were approximately 890 million visits to office-based physicians.[93]

The previously described Maryland study of EDs also examined the use of physicians to treat dental problems after the Medicaid reimbursement of dentists was eliminated.[94] Unexpectedly, after dentist reimbursement was eliminated, the rate of claims for physician office visits decreased by 7%. It seemed that patients assumed that if dental visits were no longer covered, visits to physician for dental problems would not be covered, either. Although the rate of physician office claims did not increase after the policy change, the rate of physician office visits still was greater than that reported for EDs. National data from the 2001 MEPS survey previously cited found that approximately 7% of individuals who experienced a dental problem outside of the normal dental office–based delivery system received care from a physician.[36] Patients who had dental problems were more likely to have made physician visits than ED visits. It seems, therefore, that individuals lacking a usual source of dental care prefer physician offices rather than EDs as a treatment site.

A survey of two family medicine practices found that 4.5% of their patient visits were related to oral problems.[95] Pain and mucosal ulcerations were the problems most frequently encountered. The most frequent treatment provided was advice (62%), followed by prescriptions (48%) and office treatment (20%). The authors concluded that oral problems were a common occurrence in family medicine practices and suggested the desirability of including oral medicine topics in the training and continuing education of primary care doctors. Consistent with this study, a state-wide telephone survey of Maryland residents found that approximately 6% of individuals over the age of 20 years reported seeing a physician for a dental problem sometime during the prior 12 months.[96] The problem most frequently mentioned was "toothache" (26.7%). The majority of respondents who had dental-related physician visits (80%) were satisfied with the treatment or advice they received. Approximately one third of the respondents who saw a physician (36.4%) reported that they had to see a dentist for the same problem. Respondents expressing greater dissatisfaction with their medical visit were more likely to report a follow-up visit with a dentist for the same problem. This dissatisfaction may have resulted from their expectations for obtaining relief for their dental problem not being met.[97]

The previously cited Maryland study also examined the characteristics of low-income minority adults who sought relief from toothache pain at physician offices.[44] Approximately 20% of the respondents sought relief from physicians, and approximately 83% of these respondents also subsequently contacted a dentist. Respondents' use of physicians was associated directly with both the degree to which their pain interfered with their everyday activities and the severity of their pain. The majority of respondents were told to see a dentist/oral surgeon (66.7%). Consistent with other reports of physician-related dental services,[36] respondents with higher incomes were more likely to receive prescriptions than were respondents with lower incomes, and those who had the lowest income were most likely to be told to see a dentist. This pattern of prescribing is contrary to that found with dentists,[98] who were more likely to prescribe drugs for lower-income and minority patients. It was not possible to tell if this pattern of prescribing was based on clinical need or was influenced by physicians' attitudes or biases. Awareness of racial/ethnic disparities in health care has been increasing. An Institute of Medicine report, "Unequal Treatment: Confronting Racial and Ethnic Disparities in Health Care," addressed the potential influence of provider bias, discrimination, and patient stereotyping in health disparities.[99] The percentage of respondents who received prescriptions from EDs and physician contacts for toothache was considerably smaller than comparable figures reported nationally for ED and physician visits in general (ED: 76.7%; physician: 70.5%).[100,101] This finding was particularly surprising, given that these visits were associated with toothaches. The relatively lower rates of prescribing may reflect providers' concerns about encouraging dental-related visits or their discomfort in treating dental-related problems. None of the respondents received definitive treatment for their toothache pain; rather, most were instructed to see a dentist. Surprisingly, given the absence of definitive treatment and that only a minority of the respondents received a prescription/drug sample, a majority reported that the treatment/advice helped "a lot." As with ED care, this high level of perceived effectiveness may reflect, paradoxically, a high concordance of respondent expectations with the actual care received.[47] Of special note, 16.8% of the respondents delayed dental visits because of a perceived "medical complication," that is, pregnancy. This concern was especially notable in Hispanic respondents, among whom it was the most common reason given for delaying care. Hispanics also were most likely to mention medical complications as a reason for visiting a physician. Apparently, Hispanics have misconceptions surrounding the appropriate use of dental services during pregnancy. The importance of health literacy in addressing health disparities has been gaining increasing recognition,[102] and improving dental health literacy, especially among minority groups, is an important goal.

Unfortunately, like EDs, physician offices often are not the most appropriate setting for adults to receive care for a dental problem. As discussed previously, primary health care providers are increasingly receiving training in providing preventive services to children. Unfortunately, physicians generally have received minimal if any training in the management of adult dental problems.[103–105] Several authors have provided guidance to physicians in this area.[46,81–83,85] Recognizing this deficiency, the General Medical Services Committee of the British Medical Association published guidelines on the management of dental problems.[106] Additional education and guidelines have proven beneficial in assisting physicians in dealing with dental problems.[107] The children's oral health curriculum developed by the Society of Teachers of Family Medicine Group on Oral Health, as previously cited, also contains educational modules directed at adult oral health issues.[62] More recently, family practice and emergency room residents in New Mexico were provided dental training to gain an understanding of dental anesthesia, treatment planning, diagnosis, and the management of dental trauma and infections.[108] Resident graduates were able to provide emergency dental procedures in rural EDs and practices. A similar training program was instituted in Maine, where family practice residents received training in emergency dental evaluation and treatment procedures and general oral health care. This innovative program concentrated on developing faculty skills as the basis for continued resident training. A survey of patients receiving tooth extraction services found that overall satisfaction was high.[109] Training programs such as those just described undoubtedly will enhance physicians' ability to provide effective adult emergency dental services.

ROLE OF PHARMACISTS IN CONSULTING WITH THE UNDERSERVED REGARDING TOOTHACHE PAIN

In addition to using EDs and physicians as sources of care, oral pain sufferers also may seek advice and consultation regarding their dental problems from pharmacists. Several authors have provided pharmacists with advice regarding their role in the management of dental pain.[110–113] Furthermore, international studies have documented pharmacists' role in this regard.[114–116] The role of pharmacists in dental pain relief also has been documented in the United States. For example, in one study 5% of child/adolescent patients suffering from dental pain sought a pharmacist's advice before seeking care from a dentist.[50]

Only a few studies have examined the pharmacist's role in the management of toothache pain from the perspective of the patient. A Maryland survey of toothache pain sufferers found that approximately 20% discussed their most recent toothache pain with a pharmacist.[117] This percentage was considerably greater than the 5% of children/adolescents who consulted pharmacists.[50] Pharmacists were consulted as frequently as physicians and more than twice as frequently as EDs.[44] Longer-suffering respondents, those experiencing the greatest interference with daily activities, and those with the most intense toothache pain were more likely to seek advice from pharmacists. As might be expected and consistent with other reports,[115] a majority of respondents (57.8%) who spoke with a pharmacist reported that they asked what medicine to take, and 37.9% asked what they could do to treat their toothache themselves. Only a few were seeking comfort or support (2.6%) or asked about whom to call or visit (1.7%). Approximately 56% of the respondents reported that the advice they received helped "a lot." This level of satisfaction was consistent with that reported elsewhere for advice/treatment from EDs and physicians.[44]

Pharmacists have a greater role in delivering advice about oral health problems in the United Kingdom, as demonstrated by formal inquires[118,119] and published research reports.[114,115,120–122] No comparable focus in the United States is apparent. This disparity seems to be related to differences in the health care systems, in pharmacy practice, and in reimbursement. Proposed changes in pharmacy practice in the United States concerning behind-the-counter medical authority may lead to an increased emphasis on the pharmacist's role as an oral health adviser.[123]

Pharmacists are key members of the health care team and are capable of playing an important role in alleviating toothache pain.[118,120] This role is especially relevant for low-income and minority individuals lacking ready access to dentists, because pharmacists are among the easiest health care professionals to access.[120] As is true for many physicians who have received little or no training in the management of dental problems, and as has been documented abroad for pharmacists,[114,116,124] the formal training of pharmacists in the United States regarding dental problems must be enhanced if their full potential to alleviate toothache pain is to be achieved. In a related area, the Agency for Health care Research and Quality recently developed tools to help pharmacists better assist low-income and minority patients who have limited health literacy.[125] Such efforts have obvious implications regarding pharmacists' ability to provide consultations related to dental problems.

FUTURE DIRECTIONS

The disadvantaged continue to suffer disproportionately from dental problems,[126] are more likely to have untreated oral health problems and associated pain, and also are more likely to forego dental treatment even when in pain.[12] This finding is consistent with reports that individuals who have the greatest need are least likely to receive care.[127] Additionally, minorities experience greater behavioral impact from dental pain and use higher levels of self-medication.[128] Minorities also often face additional barriers to care associated with their cultural competence.[129] The need to address these health disparities has received national attention.[21,130]

It can be assumed that many individuals lacking access to traditional dental services will continue to seek care and consultation from EDs, physicians, and pharmacists. This issue will assume increasing importance as the population continues to age and become more diverse, because the elderly and ethnic and racial minorities, in particular, face significant economic barriers to accessing private dental services.[21,131] In addition, the awareness of the importance of cultural issues in health care delivery will continue to increase.[38] The elimination of disparities in health care must consider both the cultural influences that exist in minority populations and health providers' responsibilities for providing services directed at eliminating the disparities.[132] In this context, given the changing demographic composition of the United States population, the issue of dental workforce diversity is likely to gain in importance.[133] Culturally competent clinicians are more likely to work in clinical settings that offer training in cultural diversity and culturally appropriate educational materials and that employ a higher percentage of nonwhite staff. In addition, clinicians who demonstrate cultural competence are more likely to demonstrate that they understand and respect the language, values, and beliefs of ethnic and racial minorities and that they possess the attitudes and skills to provide care in a manner that demonstrates their respect and understanding.[134] These skills will become increasingly important for pediatricians and family practitioners, as well as for dentists.

Poor access to oral health care services and growing racial and ethnic disparities in oral health require new approaches to the delivery of services to strengthen the oral health safety net. Common core elements of successful programs include involving the community in planning and implementation, building on the existing health safety net to link oral health care services with primary care, and changing public or institutional policy to support the financing and delivery of dental care.[135] Involving the community in planning must include the dental profession. As physicians' provision of oral health care services increases, it will be important to ensure the cooperation of the dental profession. Concerns have been voiced about potential encroachment, especially with the provision of children's preventive services.[136] These concerns are likely to escalate if physicians' provision of adult emergency services, including extractions, becomes more widespread.[108,109] Finally, physicians and pharmacists will need enhanced training in the management of oral health problems if their potential to help alleviate oral health disparities is to be realized fully.

REFERENCES

1. Lipton JA, Ship JA, Larach-Robinson D. Estimated prevalence and distribution of reported orofacial pain in the United States. J Am Dent Assoc 1993;124:115–21.
2. National Center for Health Statistics (NCHS). Current estimates from the National Health Interview Survey, 1996. Series 10, no. 200. Hyattsville (MD): Public Health Service; 1996.
3. Gift HC, Reisine ST, Larach DC. The social impact of dental problems and visits. Am J Public Health 1992;82:1663–8.
4. General Accounting Office. Oral health: dental disease is a chronic problem among low-income populations. Report GAO/HES-00–72. Available at: http://www.gao.gov. Accessed October 21, 2008.
5. Gross CP, Mead LA, Ford DE, et al. Physician heal thyself? Regular source of care and use of preventive health services among physicians. Arch Intern Med 2000;160:3209–14.
6. Ettner SL. The relationship between continuity of care and health behaviors of patients: does having a usual physician make a difference? Med Care 1999;37:547–55.
7. DeVoe JE, Fryer GE, Phillips R, et al. Receipt of preventive care among adults: insurance status and usual source of care. Am J Public Health 2003;93:786–91.
8. Health status of minorities and low-income groups. 3rd edition. Washington, DC: U.S. Department of Health and Human Services, Public Health Service, Health Resources and Services Administration; 1991.

9. National Findings. Oral health of United States adults: the National Survey of Oral Health in U.S. Employed adults and seniors 1985–1986. Washington, DC: National Institute of Dental Research. Publication #NIH 87-2868.
10. National Center for Health Statistics (NCHS). Third National Health and Nutrition Examination Survey (NHANES III) reference manuals and reports [CD-ROM]. Hyattsville (MD): U.S. Department of Health and Human Services, Public Health Service, Centers for Disease Control and Prevention; 1996.
11. Green BL, Person S, Crowther M, et al. Demographic and geographic variations of oral health among African Americans. Community Dent Health 2003;20: 117–22.
12. Vargas CM, Macek MD, Marcus SE. Sociodemographic correlates of tooth pain among adults: United States, 1989. Pain 2000;85:87–92.
13. Riley JL, Gilbert GH, Heft MW. Socioeconomic and demographic disparities in symptoms of orofacial pain. J Public Health Dent 2003;63:166–73.
14. Duncan RP, Gilbert GH, Peek CW, et al. The dynamics of toothache pain and dental services utilization: 24-month incidence. J Public Health Dent 2003;63: 227–34.
15. Manski RJ, Moeller JF, Maas WR. Dental services: an analysis of utilization over 20 years. J Am Dent Assoc 2001;132:655–64.
16. Health, United States, 2003. Hyattsville (MD): National Center for Health Statistics; 2003.
17. Agency for Healthcare Research and Quality. 2007 national healthcare disparities report. Agency for Healthcare Research and Quality. Available at: www. ahrq.gov/qual/qrdr07.htm. Accessed October 21, 2008.
18. Pleis JR, Coles R. Summary health statistics for U.S. adults: National Health Interview Survey, 1999. National Center for Health Statistics. Vital Health Stat 10(212). 2003.
19. Manski RJ, Brown E. Dental use, expenses, private dental coverage, and changes, 1996 and 2004. Rockville (MD): Agency for Healthcare Research and Quality; 2007. MEPS Chartbook No. 17.
20. Manski RJ, Macek MD, Moeller JF. Private dental coverage: who has it and how does it influence dental visits and expenditures? J Am Dent Assoc 2002;133: 1551–9.
21. U.S. Department of Health and Human Services. Oral health in America: a report of the Surgeon General. Rockville (MD): U.S. Department of Health and Human Services; 2000. National Institute of Dental and Craniofacial Research, National Institutes of Health.
22. Jack SS, Bloom B. Use of dental services and dental health; United States, 1986. National Center for Health Statistics. Vital Health Stat 1988;10(165).
23. Schneider D, Schneider K. Medicaid dental care for adults: a vanishing act. Presented at the National Oral Health Conference. Milwaukee (WI), April 28–29, 2003.
24. Waldrop RD, Ho B, Reed S. Increasing frequency of dental patients in the urban ED. Am J Emerg Med 2000;18:687–9.
25. Battenhouse MR, Nazif MM, Zullo T. Emergency care in pediatric dentistry. J Dent Child 1988;55:68–71.
26. Majewski RF, Snyder CW, Bernat JE. Dental emergencies presenting to a children's hospital. J Dent Child 1988;55:339–42.
27. Zeng Y, Sheller B, Milgrom P. Epidemiology of dental emergency visits to an urban children's hospital. Pediatr Dent 1994;16:419–23.
28. Silverman S, Eisenbud L. Patterns of referral of dental patients to the emergency room. J Hosp Dent Pract 1976;10:39–40.

29. Berger JL, Mack D. Evaluation of a hospital dental emergency service. J Hosp Dent Pract 1980;14:100–4.
30. Sonis ST, Valachovic RW. An analysis of dental services based in the emergency room. Spec Care Dentist 1988;8:106–8.
31. Galea H. An investigation of dental injuries treated in acute care general hospital. J Am Dent Assoc 1984;109:434–8.
32. Meadow D, Lindmer G, Needlemon H. Oral trauma in children. Pediatr Dent 1984;6:248–51.
33. Burt CW, McCaig LF. Trends in hospital emergency department utilization: United States, 1992–99. National Center for Health Statistics. Vital Health Stat 2001;13(150).
34. Lewis C, Lynch H, Johnston B. Dental complaints in emergency departments: a national perspective. Ann Emerg Med 2003;42:93–9.
35. Burt CW, Schappert SM. Ambulatory care visits to physician offices, hospital outpatient departments, and emergency departments: United States, 1999–2000. National Center for Health Statistics. Vital Health Stat 2004;13(157).
36. Cohen LA, Manski RJ. Visits to non-dentist health care providers for dental problems. Fam Med 2006;38:548–56.
37. Like R, Steiner P, Rubel A. Recommended core curriculum guidelines in culturally sensitive and competent health care. Fam Med 1996;27:291–7.
38. Formicola AJ, Stavisky J, Lewy R. Cultural competency: dentistry and medicine learning from one another. J Dent Educ 2003;67:869–75.
39. Cohen LA, Manski R, Hooper FJ. Does the elimination of Medicaid reimbursement affect the frequency of emergency department dental visits? J Am Dent Assoc 1996;127:605–9.
40. Manski R, Cohen LA, Hooper FJ. Use of hospital emergency rooms for dental care. Gen Dent 1998;46:44–7.
41. Cohen LA, Manski RJ, Magder LS, et al. Dental visits to hospital emergency departments by adults receiving Medicaid: assessing their use. J Am Dent Assoc 2002;133:715–24.
42. Cohen LA, Magder LS, Manski RJ, et al. Hospital admissions associated with nontraumatic dental emergencies in a Medicaid population. Am J Emerg Med 2003;21:540–4.
43. Mullins CD, Cohen LA, Magder LS, et al. Medicaid coverage and utilization of adult dental services. J Health Care Poor Underserved 2004;15:672–87.
44. Cohen LA, Bonito AJ, Akin DR, et al. Toothache pain: a comparison of visits to physicians, emergency departments, and dentists. J Am Dent Assoc 2008; 139:1205–16.
45. Cohen LA, Harris SL, Bonito AJ, et al. Coping with toothache pain: a qualitative study of low income persons and minorities. J Public Health Dent 2007;67:28–35.
46. Drum MA, Chen DW, Duffy RE. Filling the gap: equity and access to oral health services for minorities and the underserved. Fam Med 1998;30:206–9.
47. Dayton E, Zhan C, Sangl J, et al. Racial and ethnic differences in patient assessments of interactions with providers: disparities or measurement biases? Am J Med Qual 2006;21:109–14.
48. Burgess J, Byers MR, Dworkin SF. Pain of dental and intraoral origin. In: Bonica JJ, editor. The management of pain, 1. Philadelphia: Lea and Febiger; 1990.
49. Venugopal T, Kulkarni VS, Neruker RA, et al. Role of pediatrician in dental caries. Indian J Pediatr 1998;65:85–8.
50. Mason C, Porter SR, Madland G, et al. Early management of dental pain in children and adolescents. J Dent 1997;25:31–4.

51. Lewis CW, Grossman DC, Domoto PK, et al. The role of the pediatrician in the oral health of children: a national survey. Pediatrics 2000;106:1–7.

52. Rosenbach ML, Irvin C, Coulam RF. Access for low-income children: is health insurance enough? Pediatrics 1999;103:1167–74.

53. Mouradian WE, Wehr E, Crall JJ. Disparities in children's oral health and access to dental care. JAMA 2000;284:2625–31.

54. Institute of Medicine: Committee on the Future of Dentistry. In: Field MJ, editor. Dental education at the crossroads: challenges and change. Washington, DC: National Academy Press; 1995. p. 3–4.

55. Curriculum and clinical training in oral health for physicians and dentists: report of a panel of the Macy Study. Available at: publications@adea.org.

56. Children's dental services under Medicaid: access and utilization. publication OEI 09-93-00240. San Francisco (CA): US Dept of Health and Human Services; 1996.

57. The face of a child. The Surgeon General's Conference on Children and Oral Health. Available at: http://www.nidcr.nih.gov/sgr/children.htm. Accessed October 21, 2008.

58. Mouradian WE, Berg JH, Somerman MJ. Addressing disparities through dental-medical collaborations, part 1. The role of cultural competency in health disparities: training of primary care medical practitioners in children's oral health. J Dent Educ 2003;67:860–8.

59. Maier R. Oral health and primary care. Presented at the Hilltop Institute Symposium, Developing Comprehensive Oral Health Policy: Challenges and Opportunities for State Health Policy Makers. Baltimore, MD, June 17, 2008.

60. American Academy of Pediatrics. Oral health risk assessment timing and establishment of the dental home. Pediatrics 2003;111:1113–6.

61. Douglas JM, Douglas AB, Silk HJ. A practical guide to infant oral health. Am Fam Physician 2004;70:2113–22.

62. Smiles for life: a national oral healthy curriculum for family medicine. The Society of Teachers of Family Medicine Group on Oral Health. Available at: http://stfm.org/oralhealth/. Accessed October 21, 2008.

63. Krol DM. Educating pediatricians on children's oral health: past, present, and future. Pediatrics 2004;113:487–92.

64. Sanchez OM, Childers NK, Fox L, et al. Physicians' views on pediatric preventive dental care. Pediatr Dent 1997;19:377–83.

65. Wender EH, Bijur PE, Boyce WT. Pediatric residency training: ten years after the task force report. Pediatrics 1992;90:876–80.

66. Romano-Clarke G, Caspary G, Boulter S, et al. Oral health care training among graduating pediatric residents [abstract]. Presented at the 135th annual meeting of the American Public Health Association, Washington, DC, November 7, 2007.

67. Bader JD, Rozier RG, Lohr KN, et al. Physicians' roles in preventing dental caries in preschool children: a summary of the evidence for the U.S. Preventive Services Task Force. Am J Prev Med 2004;26:315–25.

68. dela Cruz GG, Rozier RG, Slade G. Dental screening and referral of young children by primary care providers. Pediatrics 2004;114:642–52.

69. Chu M, Sweis LE, Guay AH, et al. The dental care of U.S. children—access, use and referrals by nondentist providers, 2003. J Am Dent Assoc 2007;138:1324–31.

70. Mathu-Muju KR, Lee JY, Zeldin LP, et al. Opinions of Early Head Start staff about the provision of preventive dental services by primary medical care providers. J Public Health Dent 2008;68:154–62.

71. Rozier RG, Sutton BK, Bawden JW, et al. Prevention of early childhood caries in North Carolina medical practices: implications for research and practice. J Dent Educ 2003;67:876–85.
72. Quinonez RB, Pahel BT, Rozier RG, et al. Follow-up preventive dental visits for Medicaid-enrolled children in the medical office. J Public Health Dent 2008; 68:131–8.
73. Mouradian WE, Schaad DC, Kim S, et al. Addressing disparities in children's oral health: a dental-medical partnership to train family practice residents. J Dent Educ 2003;67:886–95.
74. Douglass JM, Douglass AB, Silk HJ. Infant oral health education for pediatric and family practice residents. Pediatr Dent 2005;27:284–91.
75. Pierce KM, Rozier RG, Vann WF. Accuracy of pediatric primary care providers' screening and referral for early childhood caries. Pediatrics 2002;109:82–94.
76. Rhodenizer K. Grant will help improve oral health for Florida's children. University of Florida, Health Science Center News; May 6, 2008.
77. King R. North Carolina's Into the Mouths of Babes Program. Presented at the Hilltop Institute Symposium, Developing Comprehensive Oral Health Policy: Challenges and Opportunities for State Health Policy Makers, Baltimore, MD, June 17, 2008.
78. Anderson L. Early dental health is the aim. Baltimore Sun; May 16, 2008. p. B1, B6.
79. Seale NS, Casamassimo PS. Access to dental care for children in the United States: a survey of general practitioners. J Am Dent Assoc 2003;134: 1630–40.
80. Casamassimo PS. Oral health in primary care medicine: practice and policy challenges. Am Fam Physician 2004;70:2074–6.
81. Baker B. Emergency dental treatment for the family physician. Can Fam Physician 1987;33:1521–4.
82. Comer RW, Caughman WF, Fitchie JG, et al. Dental emergencies, management by the primary care physician. Postgrad Med 1989;85:63–6, 69–70, 77.
83. Clark MM, Album MM, Lloyd RW. Medical care of the dental patient. Am Fam Physician 1995;52:1126–32.
84. Glaros AG, Glass EG, Hayden WJ. History of treatment received by patients with TMD: a preliminary investigation. J Orofac Pain 1995;9:147–51.
85. Pyle MA, Terezhalmy GT. Oral disease in the geriatric patient: the physician's role. Cleve Clin J Med 1995;62:218–26.
86. Goodman HS, Yellowitz JA, Horowitz AM. Oral cancer prevention; the role of family practitioners. Arch Fam Med 1995;4:585–6.
87. Anderson R, Richmond S, Thomas DW. Patient presentation at medical practices with dental problems: an analysis of the 1996 General Practice Morbidity Database for Wales. Br Dent J 1999;186:297–300.
88. Thomas DW, Satterthwaite J, Absi EG, et al. Antibiotic prescription in the primary care setting. Br Dent J 1997;181:401–4.
89. Rodriguez DS, Sarlani E. Decision making for the patient who presents with acute dental pain. AACN Clin Issues 2005;16:359–72.
90. Locker D, Grushka M. Prevalence of oral and facial pain and discomfort: preliminary results of a mail survey. Community Dent Oral Epidemiol 1987;15:169–72.
91. Riley JL, Gilbert GH, Heft MW. Health care utilization by older adults in response to painful orofacial symptoms. Pain 1999;81:67–75.
92. Schappert SM. Ambulatory care visits to physician offices, hospital outpatient departments, and emergency departments: United States, 1995. National Center for Health Statistics. Vital Health Stat 1997;13(129).

93. Woodwell DA, Cherry DK. National ambulatory medical care survey: 2002 summary. Advanced data from vital and health statistics; no 346. Hyattsville (MD): National Center for Health Statisitcs; 2004. p. 84.

94. Cohen LA, Manski RJ, Magder LS, et al. A Medicaid population's use of physicians' offices for dental problems. Am J Public Health 2003;93:1297–301.

95. Lockhart PB, Mason DK, Konen JC, et al. Prevalence and nature of orofacial and dental problems in family medicine. Arch Fam Med 2000;9:1009–12.

96. Cohen LA, Cotten PA. Adult patient visits to physicians for dental problems. J Am Coll Dent 2006;73:47–52.

97. Newsome PRH, Wright GH. A review of patient satisfaction: 2. Dental patient satisfaction: an appraisal of recent literature. Br Dent J 1999;186:166–70.

98. Wall TP, Brown J, Zentz RR, et al. Dentist-prescribed drugs and the patients receiving them. J Am Coll Dent 2007;74:32–41.

99. Institute of Medicine Committee on Understanding and Eliminating Racial and Ethnic Disparities in Health Care. Unequal treatment: confronting racial and ethnic disparities in health care. Washington, DC: National Academy Press; 2002.

100. Nawar EW, Niska RW, Xu J. National Hospital Ambulatory Medical Care Survey: 2005 emergency department summary. Advance data from vital and health statistics; no. 386. Hyattsville (MD): National Center for Health Statistics; 2007.

101. Cherry DK, Woodwell DA, Rechtsteiner EA. National Ambulatory Medical Care Survey: 2005 summary. Advance data from vital and health statistics; no. 387. Hyattsville (MD): National Center for Health Statistics; 2007.

102. The invisible barrier: literacy and its relationship with oral health. A report of a workgroup sponsored by the National Institute of Dental and Craniofacial Research, National Institutes of Health, U.S. Public Health Service, Department of Health and Human Services. J Public Health Dent 2005;65:174–82.

103. Pennycook A, Makower R, Brewer A, et al. The management of dental problems presenting to an accident and emergency department. J R Soc Med 1993;86:702–3.

104. Graham DB, Webb MD, Seale NS. Pediatric emergency room visits for nontraumatic dental disease. Pediatr Dent 2000;22:134–40.

105. Tapper-Jones L. A comparison of general medical and dental practitioners' attitudes to diagnosis and management of common oral and medical problems. Postgraduate Education for General Practice 1993;4:192–7.

106. British Medical Association (General Medical Services Committee). Patients presenting with dental problems. London: British Medical Association; 1994.

107. Ma M, Lindsell CJ, Jauch EC, et al. Effect of education and guidelines for treatment of uncomplicated dental pain on patient and provider behavior. Ann Emerg Med 2004;44:323–9.

108. Beetstra S, Derksen D, Ro M, et al. A health commons approach to oral health for low-income populations in a rural state. Am J Public Health 2002;92:12–3.

109. Jenkins DR. An evaluation of dental care at the Maine-Dartmouth Family Practice: a survey of patient satisfaction and resident training. Presented at the Northeast Regional Society of Teachers of Family Medicine Meeting. Danvers (MA), October 27–29, 2006.

110. Brown T. Dealing with dental disasters—a guide for community pharmacists. Pharm J 2007;278:561–2.

111. Pray WS. Dental pain. US Pharm 2007;32:18–23.

112. Peard M. Keeping teeth for a lifetime. Australian Journal of Pharmacy 2002;83:237–9.

113. Weaver S, Gill MA, Gill CL. Oral health care. California Pharmacist 1999;46: 42–55.
114. Maunder PEV, Landes DP. An evaluation of the role played by community pharmacies in oral healthcare situated in a primary care trust in the north of England. Br Dent J 2005;199:219–23.
115. Bhati B, Duxbury AJ, Macfarlane TV, et al. Analgesics recommended by dentists and pharmacists, and used by the general public for pain relief. Int J Health Promot Educ 2000;38:95–103.
116. Gilbert L. The role of community pharmacists as an oral health adviser—an exploratory study of community pharmacists in Johannesburg, South Africa. SADJ 1998;53:439–43.
117. Cohen LA, Bonito AJ, Akin DR, et al. The role of pharmacists in consulting with the underserved regarding toothache pain. J Am Pharm Assoc 2009;49:38–42.
118. Scottish Office Department of Health. The oral health strategy for Scotland. Edinburgh (UK): The Scottish Office Department of Health; 1995.
119. Pharmacy: the report of the Committee of Inquiry appointed by the Nuffield Foundation. London: Nuffield Foundation; 1986.
120. Chestnutt IG, Taylor MM, Mallinson EJH. The provision of dental and oral health advice by community pharmacists. Br Dent J 1998;184:532–4.
121. Dickinson C, Howlett JA, Bulman JS. The role of the community pharmacist as a dental health adviser. Community Dent Health 1995;12:235–7.
122. Dickinson CM, Howlett JA, Bulman JS. The community pharmacist—a dental health advisor? Pharm J 1994;252:262–4.
123. Druggists seeking enlarged care role. Baltimore (MD): The Sun; November 1, 2007. p. A1, A10.
124. Mackie IC, Blinkhorn AS, Fuller SS. Coping with dental health problems. Manchester (UK): Center for Pharmacy Postgraduate Education; 1993.
125. Agency of Healthcare Research and Quality. New AHRQ tools help pharmacies better serve patients with limited health literacy. Available at: http://www.ahrq.gov/browse/hlitix.htm. Accessed October 21, 2008.
126. Brown LJ, Wall TP, Lazar V. Trends in caries among adults 18 to 45 years old. J Am Dent Assoc 2002;133:827–34.
127. Gilbert GH, Shelton BJ, Chavers LS, et al. The paradox of dental need in a population-based study of dentate adults. Med Care 2003;41:119–34.
128. Riley JL, Gilbert GH, Heft MW. Orofacial pain: racial and sex differences among older adults. J Public Health Dent 2002;62:132–9.
129. Stewart DCL, Ortega AN, Dausey D, et al. Oral health and use of dental services among Hispanics. J Public Health Dent 2002;62:84–91.
130. U.S. Department of Health and Human Services. A national call to action to promote oral health. Rockville (MD): U.S. Department of health and Human Services; May 2003. Public Health Service, Centers for Disease Control and Prevention and the National Institutes of Health, National Institute of Dental and Craniofacial Research. NIH Publication No. 03-5303.
131. Anderson MH. Future trends in dental benefits. J Dent Educ 2005;69:586–94.
132. Thomas SB. Health disparities: the importance of culture and health communication. Am J Public Health 2004;94:2050.
133. Mitchell DA, Lassiter SL. Addressing health care disparities and increasing workforce diversity: the next step for the dental, medical, and public health professions. Am J Public Health 2006;96:2093–7.

134. Paez KA, Allen JK, Carson KA, et al. Provider and clinic cultural competence in a primary care setting. Soc Sci Med 2008;66:1204–16.

135. Formicola AJ, Ro M, Marshall S, et al. Strengthening the oral health safety net: delivery models that improve access to oral health care for uninsured and underinsured populations. Am J Public Health 2004;94:702–4.

136. Meskin L. Look who's practicing dentistry. J Am Dent Assoc 2001;132:1352, 1354, 1356, 1358.

Improving Access to Oral Health Care for Children by Expanding the Dental Workforce to Include Dental Therapists

David A. Nash, DMD, MS, EdD

KEYWORDS

- Children's oral health • Oral health disparities
- Access to care • Dental therapists • Dental workforce

Oral Health in America: A Report of the Surgeon General[1] and the subsequent *National Call to Action to Promote Oral Health*[2] contributed significantly to raising public awareness regarding the problems of providing the benefits of oral health to all Americans. Although these reports addressed the issue of oral health for both adults and children, this article focuses on the issue as specifically related to children. It documents the disparities in oral health among children, identifies barriers to access to care for children; describes the use of dental therapists internationally to improve access to care for children; documents previous efforts in the United States to train individuals other than dentists to care for children's teeth; describes the current status of the use of dental therapists in Alaska; justifies limiting the care given by dental therapists to children; suggests potential economic advantages of using dental therapists; and concludes by describing how dental therapists could be trained and deployed in the United States to improve access to care for children and reduce oral health disparities.

DISPARITIES IN THE ORAL HEALTH OF CHILDREN

A report in the journal *Pediatrics* identified dental care as the most prevalent unmet health need for children in the United States.[3] Numerous studies, many of which are cited in the *Surgeon General's Report*,[1] document the profound and significant disparities in oral health among America's children.[2] Dental caries is the nation's most common childhood disease. It affects 58.6% of children between the ages of 5 and 17 years and is, therefore, five times more common than childhood asthma and seven

Department of Pediatric Dentistry, College of Dentistry, University of Kentucky, Lexington, KY 40536-0297, USA
E-mail address: danash@email.uky.edu

Dent Clin N Am 53 (2009) 469–483
doi:10.1016/j.cden.2009.03.007
0011-8532/09/$ – see front matter
dental.theclinics.com

times more common than hay fever. By mid-childhood more than 50% of children are affected by dental caries, and by late adolescence 80% have dental caries.[2] Children lose 52 million hours of school time each year because of dental problems, and poor children experience nearly 12 times as many restricted-activity days from dental disease as do children from higher income families.[4,5] Toothaches are the single most significant health problem encountered by elementary school teachers. Decay in the primary dentition is a predictor of decay in the permanent dentition, and children who have poor oral health often continue such a pattern into adulthood, potentially affecting speech, nutrition, economic productivity, and quality of life.[6] Eighty percent of the dental disease of children is found in 20% to 25% of children (approximately 18 million children) who predominately are from African American, Hispanic, American Indian/Alaskan Native, and low-income families.[7] Seventy-nine percent of American Indian/Alaskan Native children aged 2 to 5 years have tooth decay—frequently early childhood caries that results from improper feeding habits in infancy—and 68% of the tooth decay is untreated.[8] The prevalence and severity of dental disease are linked to socioeconomic status across all age groups.

WORKFORCE BARRIERS TO ACCESSING CARE FOR CHILDREN

Multiple barriers to ensuring access to care for children have been identified.[1,2,8–10] Significant among these barriers are the limitations of the professional dental workforce, that is, an inadequate number of dentists as well as their suboptimal distribution, ethnicity, education, and practice orientations.

The dentist to population ratio is declining from its peak of 59.5/100,000 in 1990 and will drop from the current 58/100,000 to 52.7/100,000 in the year 2020—a decline of 10%.[11,12] One estimate suggests the ratio could fall as low as 45 dentists/100,000 people by 2020.[13] Beginning in 2008, more dentists will be retiring than graduating; this trend will continue until 2020.[14] The number of pediatric dentists is not sufficient to provide adequate access to care for children. Although the number of pediatric dentists has increased significantly during the past 30 years, there are only 4357 such trained specialists practicing in the United States today. In 2000, the president of the American Academy of Pediatric Dentistry stated, "Even with a Herculean increase in training positions [for pediatric dentists], improved workforce distribution, and better reimbursement and management of public programs, pediatric dentistry will never be able to solve this national problem [of disparities] alone. We need help."[15]

Compounding the issue of the number of dentists is the location of dental practices. The overwhelming majority of dentists practice in suburbia, with few practicing in rural and inner city areas where the children with the greatest need live. The number of federally designated dental shortage areas increased from 792 in 1993 to 1995 in 2002 and to 4048 in 2008, with 48 million people living in these areas.[9,16] Although Approximately 12% of the population but only 2.2% of dentists are African American. Individuals of Hispanic ethnicity make up another 10.7% of the population, but only 2.8% of dentists are Hispanic.[17] Less than 6% of entering student dentists are African American, and less than 6% are Hispanic.[18] The demographics of oral disease indicate that these two minority groups comprise a significant proportion of the problem of disparity in care.[7]

A further issue is graduating dentists' general lack of instruction and experience in treating children. The typical college of dentistry curriculum provides an average of only 177 clock hours of didactic and clinical instruction in dentistry for children.[19] A recent study found that 33% of dental school graduates had not had any actual clinical experience in performing pulpotomies and preparing and placing stainless steel crowns, common therapies required for children.[20] Official American Dental Association (ADA) policy also questions the adequacy of the dental curriculum in preparing dentists to treat children. In 2000, an ADA House of Delegates resolution called for "a review of the predoctoral education standard regarding pediatric dentistry to assure adequate and sufficient clinical skills of graduates."[21] The background statement supporting the resolution suggested that inadequate educational preparation for treating children could be a barrier to children's access to care. There is no evidence of a subsequent increased emphasis on children's dentistry in predoctoral education. In fact, in a recent study entitled "U.S. Predoctoral Education in Pediatric Dentistry: Its Impact on Access to Dental Care," the authors concluded "results suggest that U.S. pediatric dentistry predoctoral programs have faculty and patient pool limitations that affect competency achievement, and adversely affect training and practice."[20]

An additional dimension of the workforce problem is the practice orientation of many dentists. Dentists generally do not treat publicly insured children, that is, children covered by Medicaid or the State Children's Insurance Program (S-CHIP). It is difficult to discuss the issue of access to care, particularly when focusing on the disparities that exist in oral health among America's children, without referencing the public insurance system. Medicaid provides an entitlement to comprehensive dental services for children who live at or below 150% of the federal poverty level, and S-CHIP provides the entitlement to children living at or below 200% of the federal poverty level. Medicaid and S-CHIP, however, fail to meet the oral health needs of America's children. Among the several factors contributing to this failure is dentists' unwillingness to provide care in their offices for children who have publicly financed dental insurance. Dentists offer multiple reasons for this failure, including low reimbursement schedules, demanding paper work and billing requirements, and the frequent failure of the parents of these children to keep scheduled appointments. A 1996 study indicated that only 10% of America's dentists participated in the Medicaid.[22] A more recent study indicates approximately 25% of dentists received some payment from Medicaid during a given year; however, only 9.5% received $10,000 or more.[23]

AN INTERNATIONAL APPROACH FOR IMPROVING CHILDREN'S ACCESS TO CARE

In 1921, a group of 30 young women entered a 2-year training program at Wellington, New Zealand to study to become school dental nurses;[24] in 1988 the designation was changed to "school dental therapists." Recent literature in the United States has designated this position as a "pediatric oral health therapist."[25,26] School dental therapists transformed the oral health of the children of New Zealand and laid the basis for what was to become an international movement. New Zealand's School Dental Service continues to this day and has developed an enviable record in caring for the oral health of children in New Zealand (W.M. Thomson, Associate Professor of Dental Public Health, School of Dentistry. University of Otago, Dunedin, New Zealand, personal communication, May 2003, and[27]).

The traditional curriculum in dental therapy in New Zealand enrolls high school graduates who spend 2 academic years, each of 32 weeks' duration, in the dental therapist's curriculum. During the first year topics of study include the basic biomedical sciences (general anatomy, histology, biochemistry, immunology, and oral biology) as well as clinical dental sciences (dental caries, periodontal disease, preventive dentistry, patient management, radiography, local anesthesia, restorative dentistry, dental materials, and dental assisting). In the second year, the course content includes pulpal pathology, trauma, extraction of primary teeth, clinical oral pathology, developmental anomalies, health promotion/disease prevention, New Zealand society, the health care delivery system, and record keeping, as well as administrative and legal issues associated with dental therapy practice in New Zealand. Approximately 760 hours of the 2400-hour curriculum are spent in the clinic treating children; most of this experience occurs in the second year.[25,26] Graduates entering the School Dental Service must serve for 1 year in a preceptorship with another school dental therapist (W.M. Thomson, personal communication, May, 2003, and[27]).

In New Zealand 610 registered dental therapists provide care for the country's 850,000 children.[28] Ninety-seven percent of New Zealand's children are cared for by dental therapists who are assigned to every elementary and middle school in New Zealand.[29] They work under the general supervision of a district dental officer. A recent report of the oral health of New Zealand's school children documented that at the end of a given school year essentially none of New Zealand's children in the School Dental Service had untreated tooth decay (W.M. Thomson, personal communication, May 2003, and [27]).

The model developed in New Zealand has spread to 52 other countries.[28] Currently more than 1500 dental therapists provide the overwhelming majority of dental care for children in Australia.[28]

Malaysia employs dental therapists to provide free dental care for its 3 million children in 17,000 elementary schools and 2000 secondary schools through a network of 2000 public dental clinics for children. All dental care for children in Malaysia is provided by dental therapists.[28]

Dental therapists have practiced with Health Canada, Canada's Ministry of Health, since 1972 (GM Schnell, unpublished data).[29] Approximately 100 of the 300 dental therapists practicing in Canada are employed by Health Canada to treat Canada's First Nation people (L. White, National Dental Therapy Program Officer, Health Canada, personal communication, 2007).[30] The remainder practice in Saskatchewan, where dental therapists are recognized as full members of the dental team, with many practicing in dental offices, complementing the work of dentists in much the same manner dental hygienists practice in the United States. Double-blind comparisons of the work of the Canadian dental therapists and dentists indicate the quality of restorations placed by dental therapists is equal to that of restorations placed by dentists.[31–33] Econometric research has documented the cost–benefit effectiveness of the dental therapists working for Health Canada.[33,34]

Great Britain recognizes dental therapists as important members of the dental team.[28] Currently, 700 dental therapists are practicing in a variety of oral health care settings in the United Kingdom.[35] Great Britain recently expanded the training opportunities for dental therapists and now graduates more than 200 dental therapists each year from its 15 programs.[36,37]

Recently, the Netherlands adopted a combined dental therapist/hygienist model as a major dimension of its dental delivery system and now matriculates 300 individuals per year to be dually trained in their vocational schools.[38,39] At the same, time the Dutch are reducing the number of dentists accepted to their dental schools by 20% and also are adding an additional year to the education of a dentist. The justification advanced for this change is that in the future dental therapists will provide significant aspects of basic preventive and restorative care, with dentists performing more complex procedures and treating the increasing number of medically and pharmacologically compromised patients. This new policy reduces the absolute number of dentists to control the costs of dental education—a significant issue in the United States—and develops dental therapists both to improve access to care and to reduce the costs of care.

Throughout the world the use of dental therapy is growing in popularity, primarily because of a dental workforce that otherwise is to provide adequate access to oral health care.

Dental therapist training typically has been accomplished in 2 academic years. Recently, however, New Zealand, Australia, Great Britain, and now The Netherlands, have integrated their dental hygiene and dental therapy programs into programs lasting 3 or more academic years to train individuals in both hygiene and therapy.[28]

EARLY EFFORTS TO TRAIN SCHOOL DENTAL NURSES IN THE UNITED STATES

In 1949 the Massachusetts legislature passed a bill authorizing the acceptance of funding by Forsyth Dental Infirmary for Children from the Children's Bureau to institute a special 5-year program of dental research.[40,41] The research would prepare "feminine personnel" in a 2-year training program to prepare and restore cavities in children's teeth under the supervision of a dentist in a dispensary or clinic approved by the Commissioner of Health. The program was to be conducted under the supervision of the Department of Health and the Board of Dental Examiners. The passage of this legislation provided for the establishment of an experimental dental care program for children similar to the school dental nurse of New Zealand.

The reaction and response of organized dentistry was swift and strong. The ADA House of Delegates passed multiple resolutions: "deploring" the program; expressing the view that any such program concerning the development of "sub-level" personnel, whether for experimental purposes or otherwise, be planned and developed only with the knowledge, consent, and cooperation of organized dentistry; and stating that a teaching program designed to equip and train personnel to treat children's teeth cannot be given in a less rigorous course or in a shorter time than that approved for the education of dentists.[41,42] Harold Hillenbrand, Executive Director of the ADA, communicated the ADA House of Delegates' position to the Commissioner of Health of Massachusetts in October, 1949. Of interest is the response to Hillenbrand by Vlado Getting, a physician, who was the Massachusetts Commissioner of Health at the time. In a long and thoughtful letter, Getting provided considerable background information regarding the proposal and the involvement of dentists belonging to the ADA throughout its development. He challenged the ADA, asking how the organization could "logically object to a research project designed to evaluate new methods of meeting the problem of dental disease." He suggested that the ADA response might have been "hurried and therefore inconsistent with the declared objectives of the ADA," which, he went on to say, were consistent with those of the Department of Health in Massachusetts, "namely the improvement of dental health."[41] Faced with increasing pressure from organized dentistry in Massachusetts and nationally, however, Massachusetts Governor Paul Dever signed a bill in July, 1950 rescinding the enabling legislation that had been passed the year before.[42]

In February, 1972 John Ingle, Dean of the University of Southern California School of Dentistry, proposed the use of school dental nurses, as employed in New Zealand, to address the problem of dental caries among America's school children.[43] In the spring of that year Ingle authorized the submission, on behalf of the University of Southern California, of a proposal for a training grant of $3.9 million from U.S. Public Health Service to train school dental nurses, with Jay Friedman as the program director. At the same time, California Governor Ronald Reagan established a committee to study the functions of all dental auxiliaries and to make recommendations to the California legislature and the State Board of Dental Examiners. As a result of these two significant developments the two California Dental Associations then extant established a committee to study the New Zealand dental care system and the relationship of the school dental nurse to private practice; to assess the work of the school dental nurse; and to compare the New Zealand and California systems. Their report was published in April, 1973 in the *Journal of the Southern California Dental Association*[44] and subsequently was summarized in the *Journal of the American Dental Association* (*JADA*).[45] The report stated that "there is little doubt that dental treatment needs related to caries for most of the New Zealand children age [2.5] to 15 have been met." The report concluded, however, that the public of California probably would not accept the New Zealand type of school dental service, because it would be perceived as a "second-class system." Ingle and Friedman wrote sharp rebukes of the Committee's report, pointing out the inconsistencies of the objective findings of the investigation in relation to the subjective conclusions of the report, which they judged was drawn to placate the practicing profession in California.[46,47] Dunning also criticized the report's conclusions in a letter to the editor of the *Journal of the American Dental Association*;[48] and Goldhaber, in an article in the *Journal of Dental Education*, called the committee's conclusion "absurd."[49] Coincidentally, the grant application of Drs. Ingle and Friedman was not funded.

EFFORTS IN THE UNITED STATES TO TRAIN DENTAL HYGIENISTS TO PROVIDE BASIC CARE FOR CHILDREN'S TEETH

In 1970, under the leadership of John Hein, the Forsyth Dental Center initiated what subsequently was designated (and described in a book by the same title) "the Forsyth Experiment."[50] The House of Delegates of the Massachusetts Dental Association had passed a resolution favoring research on expanded function for dental auxiliaries. The Forsyth Dental Center communicated to both the Massachusetts Board of Dental Examiners and to the Massachusetts Dental Society its plans to initiate a research project to train dental hygienists in restorative procedures for children, which were typically reserved for dentists alone. According to Ralph Lobene, the program director, no problems were encountered between 1970 and 1973. In October 1973, however, the Board of Dental Examiners notified Forsyth that a hearing would be held to review the project's feasibility. Subsequently, the State Board voted unanimously that the drilling of teeth by hygienists was a direct violation of the Dental Practice Act of Massachusetts and submitted that decision to the attorney general's office for a ruling and action. In March 1974, the attorney general ruled that "drilling teeth is deemed in the act to be undertaking the practice of dentistry, and the legislature had not exempted research from this provision." Forsyth was forced to close its "experiment" in June 1974, but not before it was able to document objectively that hygienists could be taught to provide restorative dental services in an effective and efficient manner. The projected curriculum time needed for hygienists to achieve the competencies desired was 47 30-hour weeks (1400 clock hours), but the project was able to achieve its desired educational outcomes in 25 30-hour weeks (740 clock hours). The experiment was designed to teach and evaluate clinical performance in administering local anesthesia and in preparing and placing Class I, II, and V amalgam restorations and Class III and V composites. The study's investigators concluded that advanced training in restorative care for children could be accomplished in the "traditional two year dental hygiene curriculum by adding two summer sessions and condensing and combining some courses."

Between 1972 and 1974, at the University of Kentucky, another expanded-functions project, supported by the Robert Wood Johnson Foundation, took place. This project also involved the training of dental hygienists in restorative dentistry for children.

Thirty-six students who were completing a 4-year baccalaureate program in dental hygiene participated in a compressed curriculum that provided 200 hours of didactic instruction in children's dentistry as well as 150 hours of clinical practice. The program specifically addressed providing primary care for children, including the administration of local anesthesia, restoration of teeth with amalgams and stainless steel crowns, and pulp therapy. On completion of the program, the hygienists participated in a double-blind study comparing their restorative skills with those of fourth-year dental students. No significant differences were found between the quality of the hygienists' work and that of the graduating dentists (E.E. Spohn, J.R. Chiswell, D.D. Davison. The University of Kentucky experimental duties dental hygiene project. Lexington, Kentucky: University of Kentucky, 1976; unpublished report).

At the College of Dentistry at the University of Iowa, a 5-year project conducted between 1971 and 1976 and supported by the W.K. Kellogg Foundation trained dental hygienists to perform expanded functions in restorative dentistry and periodontal therapy for both children and adults. The results were the same as in the studies at Forsyth and Kentucky: hygienists could be trained effectively, in a relatively brief time period, to perform with comparable quality restorative procedures traditionally reserved for dentists.[51]

INTRODUCING DENTAL THERAPISTS IN ALASKA

Because of the prevalence of dental disease and the chronic shortage of dentists in Alaska, the Alaska Native Tribal Health Consortium (ANTHC), with the support of the Indian Health Service, sent six Alaskans in 2003 to be trained in dental therapy at the University of Otago, New Zealand's national dental school.[52,53] They returned to Alaska in 2005 to begin practicing dental therapy in rural villages, only to be met with a lawsuit by the ADA to stop what the Association considered to be the illegal practice of dentistry.[54,55] The Alaska attorney general's office issued a ruling that dental therapists in the Alaska tribal health system are not subject to the state dental practice act because they are certified under federal law.[55] The lawsuit brought by the ADA was settled in 2007.[56,57]

An independent assessment of the quality of care provided by the first cohort of Alaskan dental therapists returning from New Zealand concluded that they met every standard of care evaluated and were "competent providers."[58] Subsequent research of the competency of the Alaskan dental therapists concluded, "No significant evidence was found to indicate that irreversible dental treatment provided by DHATs [dental therapists] differs from similar treatment provided by dentists."[59] ("DHAT" is an acronym for Dental Health Aide Therapist, a term unique to the United States Public Health Service personnel classification system.) Currently, 11 dental therapists who were trained in New Zealand are practicing in Alaska. Training of dental therapists was initiated in Alaska in January 2007 in a program in cooperation with the physician's assistant program of the School of Medicine at the University of Washington.[60] The first graduates completed the program in December 2008 and began serving their preceptorships in the clinics of the ANTHC. The American Association of Public Health Dentistry and the American Public Health Association have endorsed the practice of dental therapists in Alaska.[61,62]

A major objection to the introduction of dental therapists in the United Sates is the belief that dental therapists are not adequately trained to care for children. As previously indicated, the typical dental therapy curriculum internationally is 2400 clock hours—2 academic years. Traditionally, dental therapists have provided care only for children, so curriculum time is devoted specifically to learning to care for children, with 760 of these curriculum hours spent treating children in the clinic. As also indicated, the most recent study of the curriculum hours in United States dental schools indicates an average of 177 hours are spent teaching general dentists to care for children, including hours in the classroom and in the clinic. International studies, as well as research studies in the United States, have documented the quality of care dental therapists provide children in terms of diagnostic, preventive, and technical skills.[25,31–33,43,63–68] The results are uniform in finding that the quality of care provided by dental therapists is equivalent to that provided by dentists.

FOCUSING THE CARE BY DENTAL THERAPISTS ON CHILDREN

Dental therapists practicing in Alaska provide basic care to adults because they are located in extremely remote villages; without dental therapists, no dental care would be available for adults in these villages. In the remainder of the United States, however, ethical concerns, safety considerations, international experience, and practical political reasons justify focusing the care by dental therapists on children.

Kopleman and Palumbo[69] have published a compelling article in the *American Journal of Law and Medicine* entitled, "The U.S. Health Delivery System: Inefficient and Unfair to Children." The paper explores the four major ethical theories of social justice and concludes that, no matter which theoretical stance one takes, children should receive priority consideration in receiving health care. Norman Daniels,[70] professor of bioethics and population health at the Harvard School of Public Health, argues that a just society should provide basic health care to all but should redistribute health care more favorably to children. He justifies this conclusion by the effect health care has on equality of opportunity for children, with equality of opportunity being a fundamental requirement of justice. As noted, poor and minority children, the most vulnerable individuals in the United States, have the highest prevalence of oral disease, the poorest access to oral health care, and the poorest overall oral health. Justice demands they be maximally benefited, so that they ultimately have equal opportunity to succeed. The opportunity to realize one's potential in life is affected markedly by one's childhood. In a dental workforce unable to provide adequate access to oral health, moral considerations support the use of dental therapists focusing their care on children. President John Kennedy expressed it cogently and well: "Children may be the victims of fate; they must never be the victims of neglect."

There is increasing concern that even dentists who graduate from colleges of dentistry with 4 years of professional doctoral-level education are not adequately prepared to address appropriately and safely the oral health needs of the increasing numbers of adults who are chronically ill and are biologically and/or pharmacologically compromised. In 1995, the Institute of Medicine report on dental education, *Dental Education at the Crossroads: Challenges and Change*,[71] called for enhanced curricula in clinical medicine to enable dentists to manage oral health care more effectively in the face of the changing health profiles of their patients. Advocacy previously had been made for inserting a clinical clerkship year in general medicine in the dental curriculum to help future dentists integrate the basic biomedical sciences, including pathology and pharmacology, with clinical medicine, to care for patients better.[72] A number of dentists and dental educators have called for a required postdoctoral year of training to achieve this goal.[73,74] It is not reasonable to expect that the 2-year training of a dental therapist can address the many issues of providing safe dental care for adults. Although children also have debilitating diseases, they are not as prevalent in children, nor are children generally as biologically or pharmacologically compromised as adults. Thus they do not present the same level of safety issues in providing care. Safety considerations support dental therapists focusing their care on children.

The more than 80 years of international experience in dental therapists providing basic, primary care has essentially been entirely with children, not adults. All the research on the effectiveness of care by dental therapists is in relationship to children, not adults. International experience and the results of research support dental therapists focusing their care on children.

The ADA has opposed the provision of restorative and surgical care ("irreversible surgical procedures") by any one other than a dentist. This opposition is evidenced by the aggressive stance taken against dental therapists practicing in Alaska.[54] Dentistry as a profession understands that society is becoming increasingly dissatisfied with the profession's inability to address effectively the issue of access to care for the most vulnerable population, children. Although speculative, it is possible that organized dentistry will more readily accept expanding the dental workforce with dental therapists who only care for children. Practical political considerations support dental therapists focusing their care on children.

THE ECONOMIC ISSUE

Developing and deploying dental therapists to care for children is rational economically. Society supports the education and training of general dentists in 8 years of postsecondary education and 10–11 years of postsecondary education for specialists in pediatric dentistry. General dentists are trained in complex diagnostic and rehabilitative procedures for all patients; pediatric dentists are trained in tertiary care for children—the ability to care for children who have complex developmental and medical problems—and to manage, with the aid of sedation or general anesthesia, children who either lack cooperative ability or are uncooperative in their behavior. General dentists average earnings for 2006 were $198,350.[75] The latest data available for pediatric dentists are from 2005, when the average net income was $314,400.[76] It is questionable whether the typical child receiving basic, primary preventive and restorative care requires the expertise of a dentist or pediatric dentist. In New Zealand, dental therapists with 2 years of postsecondary education treat essentially all the nation's children and earn, on average, US$40,000/year (T.B. Kardos. Deputy Dean, School of Dentistry. University of Otago, Dunedin, New Zealand, personal communication, June 6, 2008).

The division of labor principle of organizational management science suggests that procedures should be delegated to the least trained and lowest salaried individual in an organization who is able to perform the activity effectively and competently at the required level of quality. Applying this principle to the dental workforce suggests that basic preventive and restorative procedures for children should be delegated to a dental therapist, resulting in a more economical expenditure of resources. This point is particularly relevant with regard to care paid by Medicaid/S-CHIP, given significantly constrained public monies. General dentists and pediatric dentists have an important role on the dental team, focusing on problems that cannot be managed by a dental therapist and that only a dentist can address.

New Zealand has a population approximately the same size as that of Kentucky; it has comparable numbers of children. New Zealand provides basic primary preventive and restorative oral health care for essentially all its children by dental therapists trained in 2-year programs. Complex tertiary care for children, the type of care for which pediatric dentists are trained, is provided for in New Zealand by seven pediatric dentists; as specialists, they focus on tertiary care. (T.B. Kardos, personal communication, June 6, 2008). Kentucky has 63 specialist pediatric dentists who provide both primary and tertiary care for children (John R. Mink, secretary-treasurer of the Kentucky Academy of Pediatric Dentistry, personal communication, June 10, 2008).

No direct economic comparisons can be made between the United States and New Zealand because of significantly different cultural environments. In a recent year, however, New Zealand spent US$34 million caring for all of its children age 6 months through age 17 years.[77] In New Zealand, the government pays for dental care for all children from birth through age 17 years. Kentucky's expenditures that year for children receiving Medicaid and S-CHIP alone were $40 million (J. Cecil, State Dental Director, Commonwealth of Kentucky, personal communication, July, 2003), even though the use rate by eligible Medicaid/S-CHIP recipients was less than 50%. Economic considerations suggest that expensive tertiary-trained specialists should not provide care that can be delegated safely and effectively to a dental therapist.

TRAINING THERAPISTS FOR THE DENTAL WORKFORCE

Various models are possible for training dental therapists to treat children in the United States. The classic model for the world has been a training program lasting 2 academic years, similar to current 2-year dental hygiene training programs.[28] Rather than establish separate, autonomous 2-year programs to train dental therapists to care for children, it would seem more rational and prudent to use the current infrastructure for educating dental hygienists. There are 255 2-year dental hygiene programs in the United States, existing in all 50 states.[78]

Two-year dental therapy curricula could be developed and offered alongside dental hygiene programs, sharing many of the courses in the basic biomedical and clinical dental sciences. Another option would be to combine the training of dental therapists with that of dental hygienists, as is beginning to happen globally, so that on graduation from a 3-year integrated curriculum the dually trained person could practice one or the other discipline, or both.[28] It also could be possible to offer a flexible curriculum in dental hygiene/dental therapy in which both groups of students could share the first year of the curriculum; much of the curriculum of current dental hygiene programs includes the competencies of traditional international dental therapists' programs. The second year could be devoted specifically to either dental hygiene or dental therapy, depending on the individual's career choice. If individuals wanted to have credentials in both, they could spend an additional year pursuing the content of the curriculum not previously chosen for their second year. Given the expectation that many dental hygienists currently in practice would desire to expand their skills to include those of a dental therapist, a third training option is intensive, participatory continuing education.

DEPLOYING DENTAL THERAPISTS

To address the access problem effectively, practitioners must go where children are located. As in New Zealand, a logical place to capture this audience is in the school system. It is reasonable to deploy dental therapists in school-based clinics or mobile vans to provide care on the basis of financial need, for example, to all children eligible for Medicaid and S-CHIP. Such a program, begun in an incremental manner with the youngest children, who have the least experience with dental disease and the greatest potential for implementation of preventive care, would seem to be a cost-effective way of managing the oral health needs of the poorest and neediest children. In New Zealand, the school-based clinics are a dental home both for the children in school and for the preschool children in the neighborhood or district. The New Zealand school dental therapist is involved in preventive education for parents and children from birth, an essential approach if the problem of early childhood caries is to be addressed.

Public health clinics, federally qualified health centers, and not-for-profit organizations would be additional potential practice locations in the public sector for dental therapists.

Dental therapists also could practice in private sector dental offices, as they do in Saskatchewan. In such offices, therapists could work with the dentist and serve as a dentist-extender for children's care, much as dental hygienists do for adult periodontal care. Such an arrangement could enable a dentist's office to care for more children and at a lower cost.

Practice in the offices of America's pediatricians is another potential location for dental therapists. A significant percentage of America's children are seen regularly by the nation's 60,000 pediatricians. The typical infant/child has had 12 visits to the pediatrician by age 3 years; providing multiple opportunities for early intervention to effect preventive and restorative oral health care.[79] Pediatricians could expand their scope of practice and retain dental therapists to work in their offices under their supervision. Medical and dental practice acts in a number of states would permit them to do so.[80]

SUMMARY

Inadequate access to oral health care for America's children has been documented, with resultant disparities in oral health among children. Children from low-income families and minorities experience more oral disease and receive less care. The current dental workforce is inadequate in number, composition, location, education, and orientation to address this problem. Other countries have used dental therapists, individuals trained in 2-year programs of postsecondary education, to provide basic, primary preventive and restorative care for children. The care provided by dental therapists has been documented to be equivalent in quality to that of dentists and is more economical. Developing and deploying dental therapists is a potential strategy to improve access to care and to reduce disparities among America's children.

REFERENCES

1. U.S. Department of Health and Human Services. Oral health in America: a report of the Surgeon General. National Institute of Dental and Craniofacial Research, National Institutes of Health. Rockville (MD): U.S. Department of Health and Human Services; 2000.
2. U.S. Department of Health and Human Services. National call to action to promote oral health: a public-private partnership under the leadership of the Office of the Surgeon General. National Institute of Dental and Craniofacial Research, National Institutes of Health. Rockville (MD): U.S. Department of Health and Human Services; 2003.
3. Newacheck PW, Hughes DC, Hung YY, et al. The unmet health needs of America's children. Pediatrics 2000;104:989–97.
4. Gift HC, Reisine ST, Larach DC. The social impact of dental problems and visits. Am J Public Health 1992;82:1663–8.
5. General Accounting Office. Oral health: dental disease is a chronic problem among low-income populations. Report GAO/HEHS-00-72. Washington, DC: General Accounting Office; 2000.

6. Greenwall AL, Johnsen D, DiSantis TA. Longitudinal evaluation of caries patterns from the primary to the mixed dentition. Pediatr Dent 1990;12: 278–82.

7. Kaste LM, Selwitz RH, Oldakowski JA, et al. Coronal caries in the primary and permanent dentitions of children and adolescents 1–17 years of age: United States, 1988–91. J Dent Res 1996;75:631–41.

8. Gehshan S, Straw T. Access to oral health services for low-income people: policy barriers and opportunities for intervention for the Robert Wood Johnson Foundation. Washington, DC: Forum for State Health Policy Leadership/National Council of State Legislatures; 2002.

9. American Dental Education Association. Improving the oral health status of all Americans: roles and responsibilities of academic dental institutions. Washington, DC: American Dental Education Association; 2003.

10. General Accounting Office. Oral health: factors contributing to low use of dental services by low-income populations. Washington, DC: General Accounting Office; 2000. p. 41.

11. American Dental Association. Dental workforce model, 1997–2020. Chicago: American Dental Association; 1999.

12. U.S. Department of Health and Human Services Health Resources and Services Administration. Health professions shortage areas. Rockville (MD): U.S. Department of Health and Human Services Health Resources and Services Administration; 1999.

13. Solomon ES. The future of dentistry. Dent Econ 2005;95(2):132–6.

14. Beazoglou T, Bailit H, Brown J. Selling your practice: are there problems ahead? J Am Dent Assoc 2000;131(12):1693–8.

15. Cassamassimo P. We need help! Pediatric dentistry today. Chicago: American Academy of Pediatric Dentistry; 2000. p. 30.

16. Department of Health and Human Services, Health Resources and Services Administration. Available at: http://bhpr.hrsa.gov/shortage. Accessed November 24, 2008.

17. Brown LJ, Lazar V. Minority dentists—why we need them: closing the gap. Washington, DC: Office of Minority Health, U.S. Department of Health and Human Services; 1999. p. 6–7.

18. Valachovic RW. Dental workforce trends and children. Ambul Pediatr 2002; 2(Suppl 2):154–61.

19. Tedesco LA. Issues in dental curriculum development and change. J Dent Educ 1995;59(1):97–147.

20. Seale NS, Casamassimo P. U.S. predoctoral education in pediatric dentistry: its impact on access to dental care. J Dent Educ 2003;67(1):23–30.

21. American Dental Association. Resolution 59H-2000. In: 2000 transactions for the 141st annual session, October 14–18, 2000. Chicago: American Dental Association; 2000.

22. U.S. Department of Health and Human Services, Office of the Inspector General. Children dental services under Medicaid: access and utilization. San Francisco (CA): U.S. Department of Health and Human Services; 1996.

23. Gehshan S, Hauck P, Scales J. Increasing dentists' participation in Medicaid and SCHIP. Forum for state health policy leadership. Denver and Washington: National Conference of State Legislatures; 2001.

24. Fulton JT. Experiment in dental care: results of New Zealand's use of school dental nurses. Geneva, Switzerland: World Health Organization; 1951.

25. Nash DA. Developing a pediatric oral health therapist to help address oral health disparities among children. J Dent Educ 2004;68(1):8–20.
26. Nash DA. Developing and deploying a new member of the dental team: a pediatric oral health therapist. J Public Health Dent 2005;65(1):48–55.
27. National Health Committee. Improving child oral health and reducing child oral health inequalities: report to the minister from the Public Health Advisory Committee. Wellington, New Zealand: National Health Committee; 2003.
28. Nash DA, Friedman JW, Kardos TB, et al. Dental therapists: a global perspective. Int Dent J 2008;58(2):61–70.
29. Davey K. Dental therapists in the Canadian north. J Can Dent Assoc 1974;40: 287–91.
30. Saskatchewan Dental Therapists Association. Registrar report. Saskatchewan Dental Therapists Association; 2007.
31. American Dental Association. Survey of dental education, 2006. Chicago (IL): American Dental Association; 2008.
32. Crawford PR, Holmes BW. An assessment and evaluation of dental treatment in the Baffin Region. A report to the Medical Services Branch of National Health and Welfare January 25, 1989.
33. Trueblood RG. A quality evaluation of specific dental services provided by Canadian dental therapists. Ottawa (Canada): Medical Services Branch, Epidemiology and Community Health Specialties, Health and Welfare Canada.
34. Trueblood RG. An analytical model for assessing the costs and benefits of training and utilizing auxiliary health personnel with application to the Canadian dental therapy program. Montreal, Canada: Department of Health Technology, Concordia University; 1992.
35. General Dental Council. Annual report, 2005. London: General Dental Council; 2006.
36. Education and training of personal auxiliary to dentistry. London: The Nuffield Foundation, 1993.
37. British Association of Dental Therapists'. Available at: http://www.badt.org.uk. Accessed January 11, 2007.
38. Ministry of Health, Welfare and Sports. Capacity oral health care: recommendations for short and long term policy. The Hague, The Netherlands: Ministry of Health, Welfare and Sports; 2000.
39. Secretariat of the Innovation in Dental Care Committee of the Institute for Research of Public Expenditure (IOO). [Innovation in dental care: recommendations]. Leiden, The Netherlands: Secretariat of the Innovation in Dental Care Committee of the Institute for Research of Public Expenditure (IOO); 2006 [in Dutch].
40. American Dental Association. House of Delegates' action on dental nurses program questioned by Massachusetts Commissioner of Health. J Am Dent Assoc 1959;40:363–6.
41. New York Dental Association. The Massachusetts dental research project. N Y J Dent 1950;XX:378–83.
42. American Dental Association. Massachusetts dental nurse bill rescinded. J Am Dent Assoc 1950;41:371.
43. Ingle JI. American dental care—1972: a plan designed to deliver preventive and therapeutic dental care to the children of America. Paper presented at the Conference of Dental Examiners and Dental Educators. Chicago, IL, 1972.
44. Redig D, Dewhirst F, Nevit G, et al. Delivery of dental services in New Zealand and California. J South Calif Dent Assoc 1973;41(4):318–50.

45. American Dental Association. Delivery of dental services in New Zealand and California: summary of a report to the California Dental Association and the Southern California Dental Association. J Am Dent Assoc 1973;87:542–3.
46. Friedman JW, Ingle JI. New Zealand dental nurses. J Am Dent Assoc 1973;8:1331.
47. Friedman JW, Ingle JI. New Zealand dental nurse report. J Calif Dent Assoc 1973; 1:7–8.
48. Dunning JM. New Zealand summary. J Am Dent Assoc 1974;88:271–2.
49. Goldhaber P. Improving the dental health status in the United Status—putting your money where your mouth is. J Dent Educ 1977;41:50–8.
50. Lobene R. The Forsyth experiment: an alternative system for dental care. Cambridge (MA): Harvard University Press; 1979.
51. Sisty NL, Henderson WG, Paule CL, et al. Evaluation of student performance in the four-year study of expanded functions for dental hygienists at the University of Iowa. J Am Dent Assoc 1978;97:613–27.
52. Nash DA, Nagel RJ. A brief history and current status of a dental therapy initiative in the United States. J Dent Educ 2005;69(8):857–9.
53. Nash DA, Nagel RJ. Confronting oral health disparities among American Indian/Alaska native children: the pediatric oral health therapist. Am J Public Health 2005;95(8):1325–9.
54. American Dental Association. House of Delegates proceedings. ADA annual session. Chicago: American Dental Association; 2004.
55. Lyle PR. Memorandum to Robert E. Warren, Alaska Board of Dental Examiners from Paul R. Lyle, Sr. Attorney General, State of Alaska, Department of Law. Subject: State licensure of federal dental health aides. 16 pages.
56. Alaska lawsuit dropped. Anchorage Daily News July 12, 2007.
57. American Dental Association. ADA reaches settlement in Alaska litigation. ADA News July 16, 2007;8–9.
58. Fiset L. A report on quality assessment of primary care provided by dental therapists to Alaska natives. September 30, 2005. Available at: http://www.anthc/org/cs/chs/dhs/cfm. Accessed January 18, 2007.
59. Bolin KA. Assessment of treatment provided by dental health aide therapists in Alaska: a pilot study. J Am Dent Assoc 2008;139:1530–9.
60. Anchorage Daily News. Dental therapist training program opens in Alaska, January 16, 2007. p. 8.
61. American Association of Public Health Dentistry. Resolution on the need for formal demonstration projects to improve access to preventive and therapeutic oral health services. 2006.
62. American Public Health Association. Resolution on dental therapists in Alaska, 2006. p. 9.
63. Bradlaw R, Douglas THT, Roper-Hall HT, et al. Report of United Kingdom mission on New Zealand school dental service. NZ Dent J 1951;47(228):62–78.
64. Friedman JW. The New Zealand School Dental Service: a lesson in radical conservatism. J Am Dent Assoc 1972;85(3):609–17.
65. Roder DM. The effect of treatment provided by dentists and school dental therapists in the South Australian School Dental Service. Aust Dent J 1973;18(5):311–9.
66. Roder DM. The effect of treatment provided by dentists and school dental therapists in the South Australian School Dental Service. The second report. Aust Dent J 1976;21(2):147–52.
67. Roder DM. Diagnosis, treatment planning and referral by school dental therapists. Aust Dent J 1974;19(4):242–9.

68. Riordan PJ, Espelid I, Tveit AB. Radiographic interpretation and treatment decisions among dental therapists and dentists in western Australia. Community Dent Oral Epidemiol 1991;19(5):268–71.

69. Kopelman LM, Palumbo MG. The U.S. health delivery system: inefficient and unfair to children. American Journal of Law and Medicine 1999;XXIII:319–37.

70. Daniels N. Just health care. New York: Cambridge University Press; 1985.

71. National Academy of Science, Institute of Medicine. Dental education at the crossroads: challenge and change. Washington, DC: National Academy Press; 1995.

72. Nash DA. The oral physician. Creating a new oral health professional for a new century. J Dent Educ 1995;59:587–97.

73. Formicola AJ, Myers R. A postdoctoral year for the practice of dentistry: rational and progress. J Dent Educ 1991;55(8):526–30.

74. Lefever KH, Atchison KA, McCauley KR, et al. Views of practicing dentist regarding a mandatory fifth year of training. J Dent Educ 2003;67(3):317–27.

75. American Dental Association. 2006 survey of dental practice. Chicago: American Dental Association; April, 2008.

76. American Academy of Pediatric Dentistry. Broadcast e-mail, July 14, 2008, based on report from the American Dental Association Survey Center. Chicago: American Academy of Pediatric Dentistry; 2008.

77. Wright C. Keynote address: principle of oral health services planning. N Z Dent J 2000;96:87–93.

78. American Dental Hygienists' Association Web site. Available at: http://www.adha. org. Accessed July 10, 2008.

79. American Academy of Pediatrics. Recommendations for preventive practice health care. Pediatrics 2000;105:626.

80. Center for Health Services Research and Policy. The effects of state dental practice laws allowing alternative models of preventive oral health care delivery to low income children. Center for Health Services Researcgh and Policy. School of Public Health Services. George Washington University Medical Center. Available at: http://www.gwhealthpolicy.org/downloads/Oral_Health.pdf. Accessed July 30, 2003.

Public Programs, Insurance, and Dental Access

Richard J. Manski, DDS, MBA, PhD

KEYWORDS

- Dental • Use • Expenditure • Coverage • Insurance
- Public coverage

It is 1:15 in the afternoon, and Rep. Elijah E. Cummings has just challenged approximately 200 dental, dental hygiene, and dental postgraduate members of the class of 2008 to not forget those who have been left behind. He made this challenge as he reminds the class of 2008 of the consequences of dental neglect and relates the story of an unfortunate young man in Maryland who recently died as a result of a dental-related brain abscess. With a visceral and emotional oration, Rep. Cummings told the group "Dentist after dentist after dentist refused to treat him."

Across town just about 1 month later, a forum of advocates, public health experts, researchers, and clinicians gathered and spent a day together reflecting on the development of a comprehensive oral health policy. Topics included:

Achieving access and quality in dental care
Increasing the dental workforce and program participation of dental providers
Education to improve access to dental services

Three months earlier, approximately 100 dental students gathered and attended a practice management seminar, a seminar with the intended goal of teaching dentists how to market and optimize their dental practice. Midway through the seminar, the speaker told the audience that insurance is the disdain of dental practice, and most of his clients do not accept dental insurance. He continued and suggested that each and every member of the audience should also consider not accepting insurance and supported the argument with the view that dentists are well trained, work hard, deserve to be well-compensated, and therefore should be unencumbered with the nuisances of dental insurance. Just a few words in an otherwise well-presented seminar tell much. Although most of the presentation focused on preparing dental students to set up an efficient well-run practice to best serve the community, the

Division of Health Services Research, Department of Health Promotion and Policy, Dental School, University of Maryland, 650 West Baltimore Street, Room 2209, Baltimore, MD 21201, USA
E-mail address: manski@dental.umaryland.edu

Dent Clin N Am 53 (2009) 485–503
doi:10.1016/j.cden.2009.03.010
0011-8532/09/$ – see front matter © 2009 Elsevier Inc. All rights reserved.

dental.theclinics.com

feelings expressed about third-party coverage are telling of an adversarial relationship that has fomented over the years; an adversarial relationship between practitioners and the purveyors of dental care coverage both private and public alike.

Just a few years ago, Alaska native tribal health organizations responding to a paucity of dentists in rural areas developed a new solution to address the oral health needs of Alaska natives. The Dental Health Aide Therapist Initiative was designed to educate dental health aide therapists to provide dental care to Alaska natives in rural areas. The focus of the program is on prevention, pain and infection relief, and basic restorative services.[1,2] Several years later, the American Dental Association reported to its members that a licensing subcommittee of the Minnesota House of Representatives, also responding to a perceived paucity of dentist practitioners, approved the Advanced Dental Hygiene Practitioner workforce model. If enacted, this legislation would allow midlevel providers to perform surgical procedures including extractions and restorations without the supervision of a dentist.[3]

The problem of dental access, especially the availability and participation of dentists to provide care to disadvantaged children, is and has been for the last 20 years a hot topic of concern among elected officials, oral health advocates, and dental professionals. No longer just an issue of local concern, the Domestic Policy Subcommittee of the House Committee on Oversight and Government Reform recently held an oversight hearing on Reforms to Pediatric Dental Care in Medicaid. Concurrently, the Government Accountability Office (GAO) released a report showing that dental disease in children has not decreased.[4] Just a few months earlier, the Agency for Healthcare Research and Quality (AHRQ) released a report on Dental Use, Expenses, Dental Coverage, and Changes, 1996 and 2004 showing that the percentage of children who had public dental coverage increased from 1996 to 2004.[5] Additionally, children with public dental coverage had an increase in the likelihood of having a dental visit from 1996 to 2004.

Previously, Bailit and Beazoglou presented a thorough review and perspective on current trends in public and private expenditures for dental services. They summarized their discourse in part with an optimistic view of the future for middle and upper income families that have the resources to purchase dental services.[6] On the other hand, they follow that although overall use is likely to increase for the foreseeable future, the wide disparities in access to dental care may persist, with low income populations continuing to have major problems accessing dental care.

The purpose of this article is to begin where Bailit and Beazoglou finish and continue the assessment and provide a framework with which to possibly suggest improvements in the design of current programs. Whereas Bailit and Beazoglou examine and discuss person-level use and expenditures as a function of aggregate factors including the role of employer-sponsored dental coverage, federal and state financing, and workforce considerations, this assessment will examine person-level use and expenditures as a function of preferences, price, and the use of third-party coverage.

DENTAL CARE SERVICES USE

Several factors have been associated with the likelihood of having a dental visit. Age, income, race, sex, education, and dental insurance have been shown to be primary determinants of dental use. Other factors, including geographic location, employment status, marital status, and family composition also have been associated with dental use rates.[7–14]

Analyses of data from different survey sources historically have resulted in national estimates that vary.[15] Sources of data often used to depict national dental use rates include the National Health Interview Survey (NHIS), the National Health and Nutrition Examination Survey (NHANES), and the Medical Expenditure Panel Survey (MEPS). Variations among survey results may be attributable in part to differences in survey design, question format, survey procedures, and length of time asked of respondent to recall.[15] Fortunately, sociodemographic and economic trends appear to be generally consistent across surveys. Each survey has its merits, and choice of survey should be made according to the primary question of interest.[15] For the purpose of this manuscript, I will follow the lead of the US Department of Health and Human Services, which uses MEPS for the following Healthy People 2010 oral health access benchmarks:[16]

> 21-10. Increase the proportion of children and adults who use the oral health care system each year
>
> 21-12. Increase the proportion of low-income children and adolescents who received any preventive dental service during the past year

MEPS is sponsored by the AHRQ and is a survey of families and individuals, their medical providers, and employers across the United States. MEPS is the most complete source of data on the cost and use of health care and health insurance coverage.[17] Of the three surveys, MEPS also may be the least susceptible to variation resulting from survey design.[15]

Recent data available from the MEPS show that 44% (**Fig. 1**) of the community population had a dental visit during 2004. Generally, use rates have remained remarkably stable over the last 30 years.[18] On the other hand, data suggest that although the use rate for children and the elderly increased during this same period, the gap between lower- and higher-income people has widened.[18] Indeed, recent data appear to confirm Bailit and Beazoglou's gloomy outlook for low-income populations. Although 58% (**Fig. 2**) of people from a high-income family had at least one dental visit during the year, only 30% of people from a family with low income had at least one dental visit. Black non-Hispanic and Hispanic people were less likely (**Fig. 3**) to have a dental visit in 2004 than white non-Hispanics.[5]

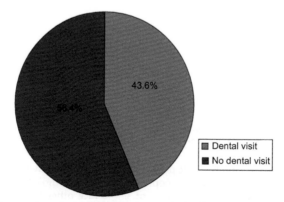

43.6%

56.4%

Dental visit
No dental visit

Fig. 1. In 2004, there were about 294 million people in the community population of the United States. Approximately 44% of the population had at least one dental visit during the year. (*Data from* Manski RJ, Brown E. Dental use, expenses, private dental coverage, and changes, 1996 and 2004. Rockville (MD): Agency for Healthcare Research and Quality; 2007. MEPS Chartbook No.17. p. 4.)

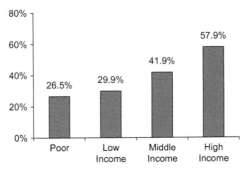

Fig. 2. Although 58% of people from a high-income family had at least one dental visit during 2004, only 30% of persons from a family with low income had at least one dental visit during the same year. Where: poor includes people in families with income less than or equal to 100% of the poverty line; low income includes people in families with income greater than 100% through 200% of the poverty line. Middle income includes people in families with income greater than 200% through 400% of the poverty line, and high income includes people in families with income over 400% of the poverty line. (*Data from* Manski RJ, Brown E. Dental use, expenses, private dental coverage, and changes, 1996 and 2004. Rockville (MD): Agency for Healthcare Research and Quality; 2007. MEPS Chartbook No.17. p. 7.)

DENTAL EXPENDITURES

Bailit and Beazoglou note that the amount of money spent on dental care is a measure of a population's use of dental services, and differences in dental expenditures among population subgroups might suggest problems of access within the United States.[6] Data available from the Centers for Medicare & Medicaid Services (CMS) sponsored National Health Expenditure Accounts (NHEA) show that dental care expenditures have been steadily increasing during the past half century.[19] In nominal terms, American spending increased from $1.96 billion in 1960 to $21.65 billion in 1985 to $81.50

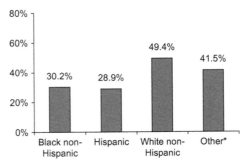

Fig. 3. Black non-Hispanic and Hispanic people were less likely to have a dental visit in 2004 than white non-Hispanic people or people of other race/ethnicity categories. *Other includes non-Hispanics who reported to be of single race other than white or black (ie, American Indian/Alaska Native, Asian, or Native Hawaiian/Pacific Islander) and non-Hispanics who reported to be of multiple races (possibly including black). (*Data from* Manski RJ, Brown E. Dental use, expenses, private dental coverage, and changes, 1996 and 2004. Rockville (MD): Agency for Healthcare Research and Quality; 2007. MEPS Chartbook No.17. p. 8.)

billion in 2004.[19] The increase has been steady and dramatic. Even adjusted for inflation, American spending has been remarkable, increasing from $12.51 billion in 1960 to $38.01 billion in 1985 to $81.50 billion in 2004.[19,20]

For comparison purposes, an expenditure amount adjusted for inflation is provided. Specifically, expenditures are adjusted to 2004 using Bureau of Labor Statistics-derived factors of 6.38 for 1960 and 1.76 of 1985 (adjustments were calculated as follows: the consumer price index is 29.6 for 1960, 107.6 for 1985 and 188.9 for 2006; so the adjustment factors are 188.9/29.6=6.38 for 1960 and 188.9/107.6=1.76 for 1985).

An annual expenditure of $81 billion is not an inconsequential amount, and represents just over 4% of all health expenditures during 2004.

Data available from the MEPS show that the total dental expense for the community population of the United States was $72 billion in 2004.

MEPS expenditure estimates are based on person-level survey data from a nationally representative sample of households in the civilian noninstitutionalized population and are linked directly to patient care events. In contrast, the NHEA estimates are constructed primarily from aggregate provider revenue data and cover a broader population and wider range of services. The NHEA cover the entire United States population, including the institutionalized population, and a full range of health care expenditures, such as public health services and research.

The average dental expense for a person with a dental visit (**Fig. 4**) increased from $374 ($450 adjusted for inflation) in 1996 to $560 in 2004.[5] For each income category except for middle income, the average expense (**Fig. 5**) (adjusted for inflation) for a person with a dental visit increased from 1996 to 2004. White non-Hispanics and Hispanics and people of other race/ethnicity categories had a statistically significant increase (**Fig. 6**) in oral health-related expenses from 1996 to 2004.

PAYING FOR DENTAL CARE

Dental care is expensive, and paying for dental care for many Americans can be difficult. Studies have shown that the cost of dental services matters.[21,22] Among the reasons given for not going to the dentist, some have reported that dental care was too expensive. On the other hand, people do pay for and receive dental care. Patients are consumers and are willing to pay for services and expect to derive a personal benefit for these payments. Utility is the term usually used to describe measure and

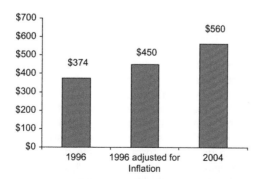

Fig. 4. Average dental expenses increased from $374 ($450 adjusted for inflation) in 1996 to $560 in 2004. (*Data from* Manski RJ, Brown E. Dental use, expenses, private dental coverage, and changes, 1996 and 2004. Rockville (MD): Agency for Healthcare Research and Quality; 2007. MEPS Chartbook No.17. p. 20.)

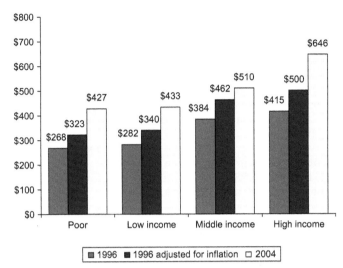

Fig. 5. For each income category except for middle income, the average expense (adjusted for inflation) increased from 1996 to 2004. Where: poor includes people in families with income less than or equal to 100% of the poverty line; low income includes people in families with income greater than 100% through 200% of the poverty line. Middle income includes people in families with income greater than 200% through 400% of the poverty line, and high income includes people in families with income over 400% of the poverty line. (*Data from* Manski RJ, Brown E. Dental use, expenses, private dental coverage, and changes, 1996 and 2004. Rockville (MD): Agency for Healthcare Research and Quality; 2007. MEPS Chartbook No.17. p. 24.)

compare differing levels of expected benefit.[23–25] Patients as consumers will allocate funds and select a set of services, or proposed treatment, that will help to maximize their overall utility. Price, or cost, is the market value that will purchase a specific set of services. Dental care demand is the quantity of services or care that a patient is willing to purchase at a specific price.[24,25] Not all dental services are alike, and the demand for dental care is not monolithic.[10] Some dental services patients want, and some dental services patients do not want but need. For some services, patients are insensitive to variations in price (price inelastic) and for other services patients will exhibit varying degrees of demand depending upon the price (price elastic). For some patients, even if the price of dental care were zero, use rates would vary, because attitudes and other demand factors differ.[24,25]

Almost two thirds (**Fig. 7**) of all Americans receive some assistance in paying for dental care through dental care coverage or dental insurance.[5] During 2004, approximately 54% of the community population had private dental coverage (see **Fig. 7**), and approximately 12% of the community population had public dental coverage only. The increase among Americans with private dental insurance has been steady since 1967, when only 4.5 million persons were covered.[5,26–29] By 2004, approximately 158 million people had some form of private dental care coverage.[5] Public coverage for dental care also has increased, especially among children. Corresponding with the advent of the State Child Health Insurance Plan (SCHIP) in 1997, the percentage of children who had public dental coverage increased from 18% in 1996 to 26% in 2004.[5,30,31] Dental care benefits lower the out-of-pocket or perceived cost of dental care, thereby stimulating demand.[12–14] In 2004, 57% (**Fig. 8**) of the

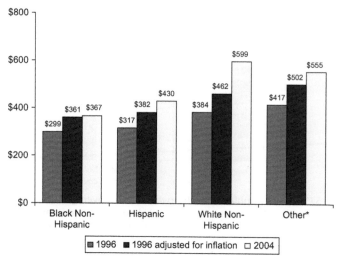

Fig. 6. White non-Hispanics and Hispanics and people of other race/ethnicity categories had a statistically significant increase in expenses from 1996 to 2004from 1996 to 2004. *Other includes non-Hispanics who reported to be of single race other than white or black (ie, American Indian/Alaska Native, Asian, or Native Hawaiian/Pacific Islander) and non-Hispanics who reported to be of multiple races (possibly including black). (*Data from* Manski RJ, Brown E. Dental use, expenses, private dental coverage, and changes, 1996 and 2004. Rockville (MD): Agency for Healthcare Research and Quality; 2007. MEPS Chartbook No.17. p. 25.)

population with private dental coverage had a dental visit; 32% of the population with public dental coverage had a dental visit, and 27% of the population without any dental coverage had a dental visit.[5] Although dental care benefits lower the out-of-pocket cost of dental care, making dental care more affordable, people from lower income families (**Fig. 9**) were less likely to have private dental coverage in 2004 than

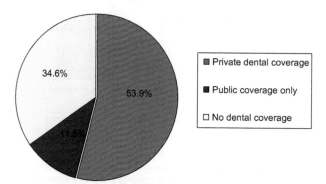

Fig. 7. In 2004, approximately 158 million people, or 54% of the community population, had private dental coverage during the year. Approximately 12% of the community population had public dental coverage only, and 35% of the community population had no dental coverage at all during the year. (*Data from* Manski RJ, Brown E. Dental use, expenses, private dental coverage, and changes, 1996 and 2004. Rockville (MD): Agency for Health care Research and Quality; 2007. MEPS Chartbook No.17. p. 10.)

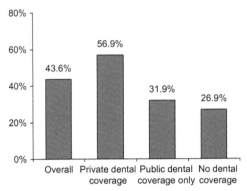

Fig. 8. In 2004, 57% of the population with private dental coverage had a dental visit; 32% of the population with public dental coverage only had a dental visit, and 27% of the population without any dental coverage had a dental visit. (*Data from* Manski RJ, Brown E. Dental use, expenses, private dental coverage, and changes, 1996 and 2004. Rockville (MD): Agency for Healthcare Research and Quality; 2007. MEPS Chartbook No.17. p. 13.)

people from a family with higher income. Additionally, although Black non-Hispanic and Hispanic persons were more likely to have public dental coverage (**Fig. 10**), they were less likely to have private dental coverage in 2004 than white non-Hispanics or people of other race/ethnicity categories. Public dental coverage is less effective than private coverage in making dental care more affordable and available. Plan design, large provider networks, efficient administrative services, and market-based fee schedules are just a few of the features that cause private plans to be more

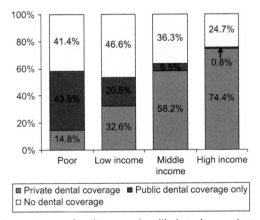

Fig. 9. People from lower income families were less likely to have private dental coverage in 2004 than people from a family with higher income. Where: poor includes people in families with income less than or equal to 100% of the poverty line; low income includes people in families with income greater than 100% through 200% of the poverty line. Middle income includes people in families with income greater than 200% through 400% of the poverty line, and high income includes people in families with income over 400% of the poverty line. (*Data from* Manski RJ, Brown E. Dental use, expenses, private dental coverage, and changes, 1996 and 2004. Rockville (MD): Agency for Healthcare Research and Quality; 2007. MEPS Chartbook No.17. p. 11.)

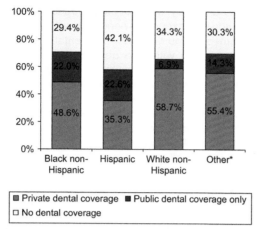

Fig. 10. Black non-Hispanic and Hispanic people were more likely to have public dental coverage and less likely to have private dental coverage in 2004 than white non-Hispanics or people of other race/ethnicity categories. (*Data from* Manski RJ, Brown E. Dental use, expenses, private dental coverage, and changes, 1996 and 2004. Rockville (MD): Agency for Healthcare Research and Quality; 2007. MEPS Chartbook No.17. p. 12.)

effective than public plans in making dental care more affordable and available. The average annual expense (**Fig. 11**) for a person with a dental visit was $612 for a person with private dental coverage, $326 for a person with public dental coverage only and $482 for a person with no dental coverage during 2004.

IS DENTAL CARE COVERAGE THE ANSWER?

Cleary, dental care coverage is an important factor in the decision to seek dental care. The difference between the 57% of the population with private dental coverage having a dental visit and the 27% of the population without any dental coverage having

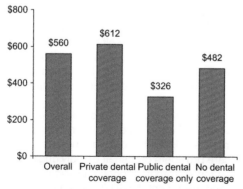

Fig. 11. The average annual expense for a person with a dental visit was $612 for a person with private dental coverage, $326 for a person with public dental coverage only, and $482 for a person with no dental coverage during 2004. (*Data from* Manski RJ, Brown E. Dental use, expenses, private dental coverage, and changes, 1996 and 2004. Rockville (MD): Agency for Health care Research and Quality; 2007. MEPS Chartbook No.17. p. 14.)

a dental visit is striking.[5] Admittedly, some of the difference is attributable to adverse selection, whereas a person who expects to need care will be more likely to sign up for dental coverage than someone who does not.[24,25] Dental benefit plan administrators attempt to mitigate the problem with plan designs that incorporate features that compensate for adverse selection, including waiting periods, exclusions for preexisting conditions, and limited enrollment periods. There is also a case to be made that the effect of adverse selection in the purchase of dental coverage is not as great as with medical coverage, however, because the cost of dental coverage and dental care is low when compared with medical coverage and medical care. When the cost of one short hospital stay can be $10,000 or more, and the cost of medical care coverage can be $1000 per month, the overall mean annual expense for dental care of $560 and the cost of a dental care plan of $50 per month for a family seems low enough to discourage significant gaming of the insurance market. On the other hand, a recent study has shown that the effect of dental care coverage on dental use may be somewhat smaller than expected.[11] This study showed that having medical insurance with or without coverage for dental care also is associated with an increased likelihood of having a dental visit.[11] If medical care coverage can stimulate the demand for dental care, even though the medical care coverage plan does not cover dental services, then one must posit that medical care coverage must proxy for some unobserved factor(s) of demand. In other words, current dental coverage modeling may result in an exaggerated interpretation of the importance of dental coverage in the decision to seek dental care.[11] As such, programs designed to improve dental access through the use of dental care coverage may offer only a modest extra improvement in use rates of dental services.

Andersen's Behavioral Model of Health Services Use provides a theoretical framework from which to suggest a rationale for this discrepancy and provide some insight into some of the factors that might mitigate some of the effect of dental care coverage.[32] Andersen's model proposes that service-specific predisposing, enabling, and need factors would explain use differentially.[32] For instance, Andersen postulates that although hospital services used in response to a serious health care problem may be explained primarily as a function of need and demographic characteristics, less serious problems including dental care more likely would be explained as a function of social structure, health beliefs, and enabling resources. As such, it would not be too surprising that dental care coverage, an enabling resource, may be diminished somewhat in effect by varying social structure and health beliefs. As such, recent studies and Andersen's Behavioral Model of Health Services Use suggest that the addition of third-party dental coverage by itself might provide less than a satisfactory or desired result. It might be argued that because the rates of coverage among the poor and disadvantaged have improved since the enactment of SCHIP, more and better dental coverage will improve use rates but not alleviate all of the problems of access.

Assistance in paying for dental care for the poor and disadvantaged in the United States has been provided primarily through Medicaid and SCHIP dental care coverage. Medicaid is a state-administered program that makes payments for health care directly to health care providers on behalf of individuals and families who fit into an eligibility group that is recognized by federal and state law. The Early and Periodic Screening, Diagnostic, and Treatment (EPSDT) service is Medicaid's comprehensive and preventive child health program for individuals under the age of 21. EPSDT legislation was enacted as part of the Omnibus Budget Reconciliation Act of 1989 (OBRA '89) and includes provisions for periodic screening, vision, dental, and hearing services.[30]

The EPSDT dental benefit, in accordance with section 1905(r) of the Act, must include:

"Dental Services—At a minimum, include relief of pain and infections, restoration of teeth, and maintenance of dental health. Dental services may not be limited to emergency services. Although an oral screening may be part of a physical examination, it does not substitute for examination through direct referral to a dentist. A direct dental referral is required for every child in accordance with the periodicity schedule developed by the state and at other intervals as medically necessary. The law as amended by OBRA 1989 requires that dental services (including initial direct referral to a dentist) conform to the state periodicity schedule, which must be established after consultation with recognized dental organizations involved in child health care."[33]

The SCHIP enacted into law as part of the Balanced Budget Act of 1997 provided for an expansion in the federal effort to extend health insurance to those children who were uninsured. Although dental services were included as an optional benefit for all children up to age 19, all states have opted to provide coverage for dental services.[30] Coverage among the poor and disadvantaged children has improved since the enactment of SCHIP. The percentage of children who had public dental coverage increased (**Fig. 12**) from 18% of all children in 1996 to just over 26% in 2004.[5] Poor, low-income, and middle-income children were much more likely (**Fig. 13**) to have public dental coverage and less likely to have no dental coverage in 2004 than in 1996.[5] Additionally, data show that in the years since SCHIP became the law of the land, children who had public dental coverage registered an increase in the likelihood of having a dental visit (**Fig. 14**), from 28% in 1996 to 34% in 2004.[5] Although much progress has been made, it is also obvious that more needs to be done. Although the rate of use among children with public dental care coverage has increased, the rate still lags behind that of the overall child population. Many plausible explanations for this lag have been provided or suggested.[11,32] Some plausible causes are commonly known and even have reached the halls of Congress. During a May 2007 hearing on the adequacy of the pediatric dental program for Medicaid-eligible children by the Domestic Policy Subcommittee of the House Committee on Oversight and Government Reform, Rep. Cummings cited low reimbursement rates, paper work burden, and failed appointments as three factors discouraging provider participation.

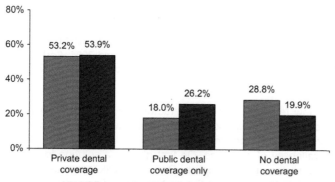

Fig. 12. The percentage of children with public dental coverage increased from 18% of all children in 1996 to just over 26% in 2004. (*Data from* Manski RJ, Brown E. Dental use, expenses, private dental coverage, and changes, 1996 and 2004. Rockville (MD): Agency for Healthcare Research and Quality; 2007. MEPS Chartbook No.17. p. 64.)

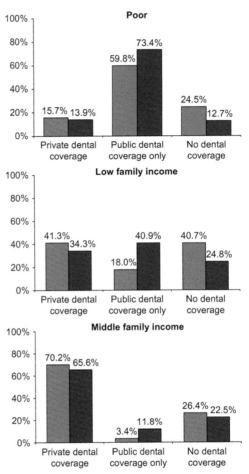

Fig.13. Poor, low-income, and middle-income children were much more likely to have public dental coverage only and less likely to have no dental coverage in 2004 than in 1996. Where: poor includes people in families with income less than or equal to 100% of the poverty line; low income includes people in families with income greater than 100% through 200% of the poverty line. Middle income includes people in families with income greater than 200% through 400% of the poverty line, and high income includes people in families with income over 400% of the poverty line. (*Data from* Manski RJ, Brown E. Dental use, expenses, private dental coverage, and changes, 1996 and 2004. Rockville (MD): Agency for Healthcare Research and Quality; 2007. MEPS Chartbook No.17. p. 66.)

No doubt that low fees are not the only factor, but clearly it is an important factor. Simple economic theory would predict that low reimbursement rates would discourage provider participation. thereby making the availability of care limited in spite of the availability of coverage. On first glance, a solution to this problem may appear simple and easy to accomplish. One might ask, why not just raise the reimbursement schedule to encourage the participation of providers. If only it were this easy. In fact, much of the problem is rooted in the well-intentioned design of the program. A program (**Figs. 15–17**) designed to provide a robust set of benefits on behalf of individuals and families that fit into an eligibility group is a program that

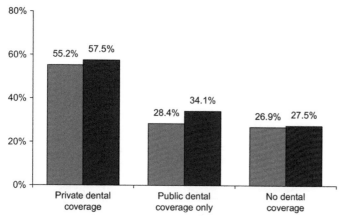

Fig. 14. Children with public dental coverage only had an increase in the likelihood of having a dental visit from 1996 to 2004. (*Data from* Manski RJ, Brown E. Dental use, expenses, private dental coverage, and changes, 1996 and 2004. Rockville (MD): Agency for Healthcare Research and Quality; 2007. MEPS Chartbook No.17. p. 52.)

must have either a very large budget or rigorous fee restrictions. Specifically, state plans direct that all eligible persons be covered and that for each person who is covered a full complement of services be made available, making programs potentially very expensive.[34] Because a budget of the size needed has not been politically viable,

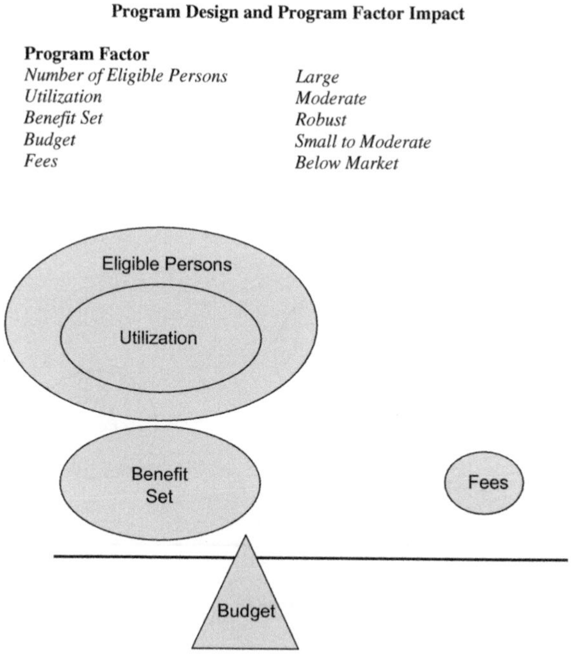

Program Design and Program Factor Impact

Program Factor
Number of Eligible Persons   *Large*
Utilization   *Moderate*
Benefit Set   *Robust*
Budget   *Small to Moderate*
Fees   *Below Market*

Eligible Persons

Utilization

Benefit Set

Fees

Budget

Fig. 15. Current program design, budget too small to support current benefit set and current use rates resulting in below market fees.

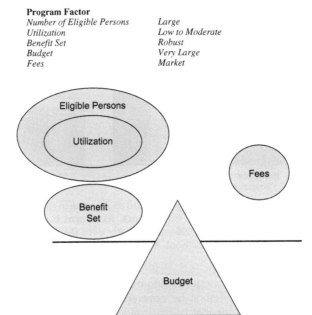

Fig. 16. Program design, large budget sufficient to support current benefit set and current use rates with at market fees.

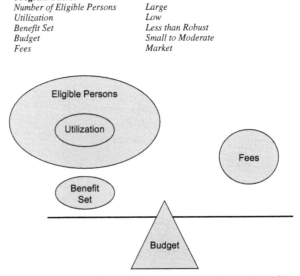

Fig. 17. Program design, current budget sufficient to support lower benefit set and lower use rates with at market fees.

in most states, below market rate fees schedules have been the result. A few states have raised fees hoping to improve provider access. In 2000, Michigan initiated a Medicaid dental program demonstration project offering dental coverage to Medicaid-enrolled children through a private dental carrier at private reimbursement rates.[35] Not surprisingly, a study of this program showed improved access to care among Medicaid recipients.[35] As such, if the political will is there to do so, similar changes are likely to result in improvements in other states also. On the other hand, if budgets are not increased or unlikely to increase in a sufficient amount to allow fees that are at least close to market rate, the only way to achieve program balance and improve access is to force providers to participate and accept below market rates, restrict the number of persons eligible to receive dental benefits, discourage use or limit the set of benefits, or some combination.

POLITICS, POLICY, AND DENTAL CARE COVERAGE

There is a reason that access and the availability of dentists to provide care to disadvantaged children have been for the last 20 years a hot topic of concern, and the reason is quite simple. It is a very difficult problem to solve, and if it were easy, it would have been worked out by now. What makes the problem so difficult is the intersection of politics, a need to ration scarce resources, and an unwillingness to make some very difficult decisions. Increasing budgetary allocations allowing fees to increase in sufficient amounts to even approach a reasonable fraction of market rates may be highly desirable, but is it is also highly unlikely. The amount needed to succeed could be substantial and would have to compete with the needs of education, public safety, and so many other needed and supported programs. In a political vacuum where no other interest competes for the attention of resources, states might be lobbied to adequately increase budgets. The likelihood of being able to increase budgets in sufficient amounts to correct market imperfections over the long term is not likely, however. This is not to suggest that budgetary improvements are not possible. In actuality, child oral health advocates have been quite successful in recent years. Maryland has made significant progress by increasing reimbursement rates, instituting loan repayment plans to encourage provide participation and establishing a fellows program to provide an alternative mode of provider care. Notwithstanding improvements made to date, an expectation that larger budget allocations will solve the problem may be overly optimistic, and the alternative of forcing providers to participate, restricting the number of persons eligible to receive dental benefits, or limiting the set of benefits are unappealing and so far difficult to achieve.

If seemingly hopeless, how then to move forward? Approximately 8 years ago in a paper titled "Access to Care: A Call for Innovation" I noted that without the will, cooperation, and support of not only providers but also of patients, of government officials, and of the public at large, the likelihood for success is probably limited.[34] Oral health child advocates and the public health community should have been included also. In addition to the suggestion that reimbursement rates be improved and administrative burden reduced, this paper focused on several possible areas for improvement including:

Designing programs to meet local or regional needs, noting that 50 states provide 50 opportunities for innovation and should encourage state-based experiments
Providing financial inducements to dental students and recent graduates to practice in targeted areas
Providing reimbursement for missed appointments

Encouraging additional efforts by caseworkers, including efforts to educate covered patients about the importance and value of oral health

Considering a reassessment of EPSDT mandates

Establishing an assessment of and prioritization of child oral health needs and a corresponding prioritization plan for care[34]

Not much has changed. On the other hand, there is now a slightly better understanding of some of the relevant issues. Today, it is known that the effect of dental care coverage on dental use may be somewhat smaller than expected, and it also is known that the effect of dental care coverage may be somewhat diminished by varying social conditions and health beliefs. Therefore, increasing the number of people who have dental care coverage or increasing the number of providers who participate will not themselves achieve the goal of improving access.

WHAT TO DO NOW

If not much has changed, then much of what was suggested 8 years ago is as valid today as it was then. Providing financial inducements to dental students and recent graduates to practice in targeted areas has been done and should continue. Designing programs that are geographically appropriate makes sense, and providing reimbursement for missed appointments should be tried. The appropriate use of community health centers should be included in this effort. Additional efforts by case workers and local communities to educate Medicaid- and SCHIP-eligible patients about the importance and value of oral health also should be undertaken. Aggressive health education promotion including the inclusion of recent advances in health literacy can alter health beliefs and counter some of the difficulties associated with a harmful social structure. Forcing providers to participate might work in the short run but is unlikely to succeed in the long run. For many Americans, dentistry not only works but works very well. Most Americans receive the care that they need and want.[34] Forcing providers to participate without correcting current problems could result in the unintended consequence of driving potential dental students into other fields and practitioners out of practice into retirement thereby exacerbating the problem. A better suggestion might be to nudge practitioners rather than force them. Dentistry is a licensed profession regulated by states. Dentists are granted the privilege as providers to participate. Most dentists understand that although the profession is primarily regulated to protect the public, the regulations also protect them and their livelihood. So, practitioners should be nudged with improvements in programs and a reminder that with the privilege of a protected profession is the responsibility to make sure that dentistry is accessible and available to each and every American. Still missing is any attempt to honestly look at EPSDT or any serious effort to prioritize child oral health needs and develop a corresponding prioritization plan for care. In addition, an effort should be made to develop a reasonable set of program goals. For instance, children from middle-income families with dental coverage on average have a use rate (**Fig. 18**) of 55%, and children from a middle-income family without dental coverage on average have a use rate of 27%. Clearly, dental care use rates among poor (15%) and low-income (16%) children are unacceptable. On the other hand, if children from a middle-income family who have dental coverage on average only have a use rate of 55%, why should one expect all children to have a dental visit each year? Just as it is time to nudge colleagues in practice it is also time to nudge oral health child advocates and public health colleagues. An honest discussion is needed about how much care patients should be expected to have. A later discussion also is needed about

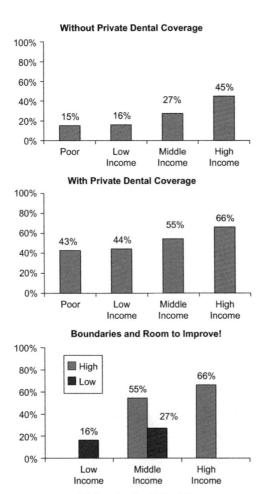

Fig. 18. Use and coverage among children in the United States.

what is a fair, equitable, and reasonable set of benefits. A discussion is needed about who needs care the most and if limits are needed how should care be prioritized. Should use be controlled in a way that directs care those with the greatest need and if so how? Recognizing that patients are consumers and recognizing that patients will attempt to maximize their overall utility, plan administrators and policy makers can design programs and benefit plans with features that will encourage patients to seek care in a way that meets program goals. All that is needed is an honest discussion and set of program goals that are realistic and in alignment with anticipated budgets.

REFERENCES

1. Available at: http://www.anthc.org/cs/chs/dhs/index.cfm. Accessed October 25, 2008.
2. Available at: http://www.phs-dental.org/depac/newfile50.html. Accessed October 25, 2008.
3. Available at: http://www.ada.org/prof/resources/pubs/adanews/adanewsarticle.asp?articleid=2928. Accessed October 25, 2008.

4. Medicaid: extent of dental disease in children has not decreased, and millions are estimated to have untreated tooth decay. GAO-08-1121. Washington, DC: Government Accountability Office; 2008.

5. Manski RJ, Brown E. Dental use, expenses, private dental coverage, and changes, 1996 and 2004. Rockville (MD): Agency for Healthcare Research and Quality; 2007. MEPS Chartbook No.17.

6. Bailit H, Beazoglou T. Financing dental care: trends in public and private expenditures for dental services. Dent Clin North Am 2008;52:281–95.

7. Douglass CW, Cole KO. Utilization of dental services in the United States. J Dent Educ 1979;43(4):223–38.

8. Kriesberg L, Treiman BR. Socioeconomic status and the utilization of dentists' services. J Am Coll Dent 1960;27:147–65.

9. Manning WG, Bailit HL, Benjamin B, et al. The demand for dental care: evidence from a randomized trial in health insurance. J Am Dent Assoc 1985;110(6):895–902.

10. Manning WG, Phelps CE. The demand for dental care. Bell Journal of Economics 1979;10(2):503–25.

11. Manski RJ, Cooper PF. Dental care use: does dental insurance truly make a difference in the US? Community Dent Health 2007;24(4):205–12.

12. Reisine ST. The impact of dental condidtions on social functioning and the quality of life. Annu Rev Public Health 1988;9:1–19.

13. Department of Health, Education and Welfare. Public Health Service, Health Resources Administration. Factors which affect the utilization of dental services. Washington, DC: US Government Printing Office; 1978.

14. Gooch BF, Berkey DB. Subjective factors affecting the utilization of dental services by the elderly. Gerodontics 1987;3(2):65–9.

15. Macek MD, Manski RJ, Vargas CM, et al. Comparing oral health care utilization estimates in the United States across three nationally representative surveys. Health Serv Res 2002;37(2):499–521.

16. US Department of Health and Human Services. Healthy people 2010. With understanding and improving health and objectives for improving health. 2nd edition. Washington, DC: US Government Printing Office; 2000.

17. Available at: http://meps.ahrq.gov/mepsweb/. Accessed October 25, 2008.

18. Manski RJ, Moeller JF, Maas W. Dental services: an analysis of utilization over twenty years. J Am Dent Assoc 2001;132(5):655–64.

19. Available at: http://www.cms.hhs.gov/NationalHealthExpendData/01_Overview.asp#TopOfPage. Accessed October 25, 2008.

20. Available at: http://www.bls.gov/cpi/. Accessed October 25, 2008.

21. Conrad DA. Dental care demand: age-specific estimates for the population 65 years of age and over. Health Care Financ Rev 1983;4(4):47–57.

22. Mueller D, Monheit AC. Insurance coverage and the demand for dental care. J Health Econ 1988;7(1):59–72.

23. McConnell, Campbell R. Economics: principles problems and policies. New York: McGraw-Hill Book Company; 1984.

24. Feldstein, Paul J. Health care economics. 3rd edition. New York: John Wiley & Sons, Incorporated; 1988.

25. Feldstein, Paul J. Financing dental care: an economic analysis. Lexington (MA): Lexington Books, D.C. Health and Company; 1973.

26. Manski RJ. The impact of not having dental insurance coverage after employment on elderly who need dental care [dissertation]. Baltimore (MD); 1993.

27. 1984/85 dental statistics handbook. Chicago (IL): Bureau of Economic and Behavioral Research, American Dental Association; 1984.

28. Source book on health insurance data. Washington, DC: Public Relations Division, Health Insurance Association of America; 1987.
29. Source book on health insurance data. Washington, DC: Public Relations Division, Health Insurance Association of America; 1990.
30. Available at: http://www.cms.hhs.gov/SCHIPDentalCoverage/. Accessed October 25, 2008.
31. Available at: http://domesticpolicy.oversight.house.gov/story.asp?ID=2192. Accessed October 25, 2008.
32. Andersen RM, Davidson PL. In: Andersen R, Rice T, Kominski J, editors. Improving access to care in America: individual and contextual indicators in changing the US health care system. Key issues in health services, policy, and management. San Francisco (CA): Jossey-Bass; 2001. p. 3–30.
33. Available at: http://www.cms.hhs.gov/MedicaidEarlyPeriodicScrn/02_Benefits.asp#TopOfPage. Accessed October 25, 2008.
34. Manski RJ. Access to dental care: an opportunity waiting. J Am Coll Dent 2001; 68(2):12–5.
35. Eklund SA, Pittman JL, Clark SJ. Michigan Medicaid's Healthy Kids Dental Program: an assessment of the first 12 months. J Am Dent Assoc 2003;134(2): 1509–15.

Dental Benefits Improve Access to Oral Care

Rene Chapin, BSJ

KEYWORDS

• Dental benefits • Coverage • Plans • Oral care • Wellness

Dental benefits have a profound, positive impact on individuals' ability to access oral health care by reducing patient costs and providing access to networks of dentists willing to treat dental plan participants. The National Association of Dental Plans' (NADP's) *2007 Consumer Survey* of 6000 respondents reveals that people with dental benefits are more likely to have a regular dentist, to visit the dentist more frequently, and to receive dental treatment.[1]

TYPES OF DENTAL BENEFIT PROGRAMS

How does dental coverage make a difference in access to care? To answer this question, it is important to have a basic knowledge about the benefit programs available. Dental benefits include insurance products and discount plans (**Fig. 1**).

Dental Preferred Provider Organizations

Dental Preferred Provider Organizations (DPPOs) are the most commonly offered dental benefit product, with 63% of the market.[2] DPPOs

- Keep out-of-pocket costs lower by negotiating discounts with dentists in their network
- Provide some payment for care from dentists that are not in their networks
- Have typical deductibles of $50[3]
- Offer annual maximums of coverage, typically ranging from $500 to $3000 with an average of $1200[3]
- Can be offered to employees without employers contributing to premiums
- Are available in some states to individuals

Amounts paid by plans usually are stated as a percentage of the allowed amount for each procedure.

National Association of Dental Plans, 12700 Park Central Drive, Suite 400, Dallas, TX 75251, USA
E-mail address: rchapin@nadp.org

Dent Clin N Am 53 (2009) 505–509
doi:10.1016/j.cden.2009.03.004
0011-8532/09/$ – see front matter © 2009 Elsevier Inc. All rights reserved.

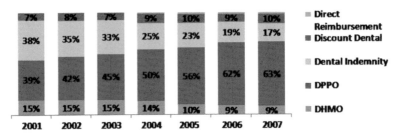

Fig. 1. Commercial dental benefits by plan type.

Dental Health Maintenance Organizations

- Have the lowest premium costs
- Use capitation (a per-patient per-month arrangement) for part or all of dentist compensation, rather than fee-for-service
- Keep out-of-pocket costs predictable with co-payments stated in specific dollar amounts
- Normally cover treatment only when provided by a network dentist
- Generally have no annual maximums or deductibles
- Can be offered to employees without employers contributing to premiums
- Are available to individuals in most states

Discount Dental Plans

- Have low monthly fees
- Provide discounts to patients seeking care from dentists in their networks
- Are not an insured product
- Require consumers to pay the full discounted cost of care out of pocket
- Can be offered to employees without employers contributing to premiums
- Are widely available to individuals

Dental Indemnity Plans

- Are traditionally benefit-rich programs
- Are a declining segment of the dental market because of the higher cost
- Have the highest premium costs
- Reimburse any dentist
- Have typical deductibles of $50[3]
- Offer annual maximums, typically ranging from $1000 to $3000[3]

AFFORDABILITY OF DENTAL PLANS

Dental benefits are affordable, with monthly premiums generally ranging from $45 to $125 for a family of three or more persons. Thus, the daily cost of dental benefits is approximately the same as that of a cup of coffee, according to the NADP *2007 Premium Trends Report*.[3] This report states national premium averages by products as follows:

Employee-only plans (including orthodontia):
DHMOs: $19.40/month, $233 annually
DPPOs: $35.02/month, $420 annually
Indemnity plans: $30.87 a month, $370 annually

Most often, individuals receive dental coverage through their employer. The NADP *2005 Purchaser Behavior Study* shows that 71% of all employers offer dental benefits. This number ranges from 40% of employers who have 6 to 24 employees to 96% of employers who have 10,000 or more employees. Ninety-seven percent of employers who have 25 or more employees consider dental benefits to be an "essential" or "differentiating" factor in attracting and maintaining talent (**Fig. 2**).

WHAT DENTAL BENEFIT PLANS TYPICALLY COVER

Group dental benefits offered through an employer generally categorize procedures as preventive, basic, or major. Most plans cover 100% of preventive care, 80% of basic care, and 50% of major procedures. Group dental plans generally cover treatment in seven categories; brief examples are given of the various procedures in each category.

1. Preventive care: cleaning and radiographs
2. Restorative care: fillings
3. Endodontic procedures: root canals
4. Oral surgery: tooth removal and tissue biopsy
5. Orthodontics: braces and retainers
6. Periodontics: treatment of gum disease
7. Prosthodontics: dentures and bridges

Although dental benefits most often are available through employment or other groups such as associations and public programs, individuals may purchase coverage on their own. Plans offered to individuals may include limits and policy riders. For instance, individual plans may cover categories 1 through 4 during the first year and add categories 6 and 7 in the second year. Orthodontia may be offered as a rider to the policy that can be selected when relevant.

Regardless of how dental benefits are obtained, individuals who have coverage respond differently to their oral health needs than do individuals lacking coverage. Following are some key findings about the "covered" versus "uncovered" individuals.

Close-up: Covered Individuals

According to the NADP *Consumer Survey*, respondents with dental benefits are

- Forty-nine percent more likely to have visited their dentist in the past 6 months
- Forty-two percent more likely to have had a check-up or cleaning in the past year
- Forty-two percent more likely to take their children to the dentist every 6 months

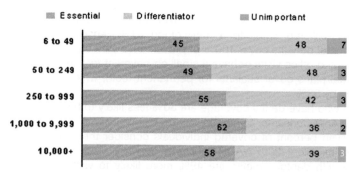

Fig. 2. Employers offering dental coverage.

In addition, respondents with dental coverage are 31% more likely to have a relationship with their "regular dentist." They also are much more likely to have had major procedures in the past 2 years. Survey findings indicate respondents with dental coverage were

- Fifty-two percent were more likely to have a root canal
- Thirty-three percent more likely to receive periodontal maintenance
- Thirty-two percent more likely to have crowns
- Eighteen percent more likely to have cavities filled

Close-up: Individuals Lacking Coverage

Conversely individuals without dental benefits are 2.5 times more likely not to visit their dentist because of their lack of coverage. They also are 16% more likely not to have had basic or major procedures in the last 2 years and are 19% more likely not to have had periodontal treatments.

In contrast, individuals who have coverage are 30% more likely not to have an extraction. This finding suggests that covered individuals' improved access to care and use of services results in the preservation of more of their original teeth, a key indicator of improved oral health.

Historically the average American over age 65 years in 1960 had only seven of his or her original teeth. Today the average is closer to 20. Baby boomers can expect to have at least 24 teeth left by age 65 years, according to the U.S. Center for Disease Control.[4]

The landmark *2000 Surgeon General's Report*[5] attributes this tremendous progress to

- The fluoridation of community drinking water
- Better awareness of the importance of dental hygiene
- The growth of dental benefits

ROLE OF DENTAL BENEFITS

The U.S. Census Bureau reports that Americans spent $86 billion for dental care in 2005[6] and that dental benefits funded half of this total. Today more than 173 million Americans, more than half the population, have dental benefits. Thus, dental benefits often are the gateway to care.

The NADP consumer white paper[7] lists 10 reasons individuals should have coverage:

1. Dental benefits pay for half of the $86 billion spent annually on dental care (U.S. Census Bureau 2005 report). In 2015, expenditures for dental care are estimated at $167.3 billion or $2076 for a family of four (U.S. Census Bureau 2005 report).
2. Most dental benefits cover 100% of preventative care such as cleanings, radiographs, and office visits or have a small co-payment for this care.
3. All dental plans cover sealants for permanent teeth, which is proven to reduce cavities by 93%.
4. People who have dental coverage are 30% less likely to have dental extractions (*2007 NADP Consumer Survey*[1])
5. Fifty-seven percent of covered individuals consider their dental health as very good or excellent (*2007 NADP Consumer Survey*[1])
6. People with dental benefits are 49% more likely to visit their dentist every 6 months and are 42% more likely to take their children to the dentist that often.

7. People with dental benefits are 31% more likely to have a regular dentist
8. Many dental plans have expanded benefits for individuals who have gum disease and serious health conditions such as diabetes and heart disease.
9. Many dental plans provide enhanced periodontal benefits for pregnant women because gum disease is associated with a 2.6-fold increase in extremely preterm births.
10. Dental plans often provide discounts for products that fight tooth decay and gum disease such as prescription-strength toothpastes and mouthwash as well as gum with a five-carbon, plant based artifical sweetner. When children who had chewed this for 2 years between the ages of 6 and 8 years were re-examined 5 years later (at the ages of 11–13 years), they were found to be 60% less likely to develop caries. Teeth that erupted after children starting chewing the gum had 93% fewer caries. Expectant women who chewed the gum did not pass the bacteria to their infants, resulting in better early childhood dental health.[5]

SUMMARY

In conclusion, dental coverage provides a means to obtain oral care, which is an important component of overall health.

REFERENCES

1. 2007 Consumer survey, July 2008. Dallas (TX): National Association of Dental Plans; 2008. p. 4.
2. 2007 Joint dental benefits report: enrollment, August 2008. Dallas (TX): National Association of Dental Plans/Delta Dental Plans Association; 2008. p. 8.
3. 2004–2008 Dental benefits report: premium trends, October 2008. Dallas (TX): National Association of Dental Plans; 2008. p. 11–16, 27.
4. Center for Disease Control. National Center for Health Statistics. Health, United States, 1999. Achievements in public health, 1900–1999: fluoridation of drinking water to prevent dental caries. MMWR Morb Mortal Wkly Rep October 1999.
5. Oral Health America. A report of the Surgeon General. National Institutes of Health; 2000.
6. 2005 U.S. Census Bureau. Table 8.1, Health care and social assistance. 9NAICS 62.
7. National Association of Dental Plans. Dental benefits: a wise investment in your family's health. Available at: http://www.nadp.org. Accessed March 2008.

Managing Clinical Risk: Right Person, Right Care, Right Time

Council on Dental Practice, American Dental Association,
Frank J. Graham, DMD, ABO*

KEYWORDS

- Clinical risk factors • Dental risk factors • Clinical risk
- Risk assessment • Risk management • Oral health risk
- Oral health policy

Clinical risk assessment indirectly affects access to care and so bears discussion when considering the topic of access. Practicing dentists and those in the health policy arena have renewed interest in clinical risk assessment and management. This interest lies in the potential to identify a patient's clinical needs for oral health care more specifically, to intervene early and maximize prevention, and to educate patients to become more informed consumers of oral health care. All of these actions could contribute to more efficient allocation of oral health care resources, that is, directing resources where they are most needed and producing the greatest value from them. The realization of this potential depends on the accuracy with which risk can be estimated and communicated and requires that risk assessment be applied appropriately.

To explore this potential and its ramifications for access to care, the current status of formal clinical risk assessment is described and ideas for appropriate application are discussed. It is recognized that

- Clinical risk assessment, management, and communication are essential to the practice of dentistry
- Valid and reliable risk assessment instruments are needed
- Risk assessment can contribute indirectly to expanded access to care
- Risk assessment should be applied to identifying and meeting patients' clinical needs

---

Council on Dental Practice, American Dental Association, 211 E. Chicago Avenue, Chicago, IL 60611, USA
* Corresponding author.
E-mail address: dentalpractice@ada.org

Dent Clin N Am 53 (2009) 511–522
doi:10.1016/j.cden.2009.03.015
0011-8532/09/$ – see front matter © 2009 Elsevier Inc. All rights reserved.

- Patients' preferences and values are integral to risk assessment
- Ongoing risk communication among dentists, policy-makers, and payers is essential.

These ideas highlight the multiple ramifications of clinical risk assessment for access to care. They also are discussed within a broad definition of clinical risk.

Clinical risk refers to the chance that a patient will develop an oral health condition or that an existing oral health condition will progress. It also implies some degree of cost, whether the cost is monetary and/or an effect on the quality of life. The management of clinical risk incorporates risk assessment and also lays the groundwork for the implementation of interventions to prevent or to slow down the onset or progression of disease or to lessen the impact of the disease or its progression. It also implies some level of benefit or effectiveness, which may be monetary and/or improvement in the quality of life.

Clinical risk assessment data are generally used by dentists and policy-makers in making decisions that have an impact on patients' health outcomes. The dentist forges the most basic link between clinical risk and access to care when he/she assesses the clinical risks of a patient and then recommends treatment based on that assessment. The relationship is expanded further by the actions of health planners, policy-makers, and payers who utilize data on clinical risks to establish targeted public policies and programs, and to design benefit plans and clinical service delivery structures. These decisions may have an indirect impact on access to care. Access afforded through policy decisions is illustrated in recent policies, such as benefit plans providing more prophylaxis for patients at higher risk for certain oral health conditions, pay-for-performance programs using risk-adjusted data in measuring performance, and evidence-based clinical recommendations advising the practitioner to consider particular recommendations in the context of patient risk levels.

The potential impact of clinical risk assessment on access to specific care, on the efficient delivery of care, and on the well-being of the patient is evident. To reap the benefits of clinical risk assessment at both the clinical and policy levels, clinical risk assessment must be applied appropriately. The dental profession has the primary responsibility for evaluating data and generating information on clinical risks and must continually expand its knowledge and skills in clinical risk assessment and management. Thus, understanding clinical risk assessment and managing it appropriately begins with the dental profession.

UNDERSTANDING RISK IS ESSENTIAL TO THE PRACTICE OF DENTISTRY

Clinical risk assessment is central to dental practice. Dentists routinely gather information regarding a patient's medical and dental histories, and clinical findings are included in the patient's record. A dentist's professional judgment and ability to integrate clinical findings with knowledge of oral disease processes, range of treatment possibilities, evidence-based treatment recommendations, experience with those treatments, and the needs of the patient are all part of clinical risk assessment and contribute to the identification of appropriate treatment. When the appropriate treatment can be delivered correctly to the patient, at the correct time, risk for a disease or condition can be lessened. The benefit can be measured in terms of improved health and perhaps in terms of decreased cost as well.

Clinical risk includes three distinct functions: risk assessment, risk management, and risk communication. Risk assessment is the determination of the likelihood that an adverse outcome will occur, based on the identification and weighting of risk factors. Risk management is the action taken to mitigate adverse outcomes. Risk communication is the sharing of risk information with the patient. Together, these three functions present an opportunity for more "individualized" oral health care, more consumer participation in clinical decision-making, and more efficient use of oral health care resources.

The focus of the dental profession is disease prevention, and risk assessment and management are integral to disease prevention. The tools and resources with which to assess and manage risk continue to develop. Deeper understanding of risk factors leads the practitioner to move toward care that is based on risk assessment. The risk of periodontal disease and its connection to systemic diseases compels the profession to expand its knowledge of risk factors for oral disease. The understanding and management of caries risk continues to develop. Although it always will be necessary to address active disease, risk assessment will become an ever-growing dimension of oral health care that will aid the practitioner in moving patient care to prevention and early intervention.

VALID AND RELIABLE RISK ASSESSMENT INSTRUMENTS ARE NEEDED

How can a dentist predict future disease or need for care, based on information that can be collected today? Formal assessment of risk factors helps in making this judgment. Formal clinical risk assessment tools are relatively recent developments in dentistry, however, and validation studies are still in the early stages.[1] Risk assessment instruments now available tend to focus on caries, periodontal disease, and oral cancer. Risk factors for caries, periodontitis, and oral cancer have been studied most extensively, because caries and periodontitis are widespread and oral cancer often can be life threatening.

Dental caries and periodontal disease are highly prevalent conditions, so prevention and treatment of these two diseases is a priority. Although the prevalence of caries has declined in much of the United States population, it still is highly prevalent in people of low socioeconomic status. Its prevalence also is increasing among older adults, because they are remaining dentate throughout their lives. Recent data also indicate an increase in caries incidence in very young children.

The ramifications of periodontal disease now are thought to be greater than in previous years because of their associations with some systemic conditions. Twelve percent of adults aged 25 to 34 years have at least one site of a 4-mm attachment loss, and this percentage increases with age.

Oral cancer is relatively rare, but it presents a serious impact on patients' quality of life and survival. There are few formal risk assessment instruments for oral cancer at this time, but there are a number of screening tools. The profession places a high priority on prevention and treatment of oral cancer, and dentists are urged to evaluate patients carefully for oral cancer.

Formal assessment instruments make it easier to discuss risk factors because they present a common vocabulary and conceptual model. Instruments group risk factors that are similar, describe their action in the disease process, and sometimes weight risk factors. They also tend to increase objectivity in the evaluation process.

There are many models, but risk factors generally fall into hierarchies or categories that describe how directly they are related to the cause of disease and how they act independently or synergistically with other risk factors. The categorization of a risk factor is fluid as evolving evidence-based scientific study provides more data about how a risk factor contributes to the disease process. For example, the understanding of how oral pathogens act in the development of periodontitis changed as scientific data showed that specific pathogens are more important in the development of periodontitis than the quantity of numerous pathogens.[2] Risk factors may be categorized as direct factors, which may be causes of disease, potentiators of disease, and markers of disease.

A direct risk factor is considered to be a major factor of a given disease and may have an independent effect in the development of a specific disease. A high level of the oral pathogen *Streptococcus mutans* is a strongly associated risk factor for caries. This risk factor is documented in the scientific literature as being a direct causative factor of caries.[3]

In other instances, risk factors are suspected of having a link to oral disease because they have very strong statistical associations with it, but causality has not yet been established. For example, an association between oral disease and some systemic processes, such as chronic inflammation, has been found. Direct risk factors also can act synergistically to increase the risk of disease.

Potentiators of disease are factors that are known either to act upon the direct or major risk factors to increase their effect or act upon the patient in a way that increases the patient's susceptibility. In either case the potentiator increases the risk of disease or further predisposes the patient to disease. Although potentiating factors tend to be lifestyle habits such as poor oral hygiene and diet, they are not exclusively lifestyle factors. For example, a symptom of Sjögren's syndrome is a dry mouth; and a dry mouth can act to potentiate the development of caries.

Risk factors also may include markers of disease, such as incipient caries, restored lesions, mobile teeth, missing teeth, and biochemical characteristics of saliva, blood, or other bodily fluids that are associated with disease. Markers are not necessarily causes of the disease but show that the disease is or has been present.

The interaction of risk factors can have a substantial effect on the development or progression of disease, and risk assessment models suggest that an estimation of risk should be based on the combination of both independent and associated factors. Acting synergistically, risk factors may increase the patient's absolute risk of disease. An example is the interaction between high levels of *Streptococcus mutans*, a diet high in simple carbohydrates, inadequate exposure to fluoride, and the susceptibility of the tooth, resulting in caries. These factors can be potentiated or modified by a host of behavioral and environmental factors, such as oral hygiene practices, smoking, socioeconomic status, access to fluoridated drinking water, and patient attitudes and knowledge about health and disease.

The dental profession currently has a better understanding about what risk factors are than about what their interactions are. For estimating a patient's total level of risk, dental risk assessment forms, developed to date, use a simple listing of risk factors. A patient's risk level is classified as high, medium, or low, based on educated approximations of the threshold number of risks that could separate each category. Some assessment forms attempt to weight each risk factor, giving greater weight to factors that are known to play a more direct role in the development of disease. The limitation of weightings is that they generally are based only on a consensus of expert opinion regarding the strength of a particular risk factor relative to the other risk factors. At this time quantification of risk often is subjective (and this subjectivity is one reason why no single form is universally accepted for risk assessment).

Risk generally is applied very narrowly by third-party payers, who frequently assign benefits for caries by the evidence of previous caries activity, without taking the broad range of risk factors into account. Because the disease already is present or has been present, the risk captured by third-party payers is the progression of caries, rather than the prevention of the disease. Some would argue that planning to address risk from this perspective is too little, too late.

Caries risk assessment tools have been developed by various organizations, agencies, and proprietary vendors. The multivariate nature of the risk of caries has led to several unique approaches. There are at least five clinical caries risk assessment protocols in somewhat widespread use. Each of these protocols emphasizes different aspects of caries risk assessment.

The American Dental Association/Food and Drug Administration Radiographic Guidelines (A/FRG), first developed in 1985 and revised in 2004, include advice on caries risk assessment.[4] This information can be integrated into the necessity for radiographic evaluation and is not formatted into a concise tool or form that can be used to document patient risk factors. Its main advantage is the flexibility in assessment given to the dentist when determining a patient's risk level.

The Caries Assessment Tool (CAT) was developed by the American Academy of Pediatric Dentists. It was introduced in 2002 and was developed for risk assessment of infants, children, and adolescents. The tool was revised in 2006 and incorporates risk factors and levels or degrees of risk in a chart form. Some factors that apply mainly to adults, such as tobacco use, are not included in the CAT.[5]

Caries management by risk assessment was developed by John Featherstone at the University of San Francisco. Two assessment forms are used, one for children under 6 years of age and one for all other patients. This risk assessment strategy includes documentation of protective factors and has been implemented at the University's dental clinics. The major disadvantage of these forms for dentists in private practice is that some of the assessment parameters, such as bacteriologic identification and measurement of salivary flow, are not typically performed in most private dental offices. The incorporation of protective factors as part of the assessment adds another layer of complication in assessing risk.[6,7]

A computerized caries risk assessment program, the Cariogram. was developed at the University of Malmo.[8] This program is available on the Internet and is not dependent on age to determine caries risk. All risk factors are graded on a continuum of 0 (low risk) to 3 (high risk). The assessment is presented graphically as a pie chart and can include a written assessment. Assessments of the population are required before individual risk factors can be entered into the program. The program requires assessments about populations before individual risk factors are entered. Three of the nine elements that are assessed are not commonly performed in private dental offices in the United States: levels of *Streptococcus mutans*, the buffering capacity of the patient's saliva, and saliva secretion rate.

A proprietary software program, PreViser™, that assesses risks for caries, for fracture, and for the development of root surface caries is available.[9] The software program takes into account the patient's age. Required risk parameters are submitted to the company over the Internet, and the company then generates a risk profile. Risk is assessed as low, moderate, or high. Individualized recommendations for prevention, oral hygiene, visits to the dental office, and communications with the patient also are provided with the risk assessment.

In 2004, the American Dental Association formed a Caries Risk Assessment Workgroup that evaluated the publicly available caries risk tools and found that none of the existing tools was adequate to assess caries risk simply in general dental practices. The A/FRG advice was not available in a form for purposes of documentation; the CAT was not designed to be used for an all-inclusive population; the caries management by risk assessment and Cariogram included risk factors that most general dentists in practice would not likely record; and the risk basis for the PreViser tool is not clear. In December 2008 the American Dental Association's Board of Trustees approved two caries risk assessment forms that were designed to record risk factors and to be used as patient communication tools.

There are two major tools available to assess the risk for periodontal disease. The first, from the American Academy of Periodontology, is Internet based.[10] Following submission of 12 self assessments, a report is generated with an assessment of the risk level (low, medium, or high) for developing periodontal disease.

An Internet-based periodontal risk and disease assessment also is available from PreViser.[9] In addition to assessing the level of risk from very low (1) to very high (5), this program provides an assessment of disease from healthy (1) to severe gum disease (100) that is based on the clinical findings of the dental office. A report with interventions, possible treatments, and the frequency for prevention and maintenance is transmitted to the dental office along with the assessment.

An oral cancer risk assessment tool is included in the PreViser suite of products, with risk reported on a scale of 1 (less risk) to 5 (greater risk). The individualized risk value seems to be based on the reported demographic characteristics and social habits of the patient.

Salivary testing may provide objective measures of oral disease. There is some evidence that it may help with the risk assessment data for oral cancer. The analysis of oral bacteria and other oral biochemical factors offer more measurable risks for developing oral disease. Colony counts of *Streptococcus mutans* and measures of salivary acidity provide risk assessment data for caries. Analysis of oral bacteria, subgingival temperature, and crevicular fluid may provide an indication of risk for periodontitis. At this time, however, most dentists do not perform such analyses on a routine basis to detect signs of disease.

Dentists usually assess risk informally and intuitively by looking for early symptoms of disease and rely on the patient to provide accurate information about lifestyle, medical history, and other risk factors. Risk can be a moving target, because a patient's risk of disease can change over time, sometimes in a matter of months. The dentist can reassess risk at every visit by asking the patient if there has been any change in lifestyle and habits and by conducting an oral examination.

In addition to their clinical usefulness, formal risk assessments can serve as educational tools. The dentist can use them in talking with the patient and provide anticipatory guidance. They provide an organized and tangible format for helping the patient understand factors that contribute to the disease process and the relative importance of those factors. Assessments also can point out the difference between factors that can be controlled directly by the patient and those that must be managed through professional care, showing the degree to which dental disease can be controlled. This explanation may help clarify for the patient what periodic visits accomplish and may motivate the patient to be more compliant with ongoing care.

CLINICAL RISK MANAGEMENT, APPROPRIATELY APPLIED, CAN CONTRIBUTE TO EXPANDED ACCESS TO CARE

An important health policy goal in the United States today is expanded access to oral health care. If overall healthcare costs can be reduced while maintaining or increasing quality of dental care, health care resources could be distributed more effectively. Clinical risk management could support that goal if it is appropriately applied.

To illustrate the possibility, consider the interest in clinical risk management and oral–systemic disease links. Recent scientific studies have shown associations between oral disease and systemic illness, such as connections between periodontal infections and diabetes control, arterial inflammation, and preterm, low birth weight babies.[11] These recent studies prompted a swift response from the benefits industry, which recognized that better control of oral infections may reduce the financial risks of insuring long-term medical illnesses, such as diabetes and cardiovascular disease.[12] Some benefit plans already have incorporated this emerging information in the design of dental benefits, allowing additional benefits for dental cleanings for pregnant women and patients who have diabetes. Risk assessment could increase costs on the dental benefit side but decrease costs on the medical benefit side, most likely decreasing overall health care costs.

Clinical risk management, based on careful risk assessment, emphasizes prevention and early intervention, which further expands the range of appropriate care. For example, the possibility of detecting incipient caries and of halting or reversing the development of carious lesions with a variety of treatment modalities such as sealants, fluoride treatments, xylitol, chlorhexidine, and other treatments, rather than providing more extensive restorative treatment, presents an expanded range of treatment intervention as well as a less costly one. Some benefit plans also have expanded the benefits for radiographs for patients at high risk of caries to aid in early caries detection.

CLINICAL RISK DATA SHOULD BE APPLIED FOREMOST TO IDENTIFYING AND MEETING PATIENTS' CLINICAL NEEDS

The dental profession, payers, and health policy planners each have obligations to meet patients' needs for care in providing direct care, providing for public health needs, or financing benefits to meet the oral health needs of plan enrollees. Each also has financial and political objectives to achieve as well. Clinical risk data are necessarily incorporated into financial or political analyses, such as estimating future claims costs and savings. Care is needed, however, to avoid using risk data to rationalize financial or political decisions or extrapolating data erroneously to justify financial or political decisions. This precaution is particularly difficult because the boundary between financial and political objectives and patients' clinical needs can be difficult to clarify and separate.

For example, payers confront potential conflicts in meeting their multiple objectives. Private payers seek to provide the best benefit plan for enrollees, at a fair price; they also seek to generate revenue to pay salaries and business costs, to compete successfully within the industry, to maintain adequate reserves to cover at-risk claims, and to enter into new insurance markets. Any additional benefit to the enrollee is likely to create additional costs and thus will impact the financial objectives of the payer directly.[13] There is potential for misapplication of risk data when clinical risk data are applied only to the extent that they will facilitate the achievement of financial objectives and are dismissed or even challenged when they do not. Over the long run, this misuse of data distorts the understanding and meeting of patients' clinical needs and could decrease the value of dental benefit programs.

Of equal concern would be a policy formulated from risk data that, for example, concludes that benefits to lower-risk patients should be diminished because scientific evidence of risk factors substantiates the need for an increase in benefits to higher-risk patients. Implementing such policy, over time, essentially directs benefit dollars to the group that will most benefit from it (the high-risk patients) but does so at the expense of making those patients at low risk worse off (in terms of benefits) than they had been. This approach exemplifies a rationalization for diminishing the benefits to some when the research does not suggest that the low-risk group needs fewer benefits. The research only suggests that the high-risk group needs more benefits. Scientific research will raise valid ethical questions about how benefits should be distributed, and such questions must be addressed.[14] All parties in the oral health care delivery system have multiple objectives that include providing access to care, delivering the best quality of care, and allocating resources to meet clinical needs and produce value. Care must be taken to apply risk assessment data correctly and transparently.

ORAL HEALTH CARE NEEDS ARE IDENTIFIED THROUGH THE EVALUATION OF CLINICAL RISK FACTORS AND OTHER CLINICAL DATA, AS WELL AS THROUGH CONSIDERATION OF PATIENT PREFERENCES AND VALUES

Although risk assessment data may support efficient allocation of care, efficient allocation has been a complex, imperfect endeavor in health care. Strategies, to date, have had significant limitations.[15] Strategies commonly center on educating patients to be value-sensitive consumers of care so that they will have the necessary information to demand care that is congruent with clinical needs; developing and disseminating performance criteria and clinical guidelines to specify the appropriate care for meeting clinical needs to providers and patients; and creating incentives for providers to adhere to performance criteria and clinical guidelines through various reimbursement structures. Much distinction is made between the need for care and the demand for care, and need often is thought to be a more accurate basis on which to allocate care. It can be argued, however, that demand is driven by legitimate patient preferences and values expressed by informed consumers of care.

The need for care is defined in numerous ways but generally refers to "a disturbance in health or well-being which should receive health care attention."[16] This broad-brush definition of need then is qualified with ethical and economic debates about what constitutes true disease and minor deviations from full health and where the line should be drawn in making these distinctions.[17] Despite the murkiness of where need begins and ends, it is commonly based on clinical signs and symptoms of disease or, in the case of populations of patients, on the incidence and prevalence of disease. From this standpoint it is considered an objective basis on which to allocate care.

In contrast, the demand for care is driven not only by objective signs and symptoms of disease but also by intangible factors such as the patient's emotional, intellectual, and social make-up, commonly expressed as patient preferences and values. From the payer perspective, intangible factors and the possibility of provider-driven demand often are thought to reflect a bias toward unnecessary care that results in wasted resources. Further, patient preferences and values are believed to increase the variability and unpredictability in the utilization of health care resources among clinically similar patients.[18]

Although risk assessment and management adds to the objectivity and accuracy of identifying clinical needs, risk communication about the uncertainty of risks and their impact encourages informed patient choice and informed patient consent. The patient becomes an essential party in preventing or delaying many oral diseases, and the dentist must enlist the cooperation of the patient to implement risk management fully. To do so, the dentist must communicate with the patient about risks of illness and alternative treatments and elicit the patient's initiative to make informed choices and provide informed consent for care.

There is little conclusive information about how the uncertainty of risk affects individual patient or provider decision-making, except that emotional and intellectual factors and social values play a significant role, especially when there is uncertainty about the diagnosis or the effectiveness of alternative treatment choices or when the impact of risks is high.[19] Dentists have intuitively known about the influence of these factors for a long time and take it into account on a daily basis. So, although risk assessment and management contribute to the objective identification of patient needs, risk communication compels the consideration of patient preferences and values in the identification of patient needs.

Allocation strategies that center on evidence-based clinical guidelines and performance measures also have limitations. The development and dissemination of clinical guidelines and performance criteria typically do not address risk assessment adequately. Most guidelines and performance criteria note the consideration of risk by stating something like "depending on the level of risk" or "based on clinical judgment." Patient preferences and values elude inclusion because they are subjective, are highly individual, and there is little evidence about exactly how or to what extent they affect the clinical need for care.

Financial incentives to providers to adhere to guidelines and performance criteria have demonstrated some effectiveness in containing the costs of care and in encouraging providers to provide care within the parameters of the guidelines and criteria. These financial incentives, however, may counteract incentives for quality of care, especially because patient preferences and values are ignored. Finally, performance criteria and guidelines do not yet assure the best outcomes of care, and the evidence base from which valid and reliable performance measures and risk assessment instruments can be developed is still in early stages of development.

Thus, the strategies that are applied to guide more efficient allocation of health care resources are useful, but to a limited degree. Although clinical risk factors and assessment could contribute to more accurate identification of clinical oral health care needs, the application of subjective elements, such as patient preferences and values, is still somewhat a black box of clinical care and, at this time, these considerations are not incorporated into clinical guidelines and performance measures in a meaningful way. Nonetheless, most practitioners have a sense that these factors cannot be ignored.

RISK COMMUNICATION IS AN ESSENTIAL PART OF RISK MANAGEMENT, REQUIRING CONTINUING DIALOGUE AMONG PATIENTS, DENTISTS, PAYERS, AND POLICY-MAKERS

The increasing complexity of oral health care delivery requires the dentist to develop greater communication skills than ever before and a more in-depth understanding of clinical risk. There must be a continuous dialogue among payers, dentists, patients, and policy-makers both to keep abreast of emerging information and to use it appropriately to expand access to care.

To participate fully in prevention and treatment strategies, patients must understand what they are being told about their individual risk of dental disease and its potential impact. The dentist should facilitate an ongoing dialogue with the patient, continually assessing what the patient understands, why the risk is important to the patient, and how the patient would be willing and able to manage the risk. "Oral health literacy" is the term used to describe this dynamic between the patient's understanding of health habits, risks, and prevention and his/her cooperation with the dental team.

Oral health literacy is defined by the American Dental Association as "the degree to which individuals have the capacity to obtain, process, and understand basic health information and services needed to make appropriate oral health decisions."[20] Evidence indicates that those patients who cannot fully understand their health risks and their role in preventing disease are at a tremendous disadvantage in navigating the health care system. They cannot successfully gain access to needed care, and they suffer negative health outcomes. Patient oral health literacy has become another determinant of having full access to care. The groups most vulnerable to low oral health literacy are those segments of the population that have completed fewer years of education, are elderly, have lower cognitive ability, and could be classified as poor or near poor. Those with lower oral health literacy are likely to require greater help from the oral health care team in understanding their oral health risks and the available intervention strategies, in understanding the impact of disease, and in sorting through the considerations in making decisions about interventions.

Risk communication also is the area in which clashes regarding the patient's goals in managing risk and those of the payer, policy-maker, and perhaps even the dentist become most apparent. Patients who are able to pay for care out-of-pocket generally have more options available to them than those who are dependent upon third-party arrangements or government programs alone for financing care. Because many patients receive oral health care services under dental benefit plans, dentists often are faced with presenting all appropriate treatment options to the patient and the risks involved, as well as having to recognize what treatment may or may not be a covered benefit and how treatment costs for the patient would be affected.

Discussing treatment alternatives leads to discussion of differences in treatment costs and raises questions about limitations in the design of benefits and the rationale of private and public policy-making. Patients must have information about their benefit plans and receive explanations of benefits that are transparent, straightforward, and accurate. Payers and the profession need ongoing dialogue regarding how these explanations can be accurately and fairly presented to patients.

For the dentist, the obligation to discuss the range of appropriate treatment options, irrespective of covered benefits, is ethical and inseparable from informed consent. The obligation of informed consent lies in the principle that the patient should have autonomy in decisions about his/her physical well-being, participating in clinical decision-making with full information. Skillful risk communication is a way of empowering patients with the understanding about the possibilities and risks of appropriate treatment, appropriate alternatives, and no treatment. Transparency of information and decision-making can lead to greater patient trust in the dentist, which can strengthen the doctor–patient relationship. It also can give the dentist a greater sense of confidence and reassurance in proceeding with treatment.

Statutory requirements for informed consent, today, are the bare minimum for empowering patients to be informed participants in their health care decision-making. The profession recognizes that many patients need more than written, standard directions, disclaimers, and consent forms. They may need explanations in lay terms, need time for questions and discussion, and perhaps need a picture of a procedure to visualize treatment or its expected outcome. Finding out how best to communicate with a patient often means that the dentist must talk to the patient about how much he/she understands. From this discussion, the dentist may recognize how best to help the patient understand the risks of illness and treatment and sort through the information, values, and preferences that the patient may want to consider. This expanded concept of communication with patients suggests that patients have meaningful access to care only if they understand to what extent they need treatment and what steps are available and effective in controlling their risks. They get that meaningful access in part through public information and health education initiatives, but the primary source of that information is the dentist. If the patient has access to a dentist, another level of access is open up to them. The dentist becomes the patient's advocate in obtaining the most personal and effective access to care.

SUMMARY

Clinical risk assessment and management is a longstanding part of dental practice, and it has been used to achieve better oral health for patients. Increasingly, dentists are basing care on the patient's clinical risk rather than on the presence of oral disease alone, moving oral health care toward prevention and early intervention. Clinical risk assessment and management also offer the possibility of generating data that can be used to allocate oral health care resources more efficiently. This improved allocation then can lead to expanded access to oral health care.

To realize this potential, risk assessment and management must be applied appropriately, noting what can be done, limitations, and future development. An immediate goal is to apply clinical risk data to identify and meet patients' clinical needs. As the dental profession develops more valid, reliable, and scientifically based risk assessment instruments, practitioners will hone their skill and experience in formally assessing and communicating risk data and also will develop greater understanding of the role of patient preferences and values in risk management. This understanding would enable more accurate and meaningful communication about risk and more specific incorporation of clinical risk into guidelines and performance criteria.

Clinical risk data will be used increasingly in policy-making, in which patient clinical needs are balanced with financial and political objectives. Financial and political objectives should be explained transparently, however, and the use of risk data should be based on accurate interpretations of the data and its scientific underpinnings.

Finally, all sectors of the dental industry must have an accurate understanding of clinical risk and must keep this knowledge current. The dental profession will be using risk assessment and management to move to another level of preventive care. Thus, ongoing communication within the profession and among dentists, payers, planners, and patients is necessary to manage and apply appropriately the coming expansion of knowledge about risk factors and their application.

The ideas that have been presented serve to explain that clinical risk assessment, management, and its communication generate much-needed data about the need for clinical oral health care. The data must be applied fully and accurately, however, to lead to efficient allocation of care and expanded access to specific care.

ACKNOWLEDGMENTS

The members of the Council on Dental Practice, American Dental Association, 2008–2009 (Drs. Frank Graham, Teaneck, NJ, chair; Mark S. Ritz, Homerville, GA, vice-chair; Robert Ahlstrom, Reno, NV; Charles W. D'Aiuto, Longwood, FL; Jerome DeSnyder, Plattsburgh, NY; David Duncan, Amarillo, TX; H. Lee Gardner, Hartsville, SC; Stephen O. Glenn, Tulsa, OK; Michael H. Halasz, Kettering, OH; Paul Kenworthy, Essex Junction, VT; Christopher C. Larsen, Moline, IL; Roger K. Newman, Columbia Falls, MT; Jeffrey Sameroff, Pottstown, PA; Jamie L. Sledd, Maple Grove, MN; Judee Tippett-Whyte, Stockton, CA; Kent L. Vandehaar, Chippewa Falls, WI; and Mark R. Zust, Saint Peters, MO) thank American Dental Association staff members Dr. John Luther, senior vice-president, Dental Practice/Professional Affairs; Dr. Donalda Ellek, manager, Office of Quality Assessment and Improvement, Council on Dental Benefit Programs; and Dr. Pamela Porembski, senior manager, Council on Dental Practice, for their invaluable assistance with this article.

REFERENCES

1. Domejean-Orliaguet S, Gansky SA, Featherstone JD. Caries risk assessment in an educational environment. J Dent Educ 2006;70(12):1346–54.
2. Capelli DP, Mobley CC. Periodontal disease and associated risk factors. In: Prevention in clinical oral health care. St. Louis: Mosby Inc.; 2008.

3. Themsch NL, Bachman LM, Imfeld T, et al. Are mutans streptococci in preschool children a reliable predictive factor for dental caries risk? A systematic review. Caries Res 2006;40(5):366–74.

4. American Dental Association, U.S. Food and Drug Administration. The selection of patients for dental radiographic examinations. 2004. Available at: http://www.ada.org/prof/resources/topics/topics_radiography_examinations.pdf. Accessed July 2008.

5. American Academy of Pediatric Dentistry. Policy on the use of a caries risk assessment tool (CAT) for infants, children and adolescents. Pediatr Dent 2005–2006;27(7 Suppl):25–7.

6. Ramos-Gomez FJ, Crall J, Gensky SN, et al. Caries risk assessment appropriate for the age 1 visit (infants and toddlers). J Calif Dent Assoc 2007;35(10):687–702.

7. Featherstone JDB, Domejean-Oliaguet S, Wolff M, et al. Caries risk assessment in practice for age 6 through adult. J Calif Dent Assoc 2007;35(10):703–13.

8. Cariogram. Available at: http://www.db.od.mah.se/car/cariogram/cariograminfo. Accessed July 2008.

9. PreViser. Available at: http://www.previser.com/Dentists/default.htm. Accessed July 2008.

10. American Academy of Periodontology. Patient based risk assessment. Available at: http://www.perio.org/consumer/4a.html. Accessed July 2008.

11. Capelli DP, Mobley CC. Introduction: integrating preventative clinical strategies into clinical practice. In: Prevention in clinical oral health care. St. Louis: Mosby Inc.; 2008.

12. Dolatowski T. To maximize dental benefit value and oral health, it pays to choose a specialist. In: Dental in depth. Available at: http://www.dentaldental.com/DID_Chooseaspeicalist.pdf. Accessed July 8, 2008.

13. Jones S, Cohodes DM, Scheil B. The risks of ignoring insurance risk management. Health Aff Spring 1994;13:108–22.

14. Deaton A. Policy implications of the gradient of health and wealth. Health Aff 2002;21(2):13–28.

15. Aday LA, Begley CE, Lairson DR, et al. Efficiency: concepts and methods. Evaluating the medical care system: effectiveness, efficiency and equity. Ann Arbor (MI): Health Administration Press; 1993.

16. Bishop E. Dental insurance. Glossary. New York: McGraw Hill; 1983.

17. Daniels N, Light DW, Caplan RL. Benchmarks of fairness for health care reform. New York: Oxford University Press; 1996.

18. O'Connor AM, Llewellyn-Thomas HA, Flood AB. Modifying unwarranted variations in health care: shared decision making using patient decision aids. Web Exclusive. Health Aff 2004;2(Suppl):VAR63–72.

19. Edwards A, Elwyn G. Understanding risk and lessons for clinical risk communication about treatment preferences. Qual Health Care 2001;10(1 Suppl):i9–13.

20. American Dental Association. Definition of oral health literacy. Annual Reports and Resolutions 2006;1(Suppl 1):4033.

Private Sector Response to Improving Oral Health Care Access

Council on Access, Prevention and Interprofessional Relations,
Lindsey A. Robinson, DDS*

KEYWORDS

- Access to dental care • Access to oral health services
- Oral health disparities • Social determinants of health
- Collaborative action to improve oral health

Despite vast improvements in the oral health status of the United States population over the past 50 years, disparities in oral health status continue, with certain segments of the population carrying a disproportionate disease burden. In the landmark Surgeon General's report, *Oral Health in America*,[1] dental caries is identified as the most common chronic disease of childhood—five times more common than asthma, with low-income children experiencing twice as much disease as affluent children. Although the reasons for these disparities vary, a principle contributing factor remains limited access to care for certain populations.

Multiple factors are responsible for this limited access, and there is confusion as to what is meant by "access to care." Some have defined access in the broadest possible sense as "peoples' ability to receive the oral health care that they desire."[2] Others cite economic theory and the behavior of markets to describe access challenges, focusing on either supply or demand within the oral health care system.[3] The main criterion for evaluating access to care has been the percentage of members of various groups that has had a dental visit during a referenced time period. Although this percentage is an inadequate way to measure the total experience with care, it does indicate entry into the system. A measure of the adequacy of access to care for underserved groups should be that they attain the same level of access enjoyed by the general population.

This article attempts to describe the problem, discuss various frameworks for action, illustrate some solutions developed by the private sector, and present a vision for collaborative action to improve the health of the nation. No one sector of the health

Council on Access, Prevention and Interprofessional Relations, American Dental Association, 211 E. Chicago Avenue, Chicago, IL 60611, USA
* Corresponding author.
E-mail address: campbellc@ada.org

Dent Clin N Am 53 (2009) 523–535
doi:10.1016/j.cden.2009.03.016
0011-8532/09/$ – see front matter © 2009 Elsevier Inc. All rights reserved.

dental.theclinics.com

care system can resolve the problem. The private sector, the public sector, and the not-for-profit community must collaborate to improve the oral health of the nation.

NATURE OF THE PROBLEM

Any analysis of access to oral health care requires identification of those groups potentially or actually experiencing inadequate access and the contributing factors. **Fig. 1**, a schematic diagram that segments the United States population into groups, is useful in understanding the major barriers to access. Although quantification of the size of the population in each group is not given in this diagram, some estimates are available: the institutionalized population is 1.4% of the general population; those with severe medical comorbidities make up 8.7% of the population; the economically disadvantaged include 15.3% of Americans; and 1.1% of the population lives in remote areas.[4]

Data quoted in the Workforce Taskforce Report (American Dental Association, unpublished data, October 2000) based upon National Health Interview Surveys (NHIS) conducted by the National Center for Health Statistics (NCHS), show that 63.6% of those interviewed had a dental visit in 2006.[5] These persons are ambulatory, live in community settings that are not remote, are generally healthy, and have adequate financial resources to access care. They are represented by the shaded boxes in the diagram. The unshaded boxes, representing a minority of Americans, indicate the various groups within the population whose members exhibit some characteristic that potentially predisposes them to encounter access barriers. The number of differing population segments makes clear that no one solution to the problem will be successful for all, even though some groups face similar problems. Still, specific elements in targeted solutions may be effective with multiple groups.

DEFINING THE ACCESS BARRIERS

Before discussing potential solutions to improve access, it is important to understand the barriers. Some are economic and others environmental; some are direct and

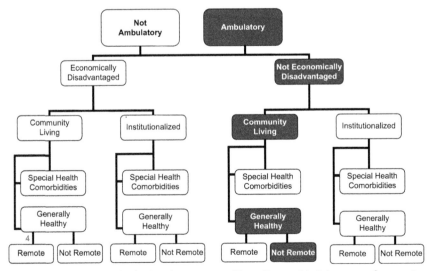

Fig. 1. Population categories by barriers to care. (*From* Brown LJ. Adequacy of current and future dental workforce. Chicago: American Dental Association, Health Policy Resources Center; 2005; with permission.)

others indirect; some are related to the individual and others to the provider. Nonetheless, use will serve as a proxy for access.

The likelihood of an individual visiting a dentist connects directly to the family income.[6] In 2004, 57.9% of individuals from high-income families, that is, families with incomes over 400% of the federal poverty level (FPL), had a dental visit. That dental visit rate decreased to 41.9% for families whose income was 200% to 400% of the FPL, to 29.9% for families whose income was 100% to 200% of the FPL, and to 26.5% for families whose income was 100% or less of the FPL.[7]

Lack of dental insurance through a benefits plan also can be an access barrier. In 2004, approximately 35% of the population had no dental coverage. Access varied directly with dental coverage; 56.9% of those with private coverage had a dental visit, as did 31.9% of those with public coverage, whereas only 26.9% of those with no coverage had a dental visit.[1] Children covered by insurance were 2.5 times more likely to receive dental care than those without coverage.[4] Employment status, because it can affect income and insurance coverage, can be a barrier to access to dental care.

The education level achieved by an individual or the family caregiver has a significant effect on access to care,[4] with low educational levels serving as a barrier. In 2004, 54.5% of college graduates had a dental visit, 37.7% of high school graduates had a visit, but only 21.9% of those with some or no schooling had a visit.[4]

Place of residence—urban, suburban, or rural—can influence access.[1] Generally, the less dense the population, the greater is the potential for access difficulties. Those in remote or frontier areas are most likely to experience access barriers. Besides geography, the type of residence also can be an important determinant of ease of access. Those in institutional settings and the homebound experience greater barriers to care than others.[1]

Beyond professional fees, significant opportunity or acquisition costs associated with accessing care may tip the balance between affordability and non-affordability. These costs include transportation costs, parking fees, childcare expenses, lost wages, office waiting time, and other factors.[3]

Age can be another barrier. It is very difficult to find a dentist who treats infants or children under the age of 2 years,[8] even though several professional associations recommend that these children have a dental visit. Considering all age categories, 25.1% of children under age 6 years receive oral health care, and 39.3% of persons beyond age 75 years have had a dental visit. Age is a barrier to obtaining care for the very young and the older population. The rate at which those between the ages of 6 years and 74 years seek oral health care fluctuates between 45% and 60%.[9]

There also are cultural barriers to gaining access to oral health care. Patients not proficient in English fear that they will be misunderstood by a dentist and that they will misunderstand information and instructions given to them by the dentist. Lack of competency in a common language by the dentist or the patient can be a barrier to access to oral health care.[10] In some cultures, dentistry is looked upon as a service that is used in response to a problem and is given little thought between problems. This attitude can be a barrier to access to on-going care.[10] In cultures where oral health care is not a priority, competing family or personal issues may relegate it as unimportant.[11]

Some families eligible for the Early Periodic Screening, Diagnosis and Treatment program do not access services for their children because they have experienced conflicts in seeking care and judge practitioners with whom they have had contact as unresponsive to their needs and disrespectful.[11] Some dentists cite negative patient behaviors are reasons for their unwillingness to treat Medicaid patients.[12]

Broken appointments and poor compliance can interfere with office routines and the success of treatment.

Immigration status also can be an access barrier. As a result of proposals in some states that would require health care providers to report undocumented immigrants and welfare reforms that affect the eligibility of that group for public programs, 39% of undocumented immigrants expressed fear about accessing medical and dental care.[13]

Fear of dental treatment and other phobias are barriers for some in accessing oral health care. This problem crosses all group categories and is not new to dentistry. It is estimated that approximately 4.3% of the population suffers from fear of dental treatment.[1] Those who have special needs, disabilities, poor functional or systemic health, or significant limitations on their mobility have difficulty accessing oral health care.[14,15]

Inability to navigate the complicated health care system, particularly for recipients of assistance programs, is another access barrier.[16] In some areas and for certain population groups, unavailability of appointments is a barrier. Some individuals cannot locate a dentist to provide care for them or are unable to schedule appointments at suitable times. They cannot establish an effective "dental home."[16] The concept of the "dental home" derives from the American Academy of Pediatrics definition of a "medical home," which states that care should be accessible, continuous, comprehensive, family-centered, coordinated, compassionate, and culturally effective. An identified dental home is recommended for all children within 6 months after the first primary tooth erupts or by 1 year of age, whichever is earlier.

Dental practices generally are located in areas where there is adequate demand for oral health care by a population with adequate economic resources. Hence a practice can be sustained in a demand-based market distribution. Where demand is insufficient, assistance programs are designed to attract practitioners and provide economic support for their practices. Economic drawbacks, however, discourage many dentists from establishing and maintaining practices in such locales—particularly new dentists who are saddled with high student debt.

Dentists report that their major reason for not treating Medicaid patients is that the low reimbursement rates sometimes do not even cover the costs of providing care. Administrative burden is a further barrier to treating Medicaid patients. Dentists cite the claims process, eligibility verification, pre-authorizations, and slow payments in this category.[12]

Individuals in minority communities are more likely to seek treatment from dentists with similar racial and/or ethnic backgrounds. Dental workforce diversity can be a significant factor in increasing overall use of oral health care.[17] The inability of minority individuals to find a practitioner of similar background can be a significant barrier to accessing care.

The "all or none" rule is a deterrent for participating in Medicaid programs for some practitioners. This rule holds that treating any Medicaid patient requires treating all Medicaid patients who seek care. Some practitioners in low-income areas would like to help but feel the need to limit their exposure to low reimbursements by limiting the number of Medicaid patients they serve. Some states are experimenting with a limited participation arrangement to overcome this barrier.

Finally one must not forget the shortcomings of the dental public health infrastructure that have contributed to the access problem. Dr. Scott L. Tomar concludes that "the U.S. dental public health workforce is small, most state programs have scant funding, and the field has minimal presence in academia."[18]

A 2001 survey indicates there were 141 dental public health specialists, a number that represents only 0.8% of all professionally active dentists.[18] Data from the Health Resources and Services Administration for Federally Qualified Health Centers indicate that in fiscal year 2007 there were 2107 full-time equivalent dentists working in that system, fewer than 2% of all practicing dentists.[19] This infrastructure plays an important role in access to care for underserved populations and has justifiably earned the title "safety net" to describe its role when all else has failed. The barriers faced by the public health infrastructure include inadequate resources, difficulty recruiting dentists, referral problems, and a low institutional priority for oral health care.[20]

This listing of the many potential barriers to access illustrates the multiple aspects to the problem and the need to understand each individual situation fully before designing programs to remediate the access problem. Generally, several barriers operating simultaneously must be addressed. Rarely will one remedy cure all. Some barriers, such as resources and reimbursement, must be overcome before any success can be realized. The resolution of these problems is necessary but not sufficient to eliminate the access problem completely.

FRAMEWORKS FOR ACTION

The American Dental Association (ADA) has a clear mission and vision for improving the oral health of the underserved as outlined in its Constitution and Bylaws (January 2007) and Strategic Plan (2007–2010).[21] The American Dental Association's *Future of Dentistry: Today's Vision Tomorrow's Reality* addressed the issue of access to care within the context of a vision statement: improved health and quality of life for all through optimal oral health.[22]

Recommendations specific to access were

- Public funding should be expanded to provide resources that would cover basic dental services for the long-term unemployed. To assure participation by providers and improve access, dentists should be reimbursed at market rates for their services. Administration should be managed using the same procedure and systems as employer-based dental prepayment plans.
- Subsidized in part by public funding, new programs should be developed in which individual employees could purchase insurance directly from risk pools if their employers do not provide it.
- Effective incentives should be offered to attract dentists to underserved areas. These incentives could include loan forgiveness, tax credits, and adequate reimbursement rates.
- The National Health Service Corps program should be expanded to help provide dental care in the underserved areas.
- A publicly funded or subsidized dental program should be developed for people who have disabilities, recognizing their special needs.
- Outreach programs at the state and local levels, which might include the establishment of specialty dental clinics, should be developed to meet the needs of patients unable to receive care in traditional dental offices.
- Deferred dental/medical saving accounts should be established in which the balances accrue over time and can be used by the elderly as needed during their retirement.

The Surgeon General's 2000 report, *Oral Health in America*, generated the *National Call to Action to Promote Oral Health: A Public-Private Partnership Under the Leadership of the Office of the Surgeon General* in 2003. It is an invitation to expand plans, activities, and programs designed to promote oral health and prevent disease, especially to reduce the health disparities that affect members of racial and ethnic groups, the economically disadvantaged, many who are geographically isolated, and others who are vulnerable because of special oral health care needs. This *National Call to*

Action to Promote Oral Health, referred to as the *"Call to Action,"* emphasized the necessity for partnership to address the oral health needs of these populations. Also following the Surgeon General's report was the updated *Healthy People 2010: Understanding and Improving Health.*[23] The section devoted to oral health has an overarching goal to "prevent and control oral and craniofacial diseases, conditions, and injuries and improve access to related services."[24]

As the nation's leading advocate for oral health, the ADA continues to build upon these existing proposals to advocate for and generate options to increase access to care. It seeks to ensure effective integration of the goals of the ADA and the profession with those of nationally accepted and established work plans.

PRIVATE SECTOR RESPONSE

In October 2004, the ADA identified five state and community models for improving access to dental care for the underserved.[25] Three state-specific and two community-level initiatives were selected as adaptable by others to improve access to care for specific populations. These models included Michigan's Healthy Kids Dental (HKD) Medicaid program, Tennessee's TennCare program, Alabama's *Smile Alabama!* initiative, a Connecticut Health Foundation effort, and a Head Start collaborative in Vermont.

In addition, a 2008 study funded by the California HealthCare Foundation ("Increasing Access to Dental Care in Medicaid: Does Raising Provider Rates Work?")[26] examined six states where the number of participating dentists and Medicaid patients rose significantly (Tennessee, Washington, South Carolina, Virginia, Alabama, and Michigan) to determine the effects of increased reimbursements and other factors on participation.

The California HealthCare Foundation confirmed that to improve dentists' participation in Medicaid, states must do three things:

- Improve the Medicaid fees
- Ease administrative burdens (to look more like the private sector)
- Involve state dental societies and individual dentists as active partners in improving the program.

Many Medicaid fees are well below what it costs the dentist to provide the care. In addition, applications to become a Medicaid provider and other paperwork requirements (such as claims submissions) often are quite different from the paperwork necessary to participate in private sector plans. All of these factors add to the cost of providing care and might result in errors that trigger costly reviews. They serve as disincentives for private practitioners to participate.

The Michigan Dental Association, the Michigan Department of Community Health, and Delta Dental of Michigan, Ohio, and Indiana joined together in 2000 and worked with Michigan's legislature and governor to develop and expand the HKD program. The program is a partnership between a state Medicaid program and a commercial dental plan, with the plan managing the dental benefit according to the standard procedure and payment mechanism it uses in its private plan. The HKD program is administered by Delta Dental of Michigan, dentists are paid usual Delta preferred provider organization fees, the child may select any participating dentist, the standard Delta claims administration is used, and there are no co-payments.[27] In other words, the program looks just like many of the private-sector plans accepted by dentists in the counties covered by the HKD program. A September 2008 study of the first 6 years of the HKD program found that there was a dramatic rise in the number of dentists participating. Before HKD, in 2000, fewer than 25% of the dentists participated in Medicaid within the counties that later were covered by the HKD program. Within 1 year of the introduction of HKD in 2002, participation rose to more than 80%, and by 2005, dental participation was more than 90% in the counties where it had been below 25% only 4 years earlier. As a consequence, the amount of time it took a Medicaid recipient to travel to the dentist's office was cut in half, equaling the travel time of patients covered by private sector Delta Dental plans. The HKD program was expanded to 61 of Michigan's 83 counties in July 2008.[27] This model demonstrates how contracting with a single commercial entity that (1) has a strong existing dental network, (2) offers competitive market-based reimbursement, (3) streamlines administration to mirror the private sector, and (4) makes participants indistinguishable from other patients based on an identification card or other identifier that reduces the stigma of a public program can substantially improve access to care for Medicaid beneficiaries.

In 2002, the legislature in Tennessee enacted a statutory carve-out of dental services, mandating a contract arrangement between the state and a private dental carrier to administer benefits for children under age 21 years. The state retained control of reimbursement rates and increased them to market-based levels. Between October 2002 and October 2006, the number of dentists participating in the TennCare dental program grew by 112% and in rural counties grew by 118%.[27] Three other states use a similar carve-out system. These examples illustrate how improving state Medicaid programs can improve access to care. Readers are referred to the ADA's *State and Community Models for Improving Access to Dental Care for the Underserved* to learn more about these and other models that have been developed to improve access. Experience has shown that increasing Medicaid reimbursement rates increases access to care significantly only if the rate is adjusted above two thirds of the average fees in an area.[12,28]

The ADA recognizes that adjustments in the dental workforce are necessary to address the oral health needs of underserved populations more effectively. To help bring about these improvements, the ADA has created and is promoting the development of a new member of the dental team—the Community Dental Health Coordinator (CDHC). The CDHC will enable the existing dental workforce to expand its reach into underserved communities.

CDHCs will be recruited from underserved dental areas and will reflect the cultural values of the communities they serve. They will be competent in developing and implementing community-based oral health prevention programs, providing individual preventive services, and performing temporization of cavitated lesions with material designed to stop caries from progressing until the patient can see a dentist. The CDHC can be employed by federally qualified health centers, the Indian Health Service (IHS), public health clinics, or private practices. These workers will be culturally competent and trained to assist individuals to navigate the dental care system, to understand the need for oral health care, and to surmount acquisition costs such as those associated with transportation and childcare. The American Dental Association Foundation has provided funding to support the development of the curriculum for the CDHC. In 2008 the ADA's House of Delegates earmarked up to $5 million dollars to continue the ADA's support for the CDHC pilot program and its evaluation.

The private sector understands it has an ethical and professional responsibility to provide care in the absence of an effective public health infrastructure and inadequate funding to support state Medicaid dental programs. Many state dental societies have joined forces with community partners to sponsor voluntary programs to deliver free or discounted oral health care to underserved children. According to the ADA's 2000

Survey of Current Issues in Dentistry,[29] approximately 7 in 10 (69.7%) dentists in private practice reported that their primary practice provided services free of charge or at a reduced rate to one or more population groups.

In light of the failure of government to provide adequate funding to support dental care through the Medicaid program and the continuing shrinkage of the dental public infrastructure, the private sector has responded by establishing and supporting meaningful volunteer programs to provide a modicum of access for underserved populations. Three examples described here are the Give Kids a Smile Program (GKAS), the American Indian/Alaska Native Volunteer Program, and the Donated Dental Services Program of the National Foundation of Dentistry for the Handicapped.

In 2003 the ADA launched what has become its signature access-to-care program for children, GKAS. The program annually reaches out to underserved communities, providing a day of free oral health services. GKAS helps educate the public and state and local policymakers about the importance of oral health care while providing needed and overdue care to large numbers of underserved children. On February 1, 2008, 1800 programs were held nationwide, with close to 500,000 children treated and 47,000 volunteers participating. The estimated value of care delivered on that day was $29.8 million.

In December 2006 the ADA Board of Trustees adopted a resolution to make GKAS "more than just a day" and to transform the initiative into a year-round effort to improve the oral health of underserved children. A National Advisory Board was established that includes representatives from industry, public health, and private practice. The Board has implemented an expanded fundraising program to provide financial and technical assistance to new and existing community-based local and regional GKAS programs, which will enable the ADA and others to advocate effectively for better access to oral health care for all children.

In 2006, the American Indian/Alaska Native Dental Placement Program was developed in response to oral health disparities experienced by American Indian/Alaska Native (AI/AN) populations and the workforce shortages at rural and frontier clinics that serve AI/AN people. The program is designed to match volunteer dentists and dental students with IHS and tribal clinics to increase access to oral health care and disease prevention services for AI/AN people; to reduce oral health disparities in AI/AN communities; to develop, pilot, and evaluate innovative, culturally responsive strategies to address the oral health needs of AI/AN communities; to support IHS efforts to fill vacant dental positions; and to create meaningful service opportunities for ADA member dentists.

The National Foundation of Dentistry for the Handicapped (NFDH), a charitable affiliate of the ADA, is committed to arranging comprehensive dental treatment and long-term preventive services to needy disabled, elderly, or medically compromised individuals through a collaborative national network of direct service programs that involve more than 12,900 volunteer dentists and 2700 volunteer laboratories.[30] The NFDH offers several distinct programs to increase access to care.

The Donated Dental Services program offers a collaborative, direct way for the dental profession to reach out to individuals who have special needs who cannot afford necessary treatment or who do not receive public aid. The Dental HouseCalls program was established to bring care to people who cannot travel easily to dental offices, including residents of nursing homes, homebound individuals, and developmentally disabled people attending day programs or living in residential centers. A fully equipped, portable dental office is transported in a van and set up at bedside or in the facilities so dentists can serve these individuals. Other programs include the Bridge Campaign of Concern and DentaCheques.

The private sector is committed to building and fostering collaborative activities to improve the oral health of all of America's children, and pediatric physicians are critical to this enterprise. At the same time, pediatricians and other physicians must complete educational programs specific to oral health to provide the best oral health guidance and care to their patients. In March 2008, the ADA Foundation awarded a 3-year $300,000 grant to the American Academy of Pediatrics to help improve the oral health of children in critical age groups, particularly children under the age of 3 years. The grant program provides up to $100,000 annually and will fund annual "train-the-trainer" oral health summits at which pediatricians will learn to conduct oral health risk assessments (including oral screening examinations), teach families about oral health and prevention, and refer children to a dental home. The grant also funds an oral health preceptorship program, which provides pediatricians in underserved areas with support to promote oral health for vulnerable children. Many states have implemented similar programs and have demonstrated outstanding results in reducing disease burden among at-risk children.

In November 2007 the ADA hosted the American Indian/Alaska Native Oral Health Access Summit.[31] A broad range of individuals and organizations was brought together to collaborate on a future vision and strategy to improve access to oral health treatment and prevention services for AI/AN people. The ADA served in a "convener" role that helped set a positive tone for the event. The participants included representatives from local tribal communities and health programs, the IHS, specialty and special-interest dental/health organizations, philanthropic organizations, state dental societies, and dental educators. At the conclusion of the summit, all participants agreed to work on activities with the following focus areas: (1) creating a new paradigm for improving the dental workforce; (2) developing collaborative strategies for lobbying, funding, and policy making, designing research, and implementing "best practices" for the prevention of oral disease, including early childhood caries; (3) fostering broader community involvement to identify oral health issues and their solutions; (4) advocating for a fully funded IHS/Tribal/Urban dental program; (5) building trust among the partners/communities of interest; and (6) encouraging meaningful tribal empowerment in oral health policy making. This summit meeting was the first of what is envisioned to be a series of efforts to build dynamic communities to improve access to care for underserved populations.

Oral health literacy is the degree to which individuals have the capacity to obtain, process, and understand basic health information and services needed to make appropriate oral health decisions. Nearly half (90 million) of adults in the United States have low functional health literacy. Low oral health literacy can affect any population group, regardless of age, race, education, or income level, and impacts an individual's ability to understand instructions on prescription drug bottles, appointment slips, educational brochures, and dentist's directions.

The ADA has established a National Oral Health Literacy Advisory Committee (NOHLAC), which is in the process of identifying the challenges and barriers to improving the nation's oral health literacy. The committee has developed focus areas to address these obstacles and has created a set of strategic goals to guide its work. The goals encompass oral health literacy in relation to dental education and practice, public awareness, research, policy development, and coalition building. Ultimately the NOHLAC will identify practical methods that can be employed by the entire dental team to minimize barriers related to limited oral health literacy.

Perhaps the most critical role the ADA plays in addressing access to care issues is serving as the nation's leading advocate for the public's oral health. The ADA and the larger dental community have worked to ensure that there is adequate funding to support the dental public health infrastructure and to support key oral health access programs within the Department of Health and Human Services (DHHS). The DHHS agencies that directly affect the oral health infrastructure include the Health Resources and Services Administration (HRSA), the Centers for Disease Control and Prevention (CDC), and the National Institute of Health's (NIH) National Institute of Dental and Craniofacial Research (NIDCR).

On an annual basis, through its advocacy efforts and in collaboration with other national dental organizations, the ADA advocates for adequate funding for HRSA's Health Professional Education and Training Programs, which play a critical role in the recruitment and retention of minority and disadvantaged students and faculty into dental schools and must be expanded to reduce oral health disparities. The ADA advocates for HRSA's Special Projects of Regional and National Significance programs through which state health departments have developed access-to-care programs targeting at-risk women and children. The Association also lobbies to support HRSA's Ryan White HIV/AIDS Dental Reimbursement Program, which increases access to oral health services for people living with HIV/AIDS and ensures that dental and dental hygiene students are trained to manage and treat patients living with HIV/AIDS. It is through these advocacy efforts that the HRSA Title VII program receives adequate funding. Title VII funds pediatric, general dentistry, and dental public health residency programs that are instrumental in training dentists to work in underserved communities and to treat populations with special health care needs. These programs are especially important, because they provide dentists with the competencies necessary to meet the needs of patients who fear dental treatment, young children, the elderly, and special-needs populations by teaching appropriate sedation and anesthesia techniques along with other skills.

The ADA advocates for increased appropriations that support HRSA's Bureau of Primary Health Care's intention to expand the number of federally qualified health centers (FQHCs) that provide dental services. As a foundational element for the dental safety net, FQHCs work diligently to address the oral health needs of the 35% of Americans who are unable to access care within the private sector. The ADA is collaborating with the National Network for Oral Health Access to encourage increased public–private partnering in support of the dental public health infrastructure.

The CDC Division of Oral Health (DOH) also benefits through the advocacy efforts and support of the ADA. The CDC's DOH supports state- and community-based programs focused on preventing oral disease, promoting oral health nationwide, and supporting applied research to enhance oral disease prevention in community settings. The CDC works with states to (1) establish oral health surveillance systems, (2) develop state oral health program infrastructure, capacity, and leadership, (3) implement, support, and monitor community water fluoridation projects, and (4) establish school-based sealant programs targeting the children at highest risk for oral disease and least likely to access care. Through the development, implementation, and evaluation of programs focused on the reduction of disease, the ADA believes there will be a concomitant reduction in treatment need and ultimately in demand for dental care.

Advocacy to ensure adequate funding for the NIDCR is a key component of the private sectors' response to the access-to-care challenges faced by the nation. The NIDCR is the only institute within the NIH that is committed to oral health research and training and remains the primary public agency that supports dental behavioral, biomedical, clinical, and translational research. The Centers for Research to Reduce Oral Health Disparities, supported through funds provided by the NIDCR, focuses on supporting community-based collaborative research on improving the oral health of populations at highest risk for oral disease.

NEXT STEPS

While remaining a leader in generating and advocating solutions to address the many issues surrounding access to care, the ADA can build upon existing proposals to ensure effective integration of the goals of the ADA and the profession with those of nationally accepted and established plans to improve the oral health of the nation. Prevention of oral disease is the bedrock upon which systems must be built to assure optimal oral health for all Americans. These systems will require a significant public policy adjustment that recognizes the need for greater investment in the public sector to address adequately what should be viewed as a societal problem.

The public and policy makers must understand that oral health is integral to sound overall health. Families must learn that a child's oral health is integral to his or her ability to grow, to thrive, to learn, to speak, and to be healthy in every sense of the word. How can the dental profession motivate parents? What are the messages that must be delivered? Who should deliver them? How can communities at highest risk be reached most effectively?

A comprehensive public prevention and awareness campaign targeting at-risk families is required. This type of campaign has been successful in the area of water fluoridation and is just beginning to bear fruit in educating the elderly about the importance of maintaining good oral health. This awareness campaign will require significant commitment, investment, and increased collaboration between the public and private sectors, which together make up the dental public health infrastructure. This campaign is not something that medicine or dentistry can address alone. Children and their families must be empowered to make healthy choices. Parents must be provided with interdisciplinary strategies to guide them in helping their children adopt healthy behaviors.

These efforts must be culturally and linguistically appropriate and cannot be accomplished within the confines of either a physician's or a dentist's office. Rather, they must come from the community and be directed back to the community.

History has demonstrated, time and again, that tragedies can be transformative and serve as tipping points for policy change. In response to the tragic death of a 12-year-old Maryland boy, Deamonte Driver, from a brain abscess attributed to untreated dental disease, the ADA elected to host a national Access to Dental Care Summit. In March 2009, the ADA convened representatives from various stakeholder groups that have a commitment and role in improving access to oral health care for the underserved to create a common vision for action. This meeting was simply the first of many next steps needed to address the access dilemma.

The time is ripe for the dental profession to move forward in partnership with other organizations and to develop new initiatives that all communities of interest can support. Making significant progress toward improving access to care for the underserved will take the commitment of a broad group of stakeholders, working together, to advance new initiatives. The 3-day summit provided another example of the private sector's willingness to convene, collaborate, and find common ground and shared solutions to problems facing the nation.

The goals for the summit included

- Creating a common vision for long-term improvement to access to oral health care
- Engaging in participatory problem solving in which the knowledge and perspectives of different sources of expertise and interests work together, so that all aspects of the challenges to improve oral health are addressed collaboratively

- Identifying and discussing new approaches and initiatives that all stakeholders can support to address oral health disparities and access for the underserved
- Developing a draft implementation plan for improving access to care.

A 12-member summit study design team, representing 12 stakeholder groups, planned the summit. A "Future Search" format was used during the summit. Future Search is a method that helps people transform their capability for action very quickly. The meeting is task-focused. Typically, the process brings people from various walks of life into the same conversation—those who have resources, expertise, formal authority, and need. Through focused activities, participants tell stories about their past, present, and desired future. Through dialogue, participants discover their common ground and then are able to make concrete action plans. The question developed by the planners to pose at the summit was "What are we going to do, in the short and long term, both individually and collectively, to assure optimal oral health through prevention and treatment for underserved people?" As we go to press, a report regarding the Access to Dental Care Summit is in development.

ACKNOWLEDGMENTS

The author acknowledges members of the Council on Access, Prevention and Interprofessional Relations, American Dental Association, 2008–2009 (Drs. Lindsey A. Robinson, Grass Valley, CA, chair; Mark A. Crabtree, Martinsville, VA, vice chair; Nolan W. Allen, Clearwater, FL; Greg L. Baber, Uvalde, TX; J. Jerald Boseman, Salt Lake City, UT; Daniel M. Briskie, Flint, MI; Gerald J. Ciebien, Riverside, IL; Gary S. Davis, Shippensburg, PA; Kevin T. Flaherty, Wausau, WI; Eleanor A. Gill, Olive Branch, MI; David R. Holwager, Cambridge City, IN; A. J. Homicz, New Castle, NH; Melanie S. Lang, Veradale, WA; Scott D. Lingle, St. Paul, MN; David J. Miller, East Meadow, NY; Lee P. Oneacre, Carrollton, TX; Leon E. Stanislav, Clarksville, TN; Jeffrey J. Stasch, Garden City, KS; and Sidney A. Whitman, Hamilton Square, NJ) thank ADA staff members Dr. Al Guay, Chief Policy Advisor; Dr. Lewis Lampiris, director, Council on Access, Prevention and Interprofessional Relations; Dr. Steve Geiermann, senior manager, Access Community Oral Health Infrastructure and Capacity; Ms. Lynne Mangan, manager, Health Promotion; and Mr. Thomas J. Spangler, Jr., Esq., director, Council on Government Affairs for their invaluable assistance with this article.

REFERENCES

1. U.S. Department of Health and Human Services. Oral health in America: a report of the surgeon general. National Institute of Dental and Craniofacial Reach, National Institutes of Health. Rockville (MD): U.S. Department of Health and Human Services; 2000. p. 81, 83, 89.
2. Mouradian WE, Wehr E, Crall JJ. Disparities in children's oral health and access to care. JAMA 2000;284(20):2625–31.
3. Guay AH. Access to dental care: the triad of essential factors in access-to-care programs. J Am Dent Assoc 2004;135:779–85.
4. Manski RJ, Edelstein BL, Moeller JF. The impact of dental coverage on children's dental visits and expenditures, 1996. J Am Dent Assoc 2001;132:1137–45.
5. National Health Interview Surveys. Available at: http://www.cdc.gov/nchs/nhis.htm.
6. Guay AH. Access to dental care: solving the problem for underserved populations. J Am Dent Assoc 2004;135:1599–605.

7. Garetto LP, Yoder KM. Basic oral health needs: a professional priority? J Dent Educ 2006;70(1):1166–9.
8. Smith RG, Lewis CW. Availability of dental appointments for young children in King County, Washington: implications for access to care. Pediatr Dent 2005; 27(3):207–11.
9. Manski RJ, Brown E. Dental use, expenses, dental coverage changes, 1996-2004. MEPS Chartbook, no. 17. Rockville (MD): Agency for Healthcare Quality and Research; 2007. p. 7.
10. Harrison RL, Li J, Pearce K, et al. The Community Dental Facilitator Project: reducing barriers to dental care. J Public Health Dent 2003;63(2):126–8.
11. Riportella-Muller R, Selby-Harrington ML, Richardson LA, et al. Barriers to the use of preventive health care services for children. Public Health Rep 1996;111(1): 71–7.
12. U.S. General Accounting Office. Factors contributing to low use of dental services by low income populations. Washington, DC: U.S. General Accounting Office; Sept 2000. GAO/HEHS-00–149.
13. Berk ML, Schur CL. The effect of fear on access to care among undocumented Latino immigrants. J Immigr Health 2001;3(3):151–6.
14. Strayer MS. Perceived barriers to oral health care among the homebound. Spec Care Dentist 1995;15(3):113–8.
15. Kujak HA, Reichmuth M. Barriers to and enablers of older adults use of dental services. J Dent Educ 2005;69(9):975–86.
16. Edelstein BL. Access to dental care for head start enrollees. J Public Health Dent 2000;60(3):221–3, 225.
17. Edmunds RK. Increasing access to care with diversity. J Dent Educ 2006;70(9): 918–20.
18. Tomar, Scott L. An assessment of the dental public health infrastructure in the U.S. J Public Health Dent 2006;66(1):5–16.
19. US Department of Health and Human Services, Health Resources and Services Administration, The Health Center Program. Uniform Data System; 2007.
20. Ramos-Rodreguez C, Schwartz MD, Rogers V, et al. Institutional barriers to providing oral health services for underserved populations in New York City. J Public Health Dent 2004;64(1):55–7.
21. American Dental Association. Constitution and bylaws, January 2007 and American Dental Association, Strategic Plan, 2007–10. Available at: http://www.ADA.org.
22. American Dental Association. Future of dentistry. Chicago: American Dental Association/Health Policy Resources Center; 2001.
23. Available at: http://wwwHealthypeople.gov/Document.
24. Available at: http://wwwHealthypeople.gov/Document/HTML/Volume2/21Oral.htm.
25. American Dental Association. State and community models for improving access to dental care for the underserved, executive summary. Chicago: American Dental Association; 2004.
26. Available at: www.nashp.org/Files/CHCF-dental-ratesd.pdf.
27. Available at: www.ada.org/prof/advocacy/test_070327_roth.pdf.
28. Naimar SMH, Tinanoff N. Effect of reimbursement rates on children's access to dental care. Pediatr Dent 1997;19(5):315–6.
29. American Dental Association, Survey Center. 2000 Survey of current issues in dentistry, charitable dental care. Chicago: American Dental Association; 2002.
30. Available at: http://nfdh.org/joomla_nfdh/content/view/121/171.
31. Available at: http://www.ada.org/prof/resources/topics/topics_accessalaska_summit.pdf.

Using Teledentistry to Improve Access to Dental Care for the Underserved

James Fricton, DDS, MS[a],*, Hong Chen, DDS, MS[b]

KEYWORDS

- Teledentistry • Craniofacial disorders • Access to care
- Temporomandibular disorder • Health disparities
- Underserved population • Information technology
- Telehealth • Telemedicine

Advances in dental care have documented that early diagnosis, preventive treatments, and early intervention can prevent or reduce the progress of most oral diseases, conditions that, when left untreated, can have painful, disfiguring, and lasting negative health consequences.[1] Unfortunately, millions of American children and adults lack regular access to routine dental care, and many of them suffer needlessly with disease that inevitably results in significant decrements in their quality of life. Problems in access to oral health care cut across economic, geographic, and ethnographic lines. Racial and ethnic minorities, people who have disabilities, and those from low-income families, particularly children, are especially hard hit. In most rural areas in this country, especially, there are many barriers to dental health care, including geographic remoteness, sparse population, adverse seasonal weather and road conditions, poor or no public transportation, poverty and lack of health insurance, a less mobile aging population, culturally specific health care needs of many groups (especially American Indian and immigrant populations); a low number of dentists relative to total population, and a scarcity of specialty and subspecialty dentists.

Teledentistry is an exciting new area of dentistry that uses electronic health records, telecommunications technology, digital imaging, and the Internet to link health care providers in rural or remote communities to enhance communication, the exchange of health information, and access to care for underserved patients. This article

[a] University of Minnesota School of Dentistry, 6-320 Moos Tower, 515 Delaware Street. SE, Minneapolis, MN 55455, USA
[b] School of Dentistry, University of North Carolina, Chapel Hill, NC, USA
* Corresponding author.
E-mail address: frict001@umn.edu (J. Fricton).

Dent Clin N Am 53 (2009) 537–548
doi:10.1016/j.cden.2009.03.005
0011-8532/09/$ – see front matter © 2009 Elsevier Inc. All rights reserved.

dental.theclinics.com

discusses how innovative health information and communication technologies can improve access to oral health care through teledentistry.

WHAT IS TELEDENTISTRY AND HOW DOES IT WORK?

Teledentistry uses electronic health records, telecommunications technology, digital imaging, and the Internet to provide teleconsultation with specialists, supervision of collaborative hygienists in remote areas, and education. Teleconsultation can take on two forms. Real-time consultation uses direct on-line computer video telecommunication between a dentist, hygienist, or patient in a remote community and a dentist or specialist in a larger community who provides support or supervision. In the "store and forward" method, electronic health records and videos store data that can be retrieved and reviewed by the specialist who renders an opinion (**Figs. 1** and **2**).

Telehealth projects, including telemedicine and teledentistry, have been implemented as models to improve education and access to care.[2–25] Telehealth has been used in various demonstration projects throughout the nation and has been shown to be particularly helpful in remote and rural areas where access to specialists is limited.[2–8] For example, Total Dental Access is the teledentistry project within the Department of Defense[2] that enables referring dentists from the US Armed Forces to consult with specialists at a medical center on the status of a patient. Total Dental Access focuses on three areas of dentistry: patient care, continuing education, and dentist–laboratory communications. This project has demonstrated increased patient access to dental care and the cost effectiveness of a Web-based system. The Children's Hospital Los Angeles Teledentistry Project, developed in association with the University of Southern California's Mobile Dental Clinic, increases and enhances the quality of oral health care provided to children living in remote rural areas of California, areas often severely underserved by dental health providers.[7] A 12-month trial of teledentistry was conducted in two general dental practices in remote sites in Scotland.[5] The dental practices had a personal computer (PC)-based videoconferencing link connected by an Integrated Services Digital Network (ISDN) at 128 kbit/s to a restorative specialist at a central hospital. Twenty-five patients were recruited into the trial. A cost-minimization analysis was undertaken by comparing the costs of teledentistry with two alternatives: outreach visits, in which the specialist regularly visited the remote communities, and hospital visits, where patients in remote communities traveled to hospital for consultation. The study found the cost savings of teledentistry were

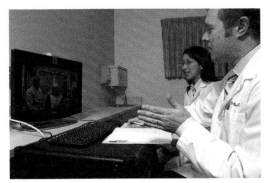

Fig. 1. Dentists and dental hygienist in remote areas can link to specialists in larger communities through teledentistry.

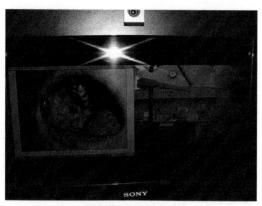

Fig. 2. Through teledentistry consultations and imaging, diagnosis of oral pathology and oral conditions in remote areas can be improved.

greatest in the remote communities, where patients otherwise would have had to travel long distances for specialist consultations.

For a typical teledentistry visit, special videoconference equipment and a video/Internet connection are set up at both the hub site and the remote site. The patient checks in at the remote clinic and before the consultation fills out questionnaires, either on paper or on line, regarding chief complaints and medical and dental history. The dentist or a member of the dental team (assistant or hygienist) at the remote clinic facilitates and records a hands-on examination (see **Fig. 2**). (This examination may take place either during the visit or earlier, when a teleconsultation is requested.) The questionnaire, examination, and any imaging or documents that are included in the dental record are transmitted to the hub (eg, to a university specialist) via the online electronic patient record system. With this information in hand and reviewed, the specialist starts a live consultation with the patient through videoconferencing (**Fig. 3**).

The live video-consultation is similar to a live in-person consultation (see **Fig. 1**). The dentist interviews the patient, asks questions, discusses the diagnosis and treatment, and educates the patient about the condition. In some situations, the dentists may ask the patient to open the mouth to determine function or measure the opening in front of the camera. In other cases, the dentist reviews the images and examination findings presented in the electronic record on a split screen with the teleconsultation and reviews this information with the patient. In all cases, patients need to feel connected to the dentist performing the consultation, as if the dentist were standing next to the patient.

A major challenge in a teledentistry visit is the collaboration between the hub site and the remote site. **Fig. 3** illustrates the process for communicating between the remote site and the specialist clinic site. Because the consultation is "remote" in nature, the dental teams at both sites must collaborate constantly for a smooth teledentistry process. The challenge begins with making the concurrent appointment at both sites, progresses through the collection of patient information and its transmittal to the specialist, facilitating the "remote" real-time examination, and ends with facilitating the plan for treatment and future care. Because the specialist cannot perform a hands-on examination, he/she must rely on the examination performed by the dental team at the remote site. Confidence and good working relationships between team members at both sites must be established. As in any other learning processes, appropriate training, practice, and patience are essential for a satisfactory result.

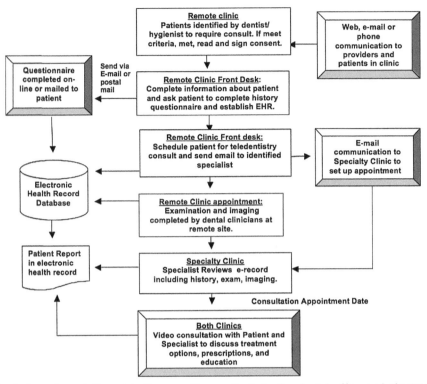

Fig. 3. Procedures followed in the recruiting patients in the dental office and obtaining consultation, illustrating the process for communicating between the remote site and the specialist clinic site.

With hands-on training and repeated practice, the dental teams at both sites can establish a reliable network for teledentistry.

THE UNIVERSITY OF MINNESOTA TELEDENTISTRY PROJECT

A teledentistry network has been established that links specialists at the University of Minnesota School of Dentistry to dentists and patients in remote rural areas where access to care is difficult. The network also increases training for dentists and dental students in the rural community in the management of orofacial disorders.[9] Minnesota traditionally has been a state with a high level of awareness regarding dental and health matters and ranks above the national average in access to health care. There are, however, special populations and several geographic areas in the state where the picture is not so bright and where barriers to quality dental care are many, including geographic remoteness and sparse population. Teledentistry has improved this situation by expanding the access of rural and underserved populations to care through electronic communication.

The teledentistry network was established in 2004 linking the University of Minnesota School of Dentistry specialists with dentists and patients in remote rural areas. The first demonstration site was implemented at the Hibbing Community College Dental Clinic. This clinic is located approximately 200 miles north of Minneapolis and is a joint venture with the Hibbing Community College. The patient population consists primarily of low-income families in St. Louis, Lake, Cook, and Carlton Counties. The clinic is staffed by dental students with supervision from faculty to provide clinical training in rural areas of Minnesota. In their junior and senior years, all dental students rotate through this clinic; at any given time, four to six students provide care to the patient population. This clinic provides care for patients who have medical assistance from states and Medicaid.

Currently, the teledentistry system provides consultations to the demonstration site for temporomandibular disorder, orofacial pain, and oral medicine. The preliminary testing and evaluation of the system revealed high levels of acceptance and satisfaction from both providers and patients. In more than 90% of the visits, specialists were satisfied with the teledentistry consultation. In 94% of the visits, providers were as confident about providing adequate diagnosis and treatment planning as in a face-to-face visit. In 83% of the cases, providers thought that patient assessment using teledentistry was as complete as in a regular visit.

One challenge in a teledentistry visit is the possible increased time needed to perform a consultation. In the majority of the visits (61%), providers reported using about the same amount of time as in a regular in-office visit, but in 33% of the visits providers thought that teledentistry visits were more time-consuming. This problem is encountered particularly when the providers are learning to use the system. With experience, skills improve, and work is performed more efficiently.

Patients expressed high levels of satisfaction with the teledentistry service. The greatest benefits that the teledentistry network offers patients are convenience and access to care. Since the program started, approximately 13 patients have made 24 teledentistry visits through the course of their care. The patient satisfaction study showed that, instead of driving 200 to 300 miles each way to the University for care, the average distance for visiting the teledentistry clinic is only 13 miles. On average, a teledentistry visit requires less than 2 hours, compared with 18 hours if the patient had to travel to Minneapolis for the visit (**Table 1**). Specialists who can treat orofacial disorders such as temporomandibular disorder, orofacial pain, and oral medicine rarely are found in local rural communities. These disorders usually are chronic conditions that require repetitive visits and ongoing care. Many patients commented on the teledentistry service as being "convenient," "effective," "saving on travel time," requiring "less time out of [the patient's]schedule," and being "easier to reach."

In addition to providing greater convenience in accessing care, teledentistry also effectively meets patients' goals in seeking care. The average rating of teledentistry in meeting a patient's goal for a visit is 9.1 (with 10 being the best possible). The patients' overall satisfaction that the teledentistry clinic met their current health care needs was rated as 6.84 on average (with 1 = not satisfied at all and 7 = completely satisfied). When considering their experience with teledentistry visits, most patients

Table 1		
Comparison between teledentistry visits and regular office visits		
Distance Traveled and Time Spent by Patient	Teledentistry Clinic	University of Minnesota School of Dentistry Specialty Clinic
Travel distance to clinic (average, one-way, in miles)	12.6	230.3
Time missing from work/school (average, in hours)	1.6	18.3

felt comfortable in visiting the doctor through the videoconference service. In fact, many patients felt that the teledentistry visit was "the same as in an office or in person," except that it was "just through the TV." When patients were asked if they would prefer to see the doctor in person, half of the participants said "no" because they perceived no need for doing so. Some patients felt that seeing the doctor in person "would always be the best" but "this [teledentistry] works well, too."

Many patients who used the teledentistry service expressed their appreciation for and satisfaction with the program. Patients commented that teledentistry is a "wonderful service to provide to patients of rural areas … to give the knowledge and expert advice of the specialists via teledentistry is such a convenience"; "thank you for giving us big city help in a rural area"; "I feel that many people would benefit from this kind of dentistry if it was available"; "I love this system. It has made getting care easier and more convenient." As a result, all participants said they would use the teledentistry service again. Some patients recommended the service to their relatives and friends.

AREAS IN WHICH TELEDENTISTRY HAS BEEN HELPFUL IN IMPROVING ACCESS TO CARE

Several areas in dentistry that are particularly appropriate for teledentistry are remote consultations for orofacial disorders, collaborative hygienists' visits in remote areas, and continuing education. Future uses of teledentistry in medicine, such as clinical decision support, consumer home use, medication e-prescribing, and simulation training, will expand as the technology and applications for dentists increase.[15-25]

Remote Consultations for Care for Orofacial Disorders

Orofacial disorders include oral cancer, temporomandibular disorders, oral mucosal disease, salivary gland disorders, orofacial pain disorders, oral neurosensory disturbances, orofacial dystonias and dyskinesias, bruxism, burning mouth, dental sleep disorders, malodor, and dental phobias. With a collective prevalence of more than 40% of the population (**Table 2**),[26-30] the need for treatment of temporomandibular disorders alone is comparable to back pain, dental caries, and periodontal disease.[27] In addition, because orofacial structures have close associations with that functions of eating, communication, sight, and hearing, as well as affecting appearance, self-esteem and expression, persistent pain of orofacial origin can adversely affect an individual's overall quality of life.[3]

Most general dentists and dental specialists feel inadequately trained to recognize and manage these problems, for several reasons, including inadequate clinical and didactic training in dental school, lack of knowledge about appropriate medical billing procedures and codes, and the different office protocols that require more time. The complexity and difficulty of managing orofacial disorders usually results in a consultation with or referral to a specialist. Teledentistry can bring the specialist in orofacial pain or oral medicine to the rural dentist or dental hygienist through remote teleconsultations. These common conditions require intense patient care and can be reimbursed by medical insurance.

If the recognition and treatment of the orofacial disorders are inadequate or inappropriate, the personal impact can be tragic, and the costs are great. Numerous studies have shown that patients who have chronic orofacial pain disorders do not receive adequate early care. When chronic pain persists, it can become entrenched in the patient's life with the development of dependent relationships, emotional disturbances, disability, and many behavioral and psychosocial problems. These disorders present a frustrating medical and dental picture with patients undergoing costly

Table 2
Common medical-dental problems that require consultation, billing with medical fees and insurance, and special treatment needs

Orofacial Disorders	Need for Treatment (%)	Treatment
Temporomandibular disorders	5–7	Splints, physical therapy, behavioral, pharmacologic, surgical
Orofacial pain disorders (neuropathic/vascular, atypical, and others)	2–3	Pharmacologic, behavioral, surgical
Benign masticatory headache	15–20	Splints, physical therapy, behavioral, pharmacologic
Sleep apnea and snoring	5	Oral and nasal appliances, surgery
Neurosensory disorders (taste and chemosensory, orofacial paresthesias)	0.1	Pharmacologic and behavioral
Orofacial dystonias/ dyskinesias	0.1	Splints, physical therapy, behavioral, pharmacologic
Bruxism and oral habits	10+	Behavioral and pharmacologic
Dental phobia/anxiety	2–5	Behavioral and pharmacologic
Oral lesion (herpes, aphthous, pre-cancer)	3–5	Biopsy and surgery
Oral mucosal disease (eg, lichen planus, *Candida*)	5–8	Biopsy, pharmacologic, and behavioral
Xerostomia and salivary gland disorders	8–10	Pharmacologic and behavioral
Burning mouth and tongue	0.5	Pharmacologic and behavioral
Malodor	5–8	Behavioral and pharmacologic
Medically compromised patients	10–15	Considerations during dental treatment

treatments, diagnostic tests, long-term medications, and an ongoing dependency on the health care system.[30] Furthermore, dissemination of scientific knowledge about these disorders to the clinical community is poor, and the need for clinical consultations is high. More effort also must be spent in clinical training to ensure these patients receive access to high-quality care. Access to care for these problems should be expanded in the community and particularly in rural and underserved areas. Teledentistry allows these patients to see a specialist in a city or university without driving for hours to the appointment.

Teledentistry and Support of Collaborative Dental Hygienists

Teledentistry also can increase access to preventive and diagnostic care for patients in remote and underserved areas by supporting community-based collaborative hygienists. Hygienists already are well trained to be frontline oral health practitioners in new models of delivery of dental care. They are optimally skilled in patient education, prevention, assessment, and triaging care as members of a collaborative oral health team. Dental hygienists in remote and underserved areas can provide local cost-effective access to dental evaluations, preventive care, and education while being supported through teledentistry by dentists and dental specialists in a nearby community. This technology allows regular communication, support, and supervision, as well as facilitating teleconsultations for orofacial disorders and referrals for restorative, periodontal, oral surgery, and other dental care.

For the patient located in an underserved or remote area, hygienists supported by teledentistry can provide more accessible and less expensive preventive dental care and education. For a dental hygienist located in a remote or underserved area, teledentistry can provide direct support and supervision by a dentist in a nearby community or by specialists to facilitate evaluation, establishing diagnoses, and recommending treatment options and/or referral to appropriate care providers. For the dentist in the nearby community, teledentistry provides an opportunity to provide care to a patient who otherwise probably would not seek care. Teledentistry enables the specialist located many miles away at a university or specialty practice to make a diagnosis, recommend treatment options, and provide prescriptions and instructions about self-care.

Teledentistry and Dental Education

The teledentistry system also can provide a unique way to deliver long-distance clinical training and continuing education. Videoconferencing and Internet technologies allow low-cost, real-time interactive, two-way communication between instructors and trainees, making long-distance education more virtual and affordable. The videoconferencing system can be used both to train dentists and dental students at remote sites in conducting clinical examinations and to train dental assistants and other clinical support staff in clinic management issues (eg, scheduling, billing, and handling insurance issues). Through the videoconferencing system, professors of dentistry can collaborate with colleagues at other universities to exchange experiences with teledentistry systems. The responses from the participants are very positive. Teledentistry is more like a telephone service that has low technical requirements at the user end. The system provides easier and clearer communication than telephones because the users at both ends can communicate face-to-face.

The teledentistry videoconferencing system can be used to help train dentists, dental students, assistants, and other office support staff at remote sites in the clinical management of orofacial disorders and other conditions. Upon seeing a patient who has a complex orofacial disorder, the dentists can be trained to review the patient's history of illness, medical and dental history, and diagnostic studies, such as digital photographs or radiographs, to perform a disease-specific clinical examination, and then to consult with the specialist via teleconferencing on the diagnosis and the best course of management and treatment. The dentists or dental student then implements the treatment plan under the guidance of the specialist at the university. The advantages of using teledentistry by dentists and dental students in a rural community and of involving dental residents at the university are the improved access to specialists for clinical training, confirming diagnosis, and formulating a treatment plan; the reduced cost of oral health maintenance through shared resources; the reduced isolation of practitioners through contact with peers and specialists; and the improved quality of care.

Teledentistry also can provide multipoint interactive continuing education courses, multicenter treatment planning conferences, and inter-residency case reviews with community dentists at remote sites. As the project grows, teledentistry can provide long-distance "hands-on" training to local therapists at remote sites through the teledentistry videoconferencing network. Teledentistry provides practitioners with links to virtual dental health clinics and the growing network of providers who subscribe to a specific Web record service. In a time of increasing consolidation throughout the health care system, this ability could create an entire new view of dentistry. Multiple providers could create virtual care groups to provide expanded clinical training and could coordinate both care and also contracts for the delivery of services. This network of providers could coordinate the care of a single patient electronically, sharing a complete multimedia chart and all the documentation therein. Teledentistry also can facilitate patient education about self-care for the problem, allow e-mail follow-up on the status of the problem, and improve doctor–patient communication.

THE USE OF ELECTRONIC RECORDS FACILITATES TELEDENTISTRY

The evolution of electronic patient records has made teledentistry an immediate reality. Because an increasing number of dental care providers can access the Internet, traditional barriers to exchanging information have been reduced. Web-based records also make cumulative, longitudinal patient records possible. Well-tested security mechanisms have ensured the integrity and confidentiality of patient information. Because Web-based systems are simple to install and configure, the cost of operating them is less. Many dental schools are adapting these technologies to expand the services offered. This component configuration at the site for teledentistry should allow a practitioner to create a multimedia electronic health record that includes intraoral and exterior images, copies of handwritten paper-based patient records, charts, and diagrams, and virtually any other type of relevant patient data. New software that can compile all this information into a single electronic patient chart, encrypt the chart for security, and transfer the chart via the Internet is part of this record. This system streamlines the process of gathering and securing data, as well as communicating it via the Internet.

TELEHEALTH EQUIPMENT AND TRANSMISSION MODES

The technology for performing video consultations and telecommunication continues to improve. For example, the Sony PCS TL-50, Polycom VC2, and Tandberg systems are for higher-quality and routine commercial use. In addition, the use of PC-based videoconferencing systems such as iChat, Skype, Windows Live Messenger, and AOL Instant Messenger provide lower-cost solutions that communicate through broadband networks. Desktop conferencing is often referred to as "PC-based video-conferencing" or sometimes even "video chatting." The average desktop conferencing system consists of the individual person's desktop or laptop computer, a separate monitor if needed or available, a microphone, headset or external speakers, a software application that is capable of coding and decoding audio and video (codec), and a Webcam. Although the quality of the picture and transmission can be lower, a desktop conferencing system typically costs significantly less than the standard room-based system, so it can be available for many dentists to use. It has some limitations, however. The most notable limitation is that, because it is based on a desktop (or similar environment), the number of users who can participate from any one end point is limited by space, the camera view, the single headset, and the surrounding environment. Normally no more than two or three people can use a desktop conferencing system, even if external speakers are used. A single patient and a dentist or hygienist should be able to participate with acceptable quality.

Teledentistry networks require encrypted transmission but can use a standard broadband Internet connection or specialized digital networks. Most networks are designed to be cost effective, to have high reliability, and are based on open architecture to allow connections between any network members as well as connections with non-network sites that use standards such as h.320 (via ISDN) or h.323 Internet Protocol (IP) standards. All teledentistry efforts need to provide sufficient security to meet Health Insurance Portability and Accountability Act (HIPAA), state, and member institution requirements. All teledentistry communications equipment should be based on h.323 IP standards for broadband residential service where available and secure.

HEALTH INSURANCE PORTABILITY AND ACCOUNTABILITY ACT AND SYSTEM SECURITY WITH TELEDENTISTRY

All members of a health care team and the teledentistry network are considered covered entities under HIPAA privacy regulations that became effective April 14, 2003. A clinic's computing hosting and facilities are considered confidential electronic patient records. A state-of-the-art computing facility is a requisite requirement for housing the databases of electronic dental records and teledentistry. The privacy, confidentiality, security, and secure back-up of data must meet HIPAA requirements and federal standards for system security. Both plans consider the storage and retrieval of patient demographic, medical history, examination, diagnosis, treatment information, and specimen storage information.

In most systems, dental records to be stored into an electronic database first must pass through several filters to get into the system. These filters provide security through firewalls and also screen data for completeness, consistency, and any irregularity. A number of methods are used to prevent unauthorized entry into the database: router filtering, user name and password protection, encryption of transferred data, internal versus external protocols, and a restricted secure file transfer protocol (SFTP). A system must serve as the initial Certificate Authority for the members of the network. Digital certificates contain a participant's identification, valid time period, public key, and other cryptographic information including the digital signature of the participant. Certificates are used to prevent hackers from entering the network by pretending to be one of the participants and must be changed periodically. The Certificates also serve to verify that the participants are authentic. The intranet system for each clinic staff uses Certificates including user log-in screens with a unique user identification and password. Once inside the intranet system, a Transaction Layer Security (TLS) or Secure Socket Layer (SSL) connection is established between each clinic and the host server to prevent outside hacking of the system. The use of digital certificates in TLS prevents eavesdroppers from monitoring data transfers. These common functions are standard in both Java and Microsoft environments. Passwords that are generated for participants are maintained as encrypted text in the database tables. Public or clinic system administrators do not have access to the security password tables. The passwords are decrypted in real time using an RD5 algorithm. Server authentication also uses the Microsoft/Microsoft Transaction Server security system, with access available via secure backdoor ports such as SFTP and direct Web scripting technologies.

SUMMARY

Teledentistry is a new area of dentistry that integrates electronic health records, telecommunications technology, digital imaging, and the Internet to improve access to care for patients in remote settings. Through collaborative hygienists in remote areas, patients have improved access to preventive dental care. Through teleconsultation with specialists in larger communities, a dentist in a nearby community can provide access to specialty care for their patients more easily. Teledentistry allows the specialist located many miles away to make a diagnosis and recommend treatment options and/or referral for patients who otherwise would find it difficult to see them. Future advances in technology will enable teledentistry to be used in many more ways, including advances seen in medicine such as clinical decision support, quality and safety assessment, consumer home use, medication e-prescribing, and simulation training.

REFERENCES

1. American Dental Association. State and community models for improving access to dental care for the underserved—A White Paper. Chicago: American Dental Association; 2004.
2. Rocca MA, Kudryk VL, Pajak JC, et al. The evolution of a teledentistry system within the Department of Defense. Proc AMIA Symp 1999;1:921–4.
3. American Academy of Orofacial Pain. Application to the American Dental Association for Specialty status. Mount Royal (NJ): American Academy of Orofacial Pain; 1998.
4. Chen JW, Hobdell MH, Dunn K, et al. Teledentistry and its use in dental education. J Am Dent Assoc 2003;134(3):342–6.
5. Scuffham PA, Steed M. An economic evaluation of the Highlands and Islands teledentistry project. J Telemed Telecare 2002;8(3):165–77.
6. Cook J, Edwards J, Mullings C, et al. Dentists' opinions of an online orthodontic advice service. J Telemed Telecare 2001;7(6):334–7.
7. Birnbach JM. The future of teledentistry. J Calif Dent Assoc 2000;28(2):141–3.
8. Bauer JC, Brown WT. The digital transformation of oral health care. Teledentistry and electronic commerce. J Am Dent Assoc 2001;132(2):204–9.
9. Chen H, Fricton J. Teledentistry: seeing the doctor from a distance. Northwest Dent 2007;86(2):27–68.
10. Schleyer TK, Dasari VR. Computer-based oral health records on the World Wide Web. Quintessence Int 1999;30(7):451–60.
11. Stephens CD, Cook J. Attitudes of UK consultants to teledentistry as a means of providing orthodontic advice to dental practitioners and their patients. J Orthod 2002;29(2):137–42.
12. Chang SW, Plotkin DR, Mulligan R, et al. Teledentistry in rural California: a USC initiative. J Calif Dent Assoc 2003;31(8):601–8.
13. Balas EA, Austin SM, Mitchell JA, et al. The clinical value of computerized information services. A review of 98 randomized clinical trials. Arch Fam Med 1996; 5(5):271–8.
14. Balas EA, Jaffrey F, Kuperman GJ, et al. Electronic communication with patients. Evaluation of distance medicine technology. JAMA 1997;278(2):152–9.
15. Bates DW, Cohen M, Leape LL, et al. Reducing the frequency of errors in medicine using information technology. J Am Med Inform Assoc 2001;8(4):299–308.
16. Bates DW, Gawande AA. Improving safety with information technology. N Engl J Med 2003;348(25):2526–34.
17. Bates DW, Teich JM, Lee J, et al. The impact of computerized physician order entry on medication error prevention. J Am Med Inform Assoc 1999;6(4):313–21.

18. Bellazzi R, Riva A, Montani S, et al. A Web-based system for diabetes management: the technical and clinical infrastructure. Proc AMIA Symp 1998;1:972.
19. Friedman CP, Elstein AS, Wolf FM, et al. Enhancement of clinicians' diagnostic reasoning by computer-based consultation: a multisite study of 2 systems. JAMA 1999;282(19):1851–6.
20. Hunt DL, Haynes RB, Hanna SE, et al. Effects of computer-based clinical decision support systems on physician performance and patient outcomes: a systematic review. JAMA 1998;280(15):1339–46.
21. Institute of Medicine. The computer-based patient record: an essential technology for health care. In: Dick RB, Steen EB, editors. Washington, DC: National Academy Press; 1991.
22. Johnston ME, Langton KB, Haynes RB, et al. Effects of computer-based clinical decision support systems on clinician performance and patient outcome. A critical appraisal of research. Ann Intern Med 1994;120(2):135–42.
23. McDonald CJ. Protocol-based computer reminders, the quality of care and the non-perfectability of man. N Engl J Med 1976;295(24):1351–5.
24. Schiff GD, Rucker TD. Computerized prescribing: building the electronic infrastructure for better medication usage. JAMA 1998;279(13):1024–9.
25. Whitlock WL, Brown A, Moore K, et al. Telemedicine improved diabetic management. Mil Med 2000;165(8):579–84.
26. Schiffman EL, Fricton JR, Haley DP, et al. The prevalence and treatment needs of subjects with temporomandibular disorders. J Am Dent Assoc 1990;120(3): 295–303.
27. Fricton JR. Recent advances in temporomandibular disorders and orofacial pain [see comments] [Review]. J Am Dent Assoc 1991;122(11):24–32.
28. Gordon M, Newbrun E. Comparison of trends in the prevalence of caries and restorations in young adult populations of several countries. Community Dent Oral Epidemiol 1986;14:104–9.
29. World Health Organization. Epidemiology, etiology and prevention of periodontal diseases: report of WHO scientific group. In: WHO Technical Report Series 621. Geneva (Switzerland): World Health Organization; 1978.
30. Locker D, Grushka M. The impact of dental and facial pain. J Dent Res 1987; 66(9):1414–7.

Social Work in Dentistry: The CARES Model for Improving Patient Retention and Access to Care

Joan M. Doris, DSW[a,b,c,]*, Elaine Davis, PhD[d],
Cynthia Du Pont, MSW[e], Britt Holdaway, MSW[e]

KEYWORDS

- Access to care • Underserved populations
- Social work in dentistry

In recent years, disparities in oral health care and difficulties in accessing oral health care have been the object of increasing public concern. Many Americans lack dental insurance, an increasing number of dentists in private practice refuse to accept Medicaid, and the escalating costs of dental care put even routine care outside the reach of a growing number of people. Although the cost of dental care provided by dental schools is typically far less than that of the same services provided by private dentists, financial concerns and difficulties with transportation, dental anxiety, mental health issues, physical health problems, and disabilities still make it difficult for many patients to complete needed dental treatment. CARES, the Counseling, Advocacy, Referral Education and Service program at the University of Buffalo School of Dental Medicine (SDM), was created to help patients overcome these difficulties, so they can receive much needed treatment. While there is no such thing as a "typical" dental patient, the following patients who were referred to the CARES program are representative of many patients treated at the University at Buffalo SDM and at other dental schools around the country.

[a] Department of Pediatric and Community Dentistry, School of Dental Medicine, University at Buffalo, 114 Squire Hall, Buffalo, NY 14214, USA
[b] School of Social Work, University at Buffalo, 114 Squire Hall, Buffalo, NY 14214, USA
[c] CARES Program, University at Buffalo, 114 Squire Hall, Buffalo, NY 14214, USA
[d] Department of Oral Diagnostic Sciences, University at Buffalo, School of Dental Medicine, 315 Squire Hall, Buffalo, NY 14214, USA
[e] CARES Program, University at Buffalo, School of Dental Medicine, 260H Squire Hall, Buffalo, NY 14214, USA
* Corresponding author. Department of Pediatric and Community Dentistry, School of Dental Medicine, University at Buffalo, 114 Squire Hall, Buffalo, NY 14214.
E-mail address: jdoris@buffalo.edu (J.M. Doris).

Dent Clin N Am 53 (2009) 549–559
doi:10.1016/j.cden.2009.03.003
0011-8532/09/$ – see front matter © 2009 Published by Elsevier Inc.

dental.theclinics.com

- Mrs. K is a veteran who is in need of extractions and dentures, and does not have the ability to pay for dental treatment. She was not eligible for treatment at the VA hospital, because her dental problems are not related to injuries sustained during her military service.
- Mrs. R is in her 50s and is disabled by a number of health conditions, including lupus, fibromyalgia, high blood pressure, hyperthyroidism, gastrointestinal problems, anxiety, and major depressive disorder. Her husband, also in his 50s, is retired. They have one adult child, who has pervasive developmental disabilities. Because of their limited income and the high cost of their other medical bills, Mrs. R has been unable to afford dental care.
- Mrs. T is 85 years of age, widowed, and suffering from angina, dementia, diabetes, arthritis, hypertension, and the sequelae of a stroke. She subsists on Social Security, which pays her $760 per month, an amount that barely covers living expenses, let alone the dental treatment she needs.

According to a 1998 survey conducted by the American Dental Association (ADA), individuals with low incomes were the most frequently reported special population receiving care at dental school clinics in the United States, followed by individuals with mental, medical, or physical disabilities. In fact, the majority of patients treated at dental school clinics came from households whose annual income was estimated to be $15,000 or less. As might be expected, many of these patients were uninsured or underinsured, 50% were covered by Medicaid or Medicare, and an additional 32% had no private dental insurance.[1]

As Haden and colleagues observe, "as providers of care, academic dental institutions are a safety net for the underserved, centers of pioneering tertiary care, and contributors to the well being of their patients through accessible oral health care services."[2] Unfortunately, the various components of this mission may be compromised when patients struggling with the difficulties presented by poverty or disability fail to comply with treatment plans or miss appointments, causing students to lose precious clinic hours. In the University at Buffalo SDM, a creative and successful solution was found to address the problem of achieving both the education and service aspects of its mission, with the creation of the CARES program.

The above considerations indicate that, in providing treatment in a dental school clinic, students, faculty, and staff are forced to deal with problems that are not limited to oral health, but rather, are psychosocial in nature. In short, dentists treat not teeth, but people. Because social workers are trained not only to deal with intrapsychic problems but also problems within social systems, they are uniquely qualified to assist patients dealing with complex psychosocial issues and to help both patients and providers navigate the complex health care and social service systems. It is this observation that inspired the development of the CARES program at the University at Buffalo SDM, which employs a social work approach to deal with issues of access to care and patient retention.

ORIGINS OF THE CARES PROGRAM

In 1999, the Dean of the University at Buffalo SDM, Louis Goldberg, DDS, PhD, and the Dean of the School of Social Work at UB, Laurence Schulman, DSW, had a conversation about the difficulty of patient retention and the barriers to care experienced by patients in the University at Buffalo SDM clinics. As Goldberg recalled, "We have social work problems, you have a school of Social Work, let's do something together."[3] This conversation became the genesis of the CARES program, an innovative collaborative effort between the two schools to address issues of access to dental care. The objective of the program was to address financial, psychological, and social needs, which create barriers to dental care. Although other, similar programs have been created in dental schools in the past, the CARES program, with a current staff of three full-time social workers and one part-time, grant-funded social worker, is one of the largest, and to our knowledge, longest running programs of it kind.

Initial funding was provided by a grant from the Community Foundation for Greater Buffalo in 2000. Some of this funding was used to conduct a needs assessment designed in part to answer the question, "Are there significant health and social concerns within the dental clinic population that indicate the need for high-risk screening and social work services?"[4] Nine hundred twenty-eight dental patients were surveyed, and results indicated that health (32%), finances (25%), medical bills, (16%) and family issues (14%) were the primary concerns identified by clinic patients. Approximately 42% of the respondents were living below the poverty level. In-depth interviews were then conducted with 157 survey respondents, and the information they provided as well as the data from the survey were used to develop the CARES program.[5]

In the fall of 2001, the program opened its doors. Funds from the community foundation grant were used to hire a part-time master's-level social worker (MSW) to work with patients seen in the dental clinic and to supervise two MSW student interns who were assigned to the CARES program for their field placement. In its first year, 27 patients were referred to the CARES program.[5]

GROWTH OF THE PROGRAM

During the second year of operation, the program expanded its initial focus on underserved older adults to include children, low-income patients, patients without insurance, and patients with complex health or mental health problems. In addition, the social worker began working with the dentists and the physical therapist in the Orofacial Pain Clinic and Temporomandibular Disorders Clinic at the University at Buffalo SDM to provide psychosocial treatment for patients experiencing temporomandibular joint disorders (TMD). Social work interventions in the clinic include progressive muscle relaxation, guided imagery, deep-breathing exercises, social skills training for anxiety and depression, and pain management skills. Finally, outreach was conducted in local senior centers to educate seniors about oral health, services offered in the University at Buffalo SDM, and how CARES staff could assist them in obtaining dental care.[5]

During this second year, the University at Buffalo SDM, assumed financial responsibility for the CARES program, which it has supported ever since. In its third year, the school increased program support to provide a full-time social worker, and by its fifth year of operations, the CARES program employed two full time master's level social workers. In 2007, a doctoral level social worker was hired as Research Director for the program; this faculty appointment is funded jointly by the Department of Pediatric and Community Dentistry in the SDM and the School of Social Work. In 2008, funding was obtained through the Dental Trade Alliance Foundation to hire a part-time social worker for the pediatric clinic at the SDM. Each year the program has also served as the field placement site for four to seven MSW students. These students, under the supervision of CARES social work staff, work with their own caseload of CARES patients, enabling more clients to receive social work services. This growth in CARES staff has been spurred by a continuous increase in the number of clients referred. Each year CARES has reached more clients in need of services from 200 in 2002, the second year of operations, to approximately 800 in 2007 (**Fig. 1**) (CARES annual report, unpublished data, 2007).

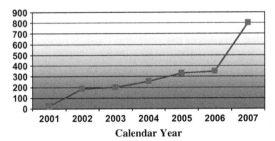

Fig. 1. Increase in new patient referrals.

The mission of the CARES program is to improve oral health by decreasing barriers to care and improving access to dental treatment for special needs and difficult-to-reach patients. As such, CARES not only addresses the needs of patients in the dental clinic, but also fills a need of the school and its students. By helping patients to access treatment at the dental school, CARES social workers provide important clinic hours for students and help the clinic to generate income for the school. CARES staff also educate students about psychosocial issues that affect a patient's ability to access care and teach dental students important skills in dentist–patient communication.

As stated above, the mission of a dental school is threefold: to educate dental professionals, to expand the knowledge base of the profession through basic and applied research, and to provide service to the community. This mission is paralleled by the roles of a social worker within a dental school as described by Levy: (1) education and training of dental professionals to improve their interactions with patients, (2) provision of social work clinical services to dental patients, and (3) research that can add to the body of knowledge on patient behaviors relevant to dental treatment.[6]

From the beginning, the leadership in the SDM recognized that the CARES program served not only the needs of the patients, but also the institution. As a result, support for the program from the leadership in the SDM has remained strong despite the vicissitudes of state funding. This support at the top echelons of leadership in the SDM has been a significant factor in the success and longevity of the program. Without the financial commitment of the Dean's office, it is doubtful that the program would have been able to continue to grow as it has.

CARES SERVICES

Typically, a dental student who is responsible for providing dental care refers a patient to the CARES program, although patients are referred through a variety of sources, including, word of mouth, community outreach events, and other social service providers. Once a patient is referred to CARES, a master's level social worker or MSW student intern will conduct a psychosocial assessment, exploring issues such as health, mental health, personal finances, transportation, and family concerns. Although the majority of referrals are made for financial reasons (ie, a patient is struggling to pay for needed dental care), difficulties in these other areas can present barriers to care, and these are often uncovered only after a thorough social work assessment. After identifying the barriers to dental care, social workers intervene to overcome the socioeconomic barriers and enable the patient to complete dental treatment.

Financial Problems

Financial concerns are responsible for an increasing number of CARES referrals. Approximately 90% of the referrals in 2007 were for financial reasons compared with only 57% in 2005. This may be in part because of a worsening economy as well as a shrinking social service net (CARES annual report, unpublished data, 2005 and 2007).

Interventions that have been used to help patients deal with financial barriers to care include:

- Donated Dental Services—a program in which the SDM donates $30,000 of dental treatment each year
- Medicaid Application—CARES social workers assess patient income and eligibility; Medicaid applications are available and social workers provide assistance in completing and returning applications
- Community Resources—Financial assistance is available through a variety of community resources, including: heating assistance (HEAP), prescription assistance, grant opportunities, and programs such as food stamps and WIC. CARES social workers link patients with appropriate resources and assist with applications when necessary. Although none of these resources are targeted toward provision of dental treatment, receiving assistance toward food or heat may free up resources to pay for dental treatment.
- CARES Fundraisers and Donations—A limited amount of money is available for dental treatment through fundraising efforts such as raffles and through donations made directly to the program

Transportation

Patients who do not drive or cannot afford a car often experience difficulty with transportation, which contributes to missed appointments. CARES social workers link patients with community van services for seniors and individuals with disabilities (available in nearly every community in Western New York to enable them to attend appointments). CARES also provides bus and metro schedules and, in the rare instance in which a patient has been treated at the SDM and has no transportation to return home, CARES has provided emergency cab fare for the patient.

Mental Health Problems

Although mental health issues are the primary reason for referral for only about 10% of CARES patients, a significantly larger percentage of CARES patients suffer from mental health problems including: depression, anxiety, obsessive–compulsive disorder, schizophrenia, substance abuse, and suicidal ideation. CARES social workers intervene by:

- Educating dental providers and acting as a liaison and educator between the dental provider and the patient
- Offering reminders of upcoming dental appointments
- Providing linkage and referral to community mental health agencies, support groups, and individual counseling
- Providing coverage in the SDM in the rare event of a mental health emergency, or to de-escalate crisis situations with patients suffering from mental illness

- Providing psycho-education regarding relaxation techniques or other coping skills
- Offering counseling or emotional support beyond that which can be provided by dental providers

Other Health Problems

Because the aged and poor are over-represented in the dental school patient population, numerous SDM patients seek assistance from the CARES program regarding their health concerns. CARES social workers provide linkages to primary care physicians, specialists, and health care clinics. They also link patients with discount prescription plans; assist patients in prioritizing and managing oral and other health care needs; educate patients regarding the connections between oral health and overall health; and refer patients to community resources that specialize in physical health needs and disabilities.

Community Outreach

The CARES program has also played an important role in promoting oral health and access to care through community outreach. Social workers participate in events such as community health fairs and the Special Olympics as well as visiting agencies, such as senior centers, to educate community members about the importance of dental care and how community members can access dental care. One regular outreach event is the Lighthouse Clinic, a free medical clinic that is staffed by University at Buffalo medical students. Dental faculty and residents also offer free dental screenings at the clinic, and CARES social workers provide patients with linkage to an appropriate dental home. Through this clinic over a course of 21 months, 80 patients consulted with a social worker, 63 of whom were referred to a community dental provider and 17 of whom became patients at the SDM.

EDUCATION

Only one member of the CARES staff holds a faculty appointment, however each of the CARES social workers is involved in teaching and training both dental students and social work students.

The CARES program provides dental students and residents with an opportunity to learn transdisciplinary methods of treating dental patients, in accordance with the recommendations of the ADA and the American Dental Education Association.[2,7] CARES social workers provide each class of dental students with information regarding the services provided by the program and the psychosocial issues that often present in a dental school patient population. Further, CARES social workers provide education through consultation regarding individual patients.

The research director is responsible for teaching content on social and behavioral sciences, including patient communication, working with older adults, and psychosocial issues in dental treatment. In addition, she teaches one course per year in the school of social work and mentors both social work and dental students conducting research on topics related to public health and psychosocial aspects of dentistry. The MSW social workers who conduct the clinical aspects of the CARES program also serve as field placement supervisors to four to seven MSW students each year. To date, the program has served as the field placement site for 36 MSW students, a remarkably high number, given the size of the program.

An important facet of the program is the coeducation of social work and dental students. Through working together to meet the needs of dental clinic patients, dental students and social work students gain understanding of and respect for the skills and knowledge base of the other's profession, helping each to work more effectively in cross- disciplinary relationships for the good of their patients.

All of the master's level social workers who have been employed by CARES (four to date) had previously completed their field placement with the program. This has benefited the program by contributing to the institutional memory as well as helping to insure continuity of care and reducing productive time lost during staff transitions, as staff members have already been trained in the purpose and workings of the program before being hired.

RESEARCH

From its beginnings, CARES program staff have participated in research to identify patients' needs. The program was initiated after a needs assessment survey was completed, and client charts have been retained on virtually all of the clients served not only for clinical purposes but also with the intent of creating a database for program evaluation. In addition to data collected during provision of services, each client is administered a client satisfaction survey conducted over the telephone after the completion of treatment.

Methodology

To date, information from almost one half of the more than 2000 patients seen since 2001 has been compiled from patient charts, interviews, and survey data and entered into a computer database. Data entry has been chronologic, so these data are not from a random sample of our patients. However, the demographic characteristics of our client population do not appear to have changed significantly over the last several years, and the services provided to clients have remained substantially the same, although financial concerns have become more common, so these data are assumed to be a fair representation of the program and the clients served. Further, the database is of sufficient size (N = 937), to allow for generalizations regarding this client population and the efficacy of CARES interventions to be made with some confidence.

Although the CARES program has been committed to research and program evaluation from its inception, a full-time research director was not hired until fall of 2007. As a result, the data gathered about clients has been collected primarily for the purposes of providing clinical services. And, given the nature of clinical charts, at times data are missing or conflicting, and some data that would provide answers to certain interesting questions are unavailable. As such, this research should be regarded as preliminary and subject to verification through continued systematic study of this and other similar programs.

Only those variables with a sufficient number of respondents to make a valid assertion regarding the data have been included in this analysis. For those variables, a frequency analysis was completed to develop a descriptive picture of the program and the clients served. Currently, CARES staff is in the process of developing new data collection methods that will enable more detailed evaluations of the program and a fuller understanding of CARES clients and their needs. The current database provides important information regarding the demographic characteristics of our clients and their needs, services provided by CARES, and client perception of the efficacy of such services.

Results

This program evaluation was undertaken using the abovementioned database, with a sample size of 937. An analysis of frequencies found the following demographic information.

Age at intake was recorded for 715 of the patients. The age of clients served by CARES ranged from 6 to 96. The mean age at intake was 57 and the mode was 78, with a median of age 53. This is, in part, a reflection of the demographics of patients at the dental school, where roughly one third of the patients are older adults, as well as the initial focus of the program. The number of older adults living in poverty and facing severe dental problems is also evident in the percentage of older patients needing social work services.[8,9] Of the 454 patients for which we have data on race, 76.4% were white, 15.6% were African American, 2.4% were Latin American, 1.3% were Asian American, 1.1% were Native American, and 3.1% were identified as "other." These figures reflect the racial composition of the Buffalo–Niagara Falls, NY area, according to 2000 census data **(Table 1)**.[10] The percentage of African-American patients seen by the CARES program is slightly higher than that in the larger population, possibly because of the number of African Americans who are also economically disadvantaged as well as the higher incidence of health problems seen in this population.

Unsurprisingly, given that many of the patients referred to CARES are referred for financial reasons, 75.2% of the patients for whom we have these data are unemployed, with only 24.8% employed. Of those who are not working, only 16% are retired, and just 15.6% are disabled or are receiving Supplemental Security Income (SSI) or Social Security Disability (SSD). Of those patients who are not currently working, only about one third (31.6%), are out of the labor force because they are unable to work or have retired. The approximately two thirds remaining are simply unable to find work. The high rate of unemployment found among CARES patients is consistent with the dismal economic picture for the region; according to census data, Buffalo is one of the poorest cities in the country.[10] It is also evidence of the difficulty many unemployed Americans have in accessing health care, as many rely on health care benefits provided through their workplace.

Only 46% of the patients had some form of health insurance and 89% had no dental insurance. Lack of dental insurance is common in America, with 66% of the population having no dental insurance; however, the percentage of CARES patients without dental coverage (almost 90%) is much larger than in the general population.[11] Obviously, this lack of dental coverage makes obtaining dental care extremely difficult for many, even given the low cost for dental procedures offered at the SDM clinics.

Just over 19% of the patients served by CARES receive Medicare, and an additional 25.9% receive Medicaid. However, Medicare does not cover dental treatment except in the rare instance in which it can be documented as an essential component of a medical procedure.[12] Although Medicaid does cover dental care for those who

Table 1
Racial composition of CARES patients compared with the racial composition of the Buffalo-Niagara Region

Race	CARES Patients (%)	Buffalo–Niagara Region (%)
White	76.4	83.3
African American	15.6	11.7
Latino	2.4	2.9
Asian American	1.3	1.3
Native American	1.1	.7
Other	3.1	1.2

are categorically eligible, for a variety of reasons, including low reimbursement rates, many dentists refuse to treat patients who are on Medicaid.[13] The SDM clinic is one of the few oral health providers in the eight-county region of western New York that does accept Medicaid, and approximately 33% of the patients treated there are treated under this program.[4]

It is unsurprising then, that the greatest number of patients referred to CARES are referred because of financial difficulties that limit ability to pay for dental care, with 52.9% falling into this category. Additionally, 15.5% are referred for chronic pain or TMD (the high percentage of TMD referrals can be attributed to the presence of the CARES social worker in the TMD Clinic once a week), and 22% are referred because of other health problems. Rounding out the top five reasons for referral are transportation difficulties (12.8%) and mental health issues (10.2%).

Although mental health may only account for 10.2% of referrals to CARES, it is worth noting that 38% of patients referred state that they have had a mental illness diagnosed. The large number of CARES patients with mental health diagnoses may be evidence of the disproportionate amount of mental health problems found in low-income populations. It also underscores the need for dentists and dental professionals to screen for mental health problems, even when other concerns appear to be more obviously pressing. Of those CARES patients with a mental health diagnosis, 19.3% have been diagnosed or treated for general anxiety, 5.5% have been diagnosed or treated for dental anxiety, and 23.2% have been diagnosed or treated for depression, with 5.9% having been suicidal. In this last category, mental health screening can prove to be life saving.

Much of this report has focused on the benefits of CARES in terms of access to dental care and educational opportunities for dental students, still, it is important to note, that CARES has had a positive financial impact on the dental school as well. Although it is difficult to access such data, results indicate that the program has generated dollars for the SDM through fees paid for dental services. One example is the number the patients that CARES generates through outreach work—to date, one in five patients who consulted CARES social workers at the Lighthouse Clinic have become patients at the SDM (CARES annual report, unpublished data, 2007). In 2005, an analysis was done to determine the approximate amount of income generated by the CARES program. Because patients who are referred to CARES are referred because barriers to care place them at risk for not continuing their dental treatment, data were collected to assess the cost of dental treatment provided to CARES patients after contact with a social worker. From 2001 through 2005 after their initial contact with a social worker, CARES patients were responsible for a total of $564,918.34 in revenue for the SDM. Although it is impossible to determine how much of that revenue is a result of CARES services, it is likely that a significant percentage of the revenue would not have been generated without CARES interventions to overcome barriers to care (CARES annual report, unpublished data, 2005). The financial impact of the CARES program on the SDM deserves special emphasis; contrary to popular misconceptions regarding the expense of social service interventions, the CARES program appears to be a significant source of revenue.

The success of the CARES program can also be measured in terms of patient satisfaction. When asked the likelihood that they would have continued dental treatment at the SDM without CARES services, 33% said that it was "not at all likely," whereas an additional 12% said it was only "a little bit" likely that they would have completed dental treatment, totaling 45.3% who were, by self report, probably not going to complete dental care before CARES intervention, who did complete it after CARES intervention. An additional 23.9% described themselves as only "somewhat" likely to complete treatment without CARES services. No one described him or herself as "very likely" to complete treatment without CARES intervention. Further, CARES patients feel positive about the program, with 89% rating the services as "better than average" to "excellent," with "excellent" being the most frequent response to this item. Finally, when asked, 95% of CARES patients stated that they would recommend the program to someone else.

SUMMARY

Social work programs in dental clinics and dental schools have been operated successfully at least since the 1940s and have been documented as contributing to patients' access to care as well as dental education.[14,15] However, unlike medical social work, with which it has much in common, social work in dentistry has failed to become a standard feature of dental schools and clinics. Despite periodic descriptions in the literature of successful programs, there has been no indication that each program is more than an isolated entity. Because many of these programs have been seen as experimental, they have disappeared when funding dried up, when the grant expired, or when the institutional supporters of the program moved on. This is unfortunate, given the demonstrated success of the CARES program. The authors hope that the CARES program serves as a model for the successful development of other programs at the intersection of social work and dentistry to the benefit of both dental patients and providers.

REFERENCES

1. American Dental Association Survey Center. 1998 Survey of Dental School Satellite Clinics. Chicago: American Dental Association; 1999.
2. Haden NK, Cattalanotto FA, Alexander CJ, et al. Improving the oral health status of all Americans: roles and responsibilities of academic dental institutions. The Report of the ADEA President's Commission. J Dent Educ 2003;67(5):563–83.
3. Mead J. Serving clinic patients: CARES works. Buffalo (NY): UB Dentist; 2007. p. 11.
4. Waldrop DP, Fabiano JA, Davis EL, et al. Coexistent concerns: assessing the social and health needs of dental clinic patients. Soc Work Health Care 2004; 40(1):33–51.
5. Zittel-Palamara K, Fabiano JA, Davis EL, et al. Improving patient retention and access to oral health care: the CARES Program. J Dent Educ 2005;69(8): 912–8.
6. Levy RI, Lambert R, Davis G. Social work and dentistry in clinical, training and research collaboration. Soc Work Health Care 1979;5:177–85.
7. American Dental Association. Principles of Ethics and Code of Professional Conduct. Available at: www.ada.org/prof/prac/law/code/interpretaion.html. Accessed December 18, 2008.
8. Waldrop DP, Fabiano JA, Nochajski TH, et al. More than a set of teeth: enhancing dental students, perceptions of older adults. Gerontol Geriatr Educ 2006;27(1): 37–56.
9. Pyle MA, Stoller EP. Health disparities among the elderly: interdisciplinary challenges for the future. J Dent Educ 2003;67:1327–36.
10. U.S. Census Bureau. Census 2000. Available at: http://censtats.census.gov. Accessed April 18, 2009.

11. National Center for Health Statistics. Dental service use and dental coverage. 1995. Available at: http://www.cdc.gov/mmrw/preview/mmwrhtm/00050448.htm. Accessed December 18, 2008.

12. Centers for Medicare and Medicaid Services. 2002. Available at: http://www.cms. hhs.gov/MedicareDentalcoverage/. Accessed April 19, 2009.

13. Waldman BH, Perlman SP. Collaboration between social workers and dentists for care of people with special needs (A commentary). Soc Health Care 2003;37(2): 101–7.

14. Wexler P, McKinley E. Function of a social worker in Walter G. Zoller Memorial Dental Clinic, University of Chicago Clinics. J Dent Educ 1953;17:59–66.

15. Board MW. Illustrations of casework in a dental clinic. J Dent Educ 1954;18:94–8.

An Introduction to Oral Health Care Reform

Kristen L. Hathaway, BS

KEYWORDS

- Oral • Dental • Access • Health care
- Health reform • Workforce

Access to dental providers is a critical issue in oral health that was recently catapulted onto the national stage by a single catastrophic event. Federal focus on dental issues has been re-engaged because of the 2007 death of Deamonte Driver. Deamonte, a 12-year-old Maryland boy, died when complications from untreated dental problems led to a fatal brain infection. Deamonte's mother struggled to find a dentist under the Maryland Medicaid system that would accept new patients and treat her two sons. Since this tragedy, Congress has held hearings on dental access issues facing families like the Drivers and others on public programs. States are looking internally and investigating if families have appropriate access to dental care to prevent what occurred in Maryland.

With new attention on oral health, there are a number of issues the dental community will need to closely monitor in the near term. The National Association of Dental Plans (NADP) actively tracks these issues for the dental benefits industry and works with partner organizations to help convey the interests of the oral health community to policymakers. Potential issues of interest to our community in the emerging health reform debate include public program expansion, proposals to increase the dental workforce, and changing the tax preferences for employer-sponsored health care coverage.

This chapter focuses on oral health from a political standpoint. It will examine how access to providers and to oral care impacts discussions throughout the dental sector. It is important to understand the variances of oral health care within public programs, as government actions can set the tone for policies, potentially affecting the private dental marketplace. Stakeholders within the dental community are promoting various workforce models, addressing the critical need for oral care of the uninsured and underinsured populations. These models are being thoroughly vetted through state pilot programs and tested on the political stage in legislative debates. As 2009 begins, the political direction and discussions on oral health access will be directly influenced by the much larger discussion of health care reform.

National Association of Dental Plans, 12700 Park Central Drive, Suite 400, Dallas, TX 75251, USA
E-mail address: khathaway@nadp.org

Dent Clin N Am 53 (2009) 561–572
doi:10.1016/j.cden.2009.03.009
0011-8532/09/$ – see front matter © 2009 Elsevier Inc. All rights reserved.

dental.theclinics.com

PUBLIC PROGRAMS: MEDICAID AND STATE CHILDREN'S HEALTH INSURANCE PROGRAM

There has been a plethora of studies, issue briefs, and reports released in 2008 questioning the availability of access to oral care by the uninsured, the underinsured, and those in public programs. Medicaid is a shared state and federal program covering health care costs for populations with limited income and assets. Although the federal government provides matching funds to finance Medicaid and sets certain coverage and benefit rules, states manage the day-to-day operation of the Medicaid program. A state can run the program directly, contract with a private insurer, or use a hybrid of the two. An additional public program is the State Children's Health Insurance Program (SCHIP) passed in 1997 as part of the Balanced Budget Act to assist in covering low-income children in families with incomes too high to qualify for Medicaid but not enough to purchase private insurance. "In general, this program builds on Medicaid by providing federal matching funds that allow states to provide health insurance coverage to certain uninsured low-income children either under Medicaid, under a separate SCHIP program, or a combination of both approaches."[1]

In 2005, one third of all children living below 200% Federal Poverty Level (FPL) did not visit a dental provider.[2] As reference, a family of four at the FPL would have an income of $21,200 (at 200% is $42,400).[3] In recent testimony to the US Congress, Centers for Medicare and Medicaid Services (CMS) explained states with lower use of children's dental services frequently require improvements in the following areas:

- Clear information for beneficiaries that is linguistically and culturally appropriate regarding the availability and importance of dental services and how to access the services
- Process to remind beneficiaries that recommended visits are due
- Updated dental provider listings
- Processes to track whether recommended visits occurred
- Availability of dental providers, particularly in more rural portions of the State
- Availability of specialists for referrals
- Availability and reliability of transportation to dental services.[4]

As CMS highlights, and states' experience confirms, it is difficult to get dentists to accept Medicaid patients, and in some geographic areas it can be very difficult to find any dentists. Dentists cite three primary reasons for their low participation in state Medicaid programs: (1) low reimbursement rates, (2) burdensome administrative requirements, and (3) problematic patient behaviors.[5] The American Dental Association (ADA) has encouraged federal legislation, which addresses dental workforce needs by providing grants to dental schools and qualified hospitals to increase the pursuit of pediatric dentistry. ADA also cites the Healthy Kids Dental program in Michigan as an example of a successful public program, as it provides Medicaid beneficiaries with the same Delta Dental private sector coverage that is widely accepted by most dentists in the states.[6] Nonetheless, access to dental services for both children and adults in low-income brackets can be difficult to attain.

In the Medicaid program, a child's EPSDT (Early Periodic Screening, Diagnosis, and Treatment) benefit requires that state programs pay for regular health items, treatment found to be medically necessary, hearing, vision screening, and comprehensive dental. SCHIP does not include the same requirements of coverage as Medicaid, and states are federally required only to include well-child services, immunizations, and emergency services. "Currently 14 states with separate SCHIP programs offer children the same benefits Medicaid provides; other states provide more limited benefits modeled after private insurance, with seven capping annual dental expenditures or limiting the number of dental services allowed per year. Today, all states except Tennessee cover some dental services under SCHIP."[7] Experts suggest that "The funding structure for SCHIP is both successful and flawed," noting that, "It has succeeded in meeting its goal of encouraging state expansions while limiting federal liability, with a matching rate sufficient to encourage all states to expand coverage. However, the program's success in enrolling children has come up against its federal funding limits. Congress has acted six times in SCHIP's brief history to modify the program's rules."[8]

In 2007, the SCHIP program was due to be reauthorized; however, the size and scope of proposals to expand the program generated controversy. Some policymakers viewed reauthorization as an opportunity to grow the program in ways that would better ensure that it reached the millions of children who remain uninsured in America. Others preferred limiting reauthorization to a simple continuation of the existing program with modest financing improvements. Ultimately, the debate centered on several points of disagreement, including how much to spend on reauthorization, how to define the upper income limit for program eligibility, and how to address the actions by some states to include parents and other adults in their SCHIP populations.

As debate on these contentious issues continued, bipartisan efforts were underway to include a provision in the reauthorization bill requiring dental coverage for children enrolled in SCHIP. The dental provision enjoyed strong support in the dental community, among children's advocates, and with bipartisan policymakers. It was adopted in the compromise bill approved by the US House of Representatives and the US Senate. However, unhappy with the outcome of several of the other more contentious issues, President Bush vetoed the bill. Congress did not have the votes to override the President's veto, and efforts to pass a full reauthorization bill were abandoned in favor of simply extending current law through early 2009. Congress is set to revisit SCHIP in 2009 with the new Obama Administration.

Amidst the SCHIP federal debate, the Director of CMS sent letters to the lead health officials of each state indicating that for states to expand SCHIP eligibility to children in families with incomes above 250% of the federal poverty level, they must guarantee that they have enrolled at least 95% of the children in their state below 200% of the federal poverty level. Some states, mainly those with higher costs of living, had begun raising their income eligibility levels for the program to 300% of poverty. As of May 2007, one state, New Jersey, had set eligibility at 350% of the FPL ($74,200).[9] Many states and children's health advocates argued that the enrollment standards established by the federal government in this directive were unattainable and therefore an attempt to forestall states' efforts to reach children in lower income families without health insurance. States with high-cost metropolitan areas such as New York City and San Francisco were extremely concerned. Others believed that the Administration's move would focus the program on its target population and reduce the threat that public program dollars would be used to replace coverage children may already have through private means, including their parents' employer-sponsored coverage.

"Crowd-out" is defined as an enrollee dropping private insurance to participate in a free or subsidized health program administered by the state. "The crowd-out of private coverage can occur through various avenues. For example, some parents who would have otherwise had family coverage through their employer might decline it for their children—or might decline coverage altogether—if their children are eligible for SCHIP. Estimates vary about the extent to which SCHIP has resulted in the reduction of private coverage. Federal law requires that the states have procedures in place to prevent people from substituting SCHIP for employer-sponsored insurance. However, on the basis of a review of the available studies, the Congressional Budget Office concluded that the reduction in private coverage among children is most probably between a quarter and a half of the increase in public coverage resulting from SCHIP. That is, for every 100 children who gain coverage as a result of SCHIP, there is a corresponding reduction in private coverage of between 25 and 50 children."[10] Although there have been extensive studies and issue briefs regarding public program expansions on employer-sponsored medical insurance, there have been no reports on how crowd-out may affect the dental marketplace. Although increasing access to oral health care is necessary, crowd-out is certainly a factor that could impact the overall oral health of the nation if adult coverage is abandoned when shifting children to public programs.

STAKEHOLDERS AND WORKFORCE MODELS

There are several key members of Congress who are actively promoting oral health care legislation, likely prompted by the Driver case and growing concern about the extent of the dental access problem in public programs like Medicaid and SCHIP. The attention of lawmakers has increased as they continue to learn about both the prevalence of dental caries (tooth decay) and the increasing evidence that oral and overall health are correlated. Tooth decay remains the most prevalent chronic disease in both children and adults, even though it is largely preventable.[11] Federal and state legislators have been investigating additional opportunities to enhance dental care. Legislation has been introduced in 2007 and 2008 to better coordinate federal efforts to improve oral health by expanding dental services to underserved populations and strengthening the dental workforce.

There are a variety of viewpoints on access to dental providers, and although stakeholders agree there currently is a severe maldistribution of dental providers, whether a shortage of dentists currently exists or will occur in the future is being debated. Whichever your viewpoint or stance, government officials are looking for solutions. Approaches to expanding access to oral health care through legislation vary; however, they tend to focus on two areas—augmenting the reimbursement of providers of oral care and increasing funding for oral health programs. Beginning in 1998, 14 states have passed legislation in which they can directly reimburse dental hygienists for services under the Medicaid program.[12] Over half of the states allow dental hygienists to initiate treatment based on the their assessment of patients' needs without the specific authorization of a dentist, and some states go further by allowing the treatment of the patients without the presence of a dentist.[13] Several of these statutes were initiated to allow dental hygienists to practice in underserved areas, such as in nursing homes or Indian reservations. Although the American Dental Hygienists Association (ADHA) has supported and likely initiated some of these statutes, lawmakers viewed these measures as a step forward in increasing access to areas in need of oral care.

NADP released a position on the access and workforce issue, taking its lead from the U.S. Surgeon General's 2000 report, "Oral Health in America." The Surgeon General's report brought national attention to the issues regarding access to dental care and the importance of dental care to overall health. "The nation's capacity to provide care that is accessible and acceptable to address the oral health needs and wants of Americans in the next century is challenged…." That report also recommended use of "public–private" partnerships to address these important issues.[14] NADP supports the principle of public–private partnerships and commits to (and its member organizations) both dialog and partnership with organized dentistry, dental education, government agencies, and organizations representing allied dental personnel to examine and implement a mix of responses to improve the nation's capacity to provide oral health care. NADP also suggests initial examination of the following mix of responses:

- Expansion of dental school classes
- Expansion of education and awareness for current and emerging members of the dental profession on ways to increase productivity of the dental workforce, particularly through the use of allied dental personnel
- Enhanced practice mobility between states, reciprocity between state licensure, and simplification of the licensure process on a national basis
- Expansion of delegated duties to qualified allied dental personnel where allowed by local laws and supported by education and accountability
- Incentives for (a) Increased availability of education and training for allied dental personnel, to insure that delegated duties are delivered without diminished quality; (b) allied dental personnel to seek that continuing education, with the goal of increased productivity and enhanced career satisfaction; (c) qualified applicants to enter dental schools, obtain relief of student debt, and obtain assistance in the formation of new practice opportunities; (d) dentists to remain in the workforce as long as they can contribute, rather than opting for full retirement; (e) quality faculty candidates to seek affiliation with dental schools; (f) research for evidence-based dentistry that can identify ways to intervene in the dental disease process before major restoration is required; (g) the development of technology that increases the productivity of a dentist in his or her practice.

NADP must play a balanced role in the access debate. Dental plans must prove to their customers (employers and other groups that provide benefits) as well as to state regulators that they provide adequate access in all areas in which the dental plan has enrollees. The plans must also provide enough business to dentists to maintain a positive relationship. Although NADP supports the availability of additional allied dental personnel, the organization has not endorsed a one-size-fits-all practitioner approach to expanding the dental workforce.

Both ADHA and ADA have introduced new models for allied dental personnel to lawmakers whom they believe would increase access to oral care. ADHA has proposed the Advanced Dental Hygiene Practitioner (ADHP), a midlevel oral health provider educated and licensed to provide both preventive and limited restorative services to meet identified patient needs. Similar to a nurse practitioner, the ADHP type of provider is used in many other countries.[15] Although both organizations have been careful in their public testimony related to the ADHP, the ADA has been opposed to the new position. Dentists cite the potential for a decrease of quality in patient care, as the yet-to-be-developed education of the ADHP may not be enough for the duties the position requires. The ADHA posits the ADA is concerned about diminishing of business from the new practitioner and notes the success of the ADHP position in other countries and similar positions in the medical community.

Although ADA states there is not a shortage of dentists, they do agree there is a maldistribution limiting the availability of dentists in certain geographic regions. ADA notes that even with an influx of dentists, providers would not necessarily practice in underserved areas. The ADA proposes the Community Dental Health Coordinator (CDHC) workforce model to remedy the need for oral care in underserved areas. The CDHC, under a dentist's supervision, will provide preventative dental services, such as basic cleanings and sealants and in addition will collect information to assist the dentist in the triage of patients and address the social, environmental, and health literacy issues facing the community population. Another facet of the CDHC will be educating community members on preventive oral health care and assisting them in developing goals to promote and manage their own personal oral health. Linking patients to avenues of oral health care will also be an important role for the CDHC in working with underserved populations going through the maize of the health and dental care systems.[16] The ADA has funded grants in three underserved areas to pilot the CDHC program.

In 2008, the Minnesota Legislature proposed a bill allowing for a new type of practitioner, similar to the ADHP. After months of debate between the Minnesota dental hygienists and the Minnesota Dental Association, the final legislation included a compromise that established a new oral health practitioner discipline, licensed by the Board of Dentistry, and working under the supervision of a dentist. The legislation created a work group (comprised of all stakeholders of the dental community) to advise the commissioner of health on recommendations and legislation to specify the training and practice details for these new oral health practitioners and report back to the 2009 Legislature.[17]

In meetings with certain lawmakers and the various dental stakeholders, ADA has fielded tough questions about how their model would address growing concerns surrounding oral health access issues. The tone of legislators comments and inquires indicates the CDHC workforce model is not viewed as an adequate solution.

As the access debate continues, the education of any new oral health provider will take time to evolve, and the American Dental Education Association (ADEA) has been involved as the voice of dental educators. As ADEA stated in Congressional testimony, "Some say we have a dental shortage. Others say we have a maldistribution of dentists to meet the nation's oral health needs. No matter how one defines it, there can be no doubt that there is a significant access problem for millions of Americans. We must acknowledge that the current dental workforce is unable to meet present day demand and need for dental care.... The math is simple on this equation. There is an increasing need and demand for dental care. There is a current shortage of dental faculty to educate and train the future dental workforce. Several new dental schools are scheduled to open across the country to meet individual state workforce and access needs. We face a crisis if resources are not dedicated to help recruit and retain faculty for the nation's dental schools."[18] This statement introduces a new facet to the access issue, a workforce shortage within dental teaching institutions.

ADEA has proposed 18 recommendations to address dental workforce challenges. The proposals range from increasing funding for oral care in Medicaid and SCHIP, including dental, in certain educational block grants, bolstering prevention and education regarding dental caries, and passing federal legislation as explained in the next section.[18]

LEGISLATIVE SOLUTIONS TO THE ACCESS ISSUE

In direct response to the death of Deamonte Driver, several Members of Congress have introduced legislation regarding oral health care.[19] The programs and funding structures of proposed legislation are important to review, because the momentum to address access to oral care has increased, and new legislation has potential for enactment. Dental stakeholders need to be working with their government officials now to shape the future legislation, whether through public programs, grants, or other arrangements. Following are the outlines of recent oral health proposals.

The *Deamonte Driver Dental Care Access Improvement Act of 2008* (H.R. 5549, S. 2723) allows for the Secretary of Health and Human Services (HHS) to award grants to:

- Schools of dentistry and hospitals with accredited training programs in pediatric dentistry to increase the number of individuals who pursue academic programs in pediatric dentistry or provide dental services to children
- Applicants to establish a pilot program for increasing access to dental care for underserved populations through the use of allied dental health professionals
- Federally qualified health centers (FQHCs) to expand and improve the provision of dental services to medically underserved populations
- Public or private entities to develop, implement, and evaluate public health and clinical strategies to prevent and manage early childhood caries.

The Act also provides a tax credit (up to $5,000) for dentists who treat Medicaid, SCHIP, and uninsured patients, and requires states to report annually information related to children's access to dental services under Medicaid and SCHIP programs. In addition, the Act requests that the Comptroller General study and report to Congress on the adequacy of payment rates for dental services provided to individuals eligible for Medicaid or SCHIP and directs the CDC to conduct a public education and awareness campaign related to pediatric dental health. Lastly, the Act requires HHS to ensure that dental health prevention and promotion activities are included in existing prenatal and maternal child health programs.

The *Essential Oral Health Care Act-2007* (H.R. 2472):

- Provides grants for improving access to dental services in underserved areas, including (a) grants for Community Dental Health Coordinators to work in clinics or private practices and (b) grants for the purchase of portable dental equipment
- Provides increased Federal Medical Assistance Percentage (FMAP) up to 90% for states that ensure Medicaid and SCHIP children have the same access to dental care as other children. States must meet requirements related to provider payments and participation rates, removal of administrative barriers, and caregiver education
- Creates tax credit up to $5,000 for dentists providing charity care to low-income persons.

The *Children's Dental Health Improvement Act-2007* (H.R. 1781, S. 739) is similar to the previous legislation in that it provides grants to states, in this case (a) through the Department of Health and Human Services (HHS) to improve dental services for SCHIP and Medicaid, (b) through the Centers for Disease Control and Prevention to improve oral health for children and their families, and produce public statistical reporting of the types of dental care services received (c) through HHS to improve primary dental services in underserved areas, including retention bonuses for dental officers in IHS. In addition, states will have the option to provide wrap-around coverage of dental services for kids with private coverage and revise the Graduate Medical Education (GME) payments for dental residency programs. The bill requires HHS create initiatives to (a) reduce disparities in oral health and (b) identify populations at risk for early childhood caries and develop prevention programs. Additionally, the legislation establishes Chief Dental Officers for Medicaid, SCHIP, Health Resources and Services Administration (HRSA) and Centers for Disease Control and Prevention (CDC), and requires CDC to collect data on oral health.

The *Oral Health Initiative Act of 2008* (S.3064) establishes a working group to review the effectiveness of and recommend improvements to existing Federal oral health programs and to develop programs to improve the oral health of and prevent dental disease in children, Medicaid-eligible adults, medically compromised adults, and other high-risk vulnerable populations.

The *Dental Health Improvement Act of 2007* (S.3067) reauthorizes a program that awards grants to states to help the states develop and implement programs to address the dental workforce needs of designated dental health professional shortage areas.

Although federal bills are prolific and receive national attention within the dental community, state legislatures also have been taking action. Vermont and Maine passed voluntary health reform programs, and Massachusetts was the first state to mandate all individuals be covered by health insurance. Included in the Massachusetts regulations was a dental component for low-income children and adults. California tried to tackle health reform, but political issues kept the legislation from passing. Many states are waiting for a clear cost–benefit analysis to emerge in Massachusetts, as early results indicate costs are much higher than budgeted. The economic crisis is also straining state budgets, leaving less room for health initiatives. However, states are examining incremental steps in medical and in dental systems. As mentioned previously, expansion of duties for dental hygienists has been a prevalent policy discussion, and many states are reimbursing dental hygienists directly through Medicaid for basic dental services to the underserved population. The trend of expanding a hygienist's duties and areas they can serve is a trend likely to continue into 2009.

THE DENTAL COMMUNITY AND HEALTH REFORM

As President Barack Obama formulates his administration, some might suggest that health care reform could take a backseat to the increasing concern over the economy. However, Bob Blendon, who studies public opinion at the Harvard School of Public Health, states "Even if the new president was tempted by the sagging economy to put off his promise to address the health care mess, he would do so at his peril. Not only did voters who cited health care as their top issue flock to Obama in huge proportions, but 60% of his voters expect that if he became president, something big would be done about this problem.... Of course, a big problem is that voters still disagree about what "something big" in health reform would look like."[20] Most of the stakeholders within the dental community have released principles on oral health care reform, with many organizations framing their statements around the larger discussion of health care reform.

The NADP released a *Position Statement on Health Care Reform* in 2008. The statement outlines NADP's five principles for expanding access to dental health benefits: (1) oral health is vital to overall health; (2) cost is a key barrier to dental care; (3) dental benefits are key to expanding access to affordable, quality dental care; (4) employers play a critical role in providing access to dental benefits; and (5) dental plans help government programs work for beneficiaries. Reports from the both the Surgeon General's Office and the National Center for Health Statistics of the CDC provide evidence that enrollees covered by private or public dental coverage will visit the dentist more frequently.[21]

In 2008, ADA adopted a resolution on Improving *Oral Health In America*. The resolution is in three parts: (1) oral health is essential for a healthy America; (2) access is a key to good oral health; and (3) we must build on current successes. The ADA stresses educating the population about oral care, making reimbursement rates and funding for public programs and dental education a priority, and supports the NADP position that private dental benefits currently work and should be used when expansion of coverage is considered.[22]

ADHA has made public their *Statement on Health Reform*, highlighting that oral health must not be neglected, disease can be avoided with preventive care, and costs should be less expensive. The statement adds that workforce must be expanded and offered in a variety of settings, and federal funding should test the ADHP model. ADEA has supported two *Main Principles for Health Care Reform*: (1) The availability of health care, including oral health, fulfills a fundamental human need and is necessary for the attainment of general health and (2) The needs of vulnerable populations have a unique priority. ADEA has also released a policy statement, adding that any comprehensive reform of the U.S. health care system must include coverage and access to affordable oral health services.[23]

There have been several nonprofit policy think tanks and consumer advocate groups that have released reports and issued briefs on oral health care; however, currently there is only one advocate group that focuses exclusively on dental—the Children's Dental Health Project (CDHP). CHDP's mission is to "forge research-driven policies and innovative solutions by engaging a broad base of partners committed to children and oral health," and they have released their key principles as the *Foundation for Health Reform in Oral Health*, including (1) affordable, comprehensive, and high-quality health coverage that includes coverage to achieve oral health for all children; (2) prevention as the most efficient strategy for avoiding costly and lifelong health and developmental consequences; (3) effective care management and professional coordination for all children and their families to achieve optimal health, including oral health; and (4) efficient systems of care that integrate emerging technologies and health professionals to improve health status and eliminate disparities.[24]

The significance of these various position statements is that these associations share very similar philosophies on oral health. The connection between oral health and overall health is the key. Many of the reform statements go into more detail, citing studies that connect dental health with heart disease and diabetes or note a correlation between poor periodontal health and premature birth and detecting the presence of oral cancer. Access to dental care cannot only identify overall health conditions but trigger their treatment, thus reducing physical and financial impacts for adults and children. Paying for dental care can reduce costs for medical care, and yet, as NADP statistics show, there are currently 173 million Americans with dental benefits, leaving two of five Americans without dental coverage. The dentally uninsured outnumber the medically uninsured by two and half times.[25]

Although there are more similarities than differences among the dental community, each organization has various priorities on how health reform should take shape and where government funding should be spent. The focus spent on advocacy and lobbying within these associations varies greatly on their scope and size, but each one has a presence in Washington D.C. And although discussions among the dental community take place often, how and when these groups will advance their priorities will depend on how health reform takes shape in the Obama Administration.

HEALTH REFORM SCENARIOS

If major health reform is to occur, it may move quickly in the new congressional session, set to begin in January 2009.[26] President Obama has created a health care transition working group, which has already begun planning and engaging the public and interest groups on health reform. Major reform could take many different shapes. It might include an expansion of public programs such as Medicaid and SCHIP. It also could include the expansion of dental coverage to Medicare, funding for dental workforce models, or other targeted components that impact dental. New political discussions also have taken place regarding the use of the tax code to support health insurance. For example, Senator Baucus (D), Chair of the U.S. Senate Finance Committee has suggested capping the amount of the health care premiums that can be excluded from employee wages for income and payroll tax purposes. There is also discussion regarding provider payments and changes to insurance regulations. All of these reforms are likely to directly impact the dental sector.

If comprehensive reform proves unachievable, incremental reform may be possible. This might include, for example, more targeted expansions of public programs such as a sizable expansion of the SCHIP program. Small does not mean insignificant; consider that both the Health Insurance Portability and Accountability Act (HIPAA) and SCHIP were "incremental" reforms after the failure of Clinton health care reform. Of course, it remains possible that health reform will not occur for several years because of factors such as the economy and the war in Iraq or the lack of political consensus.

The majority of analysts believe there will be some sort of health reform, because the consequences are too great if it is not addressed. However, action on reform will require overcoming political and fiscal challenges. Without action, employers, specifically small business, will continue to struggle with affordability of health insurance, health care costs will continue to escalate, and the uninsured population will likely expand.

The dental sector will be watching health reform very closely. Although all the dental stakeholders would applaud federal and state funding in public programs for oral care for children and low-income adults, concerns and priorities about the specific implementation of these and other policy options may differ.

Dental insurance is very different from medical insurance, and though oral health is systemic to overall health, care and coverage are handled very differently. In its current form, dental insurance works—it is cost effective, employers are pleased, and enrollees with coverage see their dentist regularly, satisfying plan providers.[27] Proposals regarding tax benefits will be scrutinized heavily, as virtually all dental coverage is provided through employers or other groups. Any proposal that has the potential to make employers re-evaluate their benefit packages and potentially drop their dental benefit or turn it into a voluntary benefit could reduce access to health care (a voluntary benefit is when the employer offers a health benefit that is priced at a group rate to their employees, but the employer is not subsidizing the cost). Other proposals, such as the various workforce models, certainly will be reviewed by the dental sector as well.

SUMMARY

Oral health care reform is made up of several components, but access to care is central. Health care reform will occur in some fashion at some point, and how it will impact the entire dental sector is unclear. In the short term, there is likely to be a dental component during the reauthorization of SCHIP in early 2009, and several federal oral health bills are expected to be introduced again. Additional public funding for new programs and program expansions remains questionable, as federal funding will be tight. Fiscal conservancy will be occurring in the states as well; however, various proposals to expand dental hygienists' duties are likely, as are proposals related to student grants for dental schools. Regardless of one's political stance, the profile of oral health care has been elevated, offering countless opportunities for improvement in the oral health of the nation.

ACKNOWLEDGMENTS

The author thanks Carole Johnson of Health Policy R&D, NADP's Federal Advisor, who contributed a great deal of information used throughout this article.

REFERENCES

1. Baumrucker E. Testimony before the Senate Finance Health Subcommittee - state children's health insurance program overview of program rules. Washington, DC: Congressional Research Service; July 25, 2006. CRS-2.
2. National Center for Health Statistics. Health, United States, 2007 with chartbook on trends in the health of Americans. Hyattsville (MD): Centers for Disease Control and Prevention; 2007.
3. National Archives and Records Administration. The Federal Register, January 23, 2008. 2008;73(15):3971–2.
4. Kuhn H. Testimony of CMS before the House Committee on oversight and government reform, subcommittee on domestic policy. Necessary reforms to pediatric dental care under medicaid September 23, 2008;4.
5. Borchgrevink A, Snyder A, Gehshan S. The effects of medicaid reimbursement rates on access to dental care. Washington, DC: National Academy for State Health Policy; March 2008. v.
6. Statement of the America Dental Association to the Subcommittee on Domestic Policy, Committee on Oversight and Government Reform. One year later: medicaid's response to the systemic problems revealed by the death of deamonte driver. February 14, 2008.
7. Gehshan S, Snyder A, Paradise J. Filling an urgent need: improving children's access to dental care in medicaid and SCHIP. Washington, DC: National Academy for State Health Policy, Kaiser Commission on Medicaid and the Uninsured The Henry J. Kaiser Family Foundation; July 2008. 4.
8. Lambrew J. The state children's health insurance program: past, present, and future. New York: The Commonwealth Fund; February 2007.
9. Georgetown University Health Policy Institute, Center for Children and Families. States affected by proposals to restrict SCHIP coverage options. Available at: http://ccf.georgetown.edu/index/states-affected-by-proposals-to-restrict-schip-coverage-options.
10. Congress of the United States Congressional Budget Office. The state children's health insurance program. No. 2970. May 2007. p. 9–10.
11. The Dental, Oral and Craniofacial Data Resource Center, the National Institutes of Health, U.S. Department of Health and Human Services. The Oral Health U.S. 2002 Annual Report. Available at: http://drc.hhs.gov/report.htm.
12. American Dental Hygienists Association. States which directly reimburse dental hygienists for services under the medicaid program. November 2008. Available at: http://www.adha.org/governmental_affairs/practice_issues.htm.
13. American Dental Hygienists Association. Direct Access States. August 2008. Available at: http://www.adha.org/governmental_affairs/practice_issues.htm.
14. U.S. Department of Health and Human Services, National Institute of Dental and Craniofacial Research, National Institutes of Health. Oral Health in America: a report of the surgeon general. Rockville (MD) 2000.
15. American Dental Hygiene Association. The advanced dental hygiene practitioner and access to oral health care. Chicago, Illinois, 2009.
16. American Dental Association. Frequently asked Questions on the CDHC. Web site: Available at: http://www.ada.org/public/careers/team/frequently_asked_questions_cdhc.pdf. Accessed 2008.
17. Minnesota Department of Health. Minnesota's health reform initiative. Oral health practitioner work group. Web site: Available at: http://www.health.state.mn.us/healthreform/oralhealth/index.html. Accessed 2008.

18. Swift J. Statement of the American Dental Educators Association Before the U.S. Senate Committee on Health Education Labor and Pensions Hearing. Addressing Health Care Workforce Issues. February 12, 2008.
19. Health Policy R&D, Legislative Grid for NADP Members. 2008.
20. Rovner J. Health Care Reform Looms Over Next Presidency. All Things Considered-National Public Radio. November 10, 2008.
21. National Association of Dental Plans. Position Statement on Health Reform. Dallas, Texas, July 2008.
22. American Dental Association. Resolution 38H-2008 Improving Oral Health in America. Chicago, Illinois, November 2008.
23. American Dental Hygienists Association. Statement on Health Reform. Chicago, Illinois, 2008.
24. Children's Dental Health Project. Health Care Reform Principles for Children's Oral Health. Washington, DC, October 2008.
25. The 2008 National Association of Dental Plans & Delta Dental Association Joint Dental Benefits Report. Dallas, Texas, August 2008.
26. Johnson C. NADP Webinar - Election 08: health care reform and the dental benefits industry. Health Policy R&D. Washington, DC, November 19, 2008.
27. NADP White Paper. Dental Benefits Deliver High Employer, Employee Dividends. Dallas, Texas, March 2008.

Why Public Policy Matters in Improving Access to Dental Care

Shelly Gehshan, MPP*, Andrew Snyder, MPA

KEYWORDS

- State health policy • Access to dental care • Medicaid
- SCHIP • Regulation of health professions
- Dental public health • Dental provider education

Given the large degree of control that the profession of dentistry has over its education, licensure, and practice, it is easy to overlook the fact that state policymakers have the primary authority and responsibility for regulating the health professions. That authority is rooted in the Tenth Amendment to the United States Constitution, which reserves for the states, or the people, any power not given by the framers to the federal government. State control over health providers is not limited to police power over activities that threaten public health and safety. In fact, states have broad authority that provides the underpinning for the health care system, performing a number of critical functions, some of which they share with federal or local governments: (1) providing and financing health care; (2) regulation of health practitioners and facilities; (3) ensuring the health of the public; (4) health workforce education and training; (5) regulation of insurance; (6) cost containment; (7) informing the public about the functioning of the health system; and (8) monitoring the system.[1] Each of these functions has been employed creatively to expand access to care for underserved populations. This article describes the authority that states have in the first four areas, where state policymaking is most visible and powerful, and how it can be used to expand access to care for low-income children **Fig. 1**.

PROVIDE AND FINANCE CARE

The first critical function of states is to provide dental health care to a large portion of Americans. State or county-employed dentists care for people who are in state custody, such as residents of state-run institutions for people who have developmental disabilities and prisoners, as well as for patients of government-operated

The Pew Charitable Trusts provided support for the preparation of this article.
Advancing Children's Dental Health Initiative, The Pew Charitable Trusts, 901 E. Street, 10th Floor, Washington, DC, USA
* Corresponding author.
E-mail address: sgehshan@nashp.org (S. Gehshan).

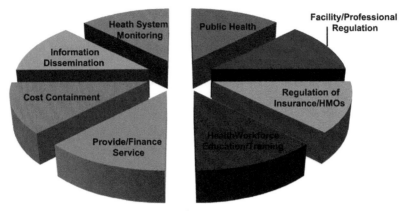

Fig. 1. Key state government roles in health care.

clinics or local health departments. The state is also a purchaser or funder of health services for children and adults enrolled in public insurance programs. In this role, the state has great power to shape incentives and disincentives for these people to obtain dental health care and for dental and medical practitioners to provide it.

Medicaid and the State Children's Health Insurance Program

Medicaid is one of the cornerstones of the American health care system. Although it covers only certain categories of low-income people, not all of them, it nevertheless is the foundation for the health care safety net. As of June 2006, Medicaid, together with the State Children's Health Insurance Program (SCHIP), covered 25.7 million children.[2] These programs are funded jointly by state and federal governments. The federal government sets broad guidelines for the program, but states have a considerable degree of flexibility in setting policy in three areas: who is eligible for the program, what benefits they receive, and how those benefits are delivered.

Medicaid generally covers four categories of low-income people: children, their parents, pregnant women, and the "aged, blind, and disabled," which includes low-income Medicare recipients and people eligible for Supplemental Security Income (SSI) and Social Security Disability Insurance (SSDI). States also can cover other groups of enrollees, such as young adults exiting foster care. SCHIP builds on Medicaid by providing states with enhanced funding to enroll children in "working poor" families (typically, those who have an income less than twice the federal poverty level) with benefits similar to those of Medicaid or private large-group insurance.

Medicaid-enrolled children are entitled to coverage of all medically necessary dental services through the Early and Periodic Screening, Diagnosis, and Treatment (EPSDT) benefit. Although the provision of dental services is not required under SCHIP, all states except one currently provide them,[3] and the proposed 2007 federal legislation to reauthorize SCHIP would have made dental coverage a requirement.[4] When states have fallen short in their obligation to provide children's dental services, advocates frequently have filed suit against them for failure to meet the federal standard that Medicaid enrollees have access to health care professionals comparable to that of other people in their community. Of 27 dental-access suits filed in 21 states, states have lost or settled all but 4.[5]

Despite the EPSDT requirement to provide dental services, states persistently have had trouble delivering these services and could do more to improve access. Data reported to the federal government show that in 2006 only one third of all children enrolled in Medicaid received any dental service. Although this percentage is an improvement from previous years **(Fig. 2)**, it still falls far below the 57% use rate among privately insured children in 2004.[6]

One of the crucial levers policymakers have for improving children's dental health is the ability to provide a meaningful Medicaid dental benefit to adults. Research has shown that coverage of a health care service for parents influences whether those parents seek that care for their children. Addressing the oral health needs of new mothers, as well as providing education and anticipatory guidance, can have positive oral health benefits for entire families.[7] A pilot program in Klamath County, Oregon, is seeking to test this hypothesis by providing home visits and intensive oral health services for pregnant women and new mothers.[8] Also, Medicaid benefits for adults change the equation for providers. It is easier for community health centers and clinics to sustain a healthy business model and to treat all comers if reimbursement is available for adults. Medicaid reimbursements to private dental providers also are very helpful in rural and underserved areas, where the population is poorer and less likely to have private dental coverage. Adult dental services are "optional" in Medicaid, however, and many states choose to limit coverage to emergency services or to provide no coverage at all.[9] This situation is in stark contrast to private dental coverage, which rarely covers children without also covering policy holders and their spouses.

Policymakers in states considering comprehensive health care reform have a variety of choices in crafting a dental benefit in their programs. To date, state health care reform efforts have not included dental benefits in any systematic way, although there have been some positive steps. For example, during comprehensive reform in Massachusetts in 2006, dental benefits were extended to children enrolled in Medicaid-style benefits through Commonwealth Care and were restored to low-income adults. The state also arranged for supplemental payments to Federally Qualified Health Centers and to some public hospitals that provided dental care to people who did not have dental benefits. An option for policymakers to consider is the design of a buy-in benefit that looks more like Medicaid, with lower cost-sharing by enrollees and more

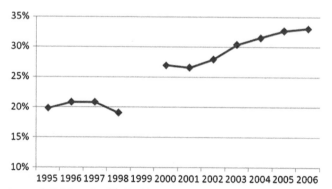

Fig. 2. Percentage of children in Medicaid receiving dental services, 1995–2006. Note that the reporting methodology for dental services changed between 1998 and 1999. (*Data from* CMS-416 annual EPSDT Use Report.)

protections for new enrollees at lower incomes, and more like state or federal employee health plans for higher-income uninsured persons.[10]

Once policymakers have determined which enrollees will have dental benefits, the state must decide how those benefits will be delivered and what resources will be allocated to deliver them.

Reimbursement Rates

The size and structure of payment is a critical policy lever. Inadequate payment is the central reason dentists cite for not enrolling as providers in state Medicaid programs. Federal Medicaid law requires states to "assure that payments are … sufficient to enlist enough providers so that care and services are available under the [Medicaid] plan at least to the extent that such care and services are available to the general population in the geographic area."[11] This federal standard has not been effectively or widely enforced, however, because, among other reasons, there is contention about what consititutes "sufficient" reimbursement. The American Dental Association's (ADA's) position is that rates set at the 75th percentile of regional fees (that is, payment rates that are as high as or higher than the retail charges of three fourths of dentists in a geographic area) is a sufficient level to attract provider participation.[12] State experience, however, shows that more modest rate increases still can generate adequate provider participation if reimbursement at least covers dentists' costs of providing the care.[13] States understand that rate increases, coupled with use increases, can cause large spending hikes; Alabama tripled its total Medicaid dental expenditures as a consequence. Still, because dental spending is less than 5% of Medicaid expenditures, and costs are shared between the state and federal government, the fiscal impact of reimbursement rate increases on state budgets is modest. For example, the increased dental expenditures in Alabama amounted to only 1.15% of total Medicaid expenditures of $3.86 billion in 2004.[14] As **Table 1** shows, increases of the reimbursement rate in three states helped them meet their goals of improving the use of services among Medicaid enrollees.[13] Advocates in states such as Wisconsin have proposed a small surcharge on sugary drinks to fund reimbursement rates that keep pace with inflationary increases.[12]

If across-the-board hikes in the reimbursement rate are not possible, strategies targeted at populations of particular interest show promise. New Mexico, for example, has used incentive payments to develop a small cadre of dentists to provide care to people who have developmental disabilities. Pennsylvania is experimenting with pay-for-performance strategies to give dentists incentives to provide a continuing "dental home" for young children, pregnant women, and people who have chronic conditions such as heart disease and diabetes.[15]

Administration

Although reimbursement rates that at least cover dentists' costs of providing care are necessary, they alone are not sufficient to increase provider participation and enrollee access to care. States need to address the "hassle factor," too. Most dental offices are small and have limited administrative capacity, and even less inclination, to navigate complex Medicaid program rules. Many dentists' offices expect full payment at the time of service and expect patients to file claims for their own insurance. Therefore, states can enhance dentists' participation if they make it easy for offices to participate in the program, to see patients in need, and to receive reimbursements in a timely fashion. Several states—Tennessee, Virginia, and Massachusetts, among others— have addressed these concerns by "carving out" dental administration and contracting with a specialized vendor for "administrative services only (ASO)," to process

Table 1
Changes in dental payments and users in three states, 2000 to 2004

Comparator	Alabama			South Carolina			Tennessee			
	2000	2004	Percent Change	2000	2004	Percent Change	2002	2004	Percent Change	
Number of enrollees using services	72,287	155,541	115	162,567	256,782	58	131,899	286,314	117	
Total dental payments ($ million)	11.5	44.4	288	48.2	89.3	85	28.7	130.3	355	
Payment per user ($)	159	286	80	296	348	18	217	455	110	

Data from CMS Medicaid Statistical Information System. Available at: http://www.cms.hhs.gov/MedicaidDataSourcesGenInfo/02_MSISData.asp. Accessed October 2007; and Borchgrevink A, Snyder A, Gehshan S. The effects of Medicaid reimbursement rates on access to dental care. Portland (ME): National Academy for State Health Policy; 2008.

claims, make determinations on coverage for services, and maintain provider and enrollee hotlines. Other states, such as Alabama, have addressed many of the same concerns through administrative improvements by the Medicaid agency. Any administrative arrangement—by managed care companies, ASOs, or directly by states—can succeed only if it has sufficient resources, dedicated staff, and leaders who are focused on dental services as a priority.[13]

Availability of Medicaid Reimbursements

In their role as purchasers of care, states can decide whether to support models of care delivery that go beyond the traditional private dental office. Because of government's purchasing power, these decisions can determine whether a new model of care is sustainable and cost effective. For example, Medicaid reimbursement was key to sustaining the fledgling "Into the Mouths of Babes" program in North Carolina, which trained—and paid—pediatricians and family practice physicians to provide children from birth to 3 years with preventive dental care services: basic oral health assessment, oral health education, and fluoride varnish.[15] Physicians were targeted because young children visit physicians earlier and more often than dentists. Because of the lessons learned from North Carolina, 26 states now use Medicaid reimbursement as a way to encourage physicians to begin attending to children's oral health as early as possible.[16]

Likewise, 14 states have decided to make Medicaid reimbursements available directly to dental hygienists, rather than having payments go first to a dentist or local health department, who then pays the hygienist. This direct payment enhances the ability of hygienists working in public health settings to reach underserved children. Although hygienists' costs in providing services are lower than dentists' costs, reimbursement rates that cover overhead costs are equally important for them. A recent study examining a model for school-based hygiene services found that reimbursement rates had to be at least 60.5% of mean national fees for the model to be sustainable and that only 5 of 13 states examined had fees that met that threshold.[17]

Finally, states can use general fund dollars to leverage the purchasing power of Medicaid (which itself leverages a federal match by state dollars). Wisconsin appropriates $632,000 annually to support a Federally Qualified Health Center with multiple clinics in rural northern areas of the state. The enhanced Medicaid reimbursements to which these clinics have access—which make up the difference between regular Medicaid payment rates and the clinics' cost of providing care—help sustain large-group dental practices that provide employment for community members and increase Medicaid enrollees' use of care by allowing them to access that care closer to home.[15]

REGULATION OF HEALTH FACILITIES AND PROFESSIONALS

The second critical function that has a significant impact on access to care for children is the regulation of facilities and health professionals. The primary vehicle for this regulation is the state dental practice act, which establishes the legal framework for the practice of dentistry. Dental practice acts define in very broad terms what constitutes the practice of dentistry and who is qualified to obtain a license to practice. This broad authority gives dentists and physicians—and no others—the right to perform any of those functions legally. Licensure for dentists began as an offshoot of medical licensure; the Alabama medical board issued the first dental license in 1841. As the science advanced and techniques and education became more standardized, practitioners sought both recognition of their profession and limits on who could practice legally. In the 1870s, local and state dental societies pressed for and won state licensure and "the elimination of charlatans" from the field.[18] As new types of providers, such as nurses, assistants, and hygienists, were developed, licensure laws were amended to recognize them, to define what services they could perform, and to give physicians and dentists the authority to supervise and delegate authority to them. Legal authority for new providers essentially was carved out of the services physicians and dentists could perform, so that only the whole package of services in the law was defined as "practicing medicine" or "practicing dentistry."

The fact that this broad authority is set in law places physicians and dentists at the top of the profession, defending its prerogatives against all comers.[19] The difficulty with this situation is that all professions evolve over time, strengthening and expanding their competency, but the law stays the same. Physicians and dentists, once licensed, need not prove their competency to perform any specific function, even though they are not all trained to perform, or are experienced or comfortable in performing, all the functions known to medicine and dentistry. Not everyone who is a dentist can perform complex oral surgery, or do orthodontics, or care for a very young child or a patient who has special needs. Yet, dental hygienists or assistants, or new providers, who seek legal authority to perform specific procedures they have been trained to do— and may be allowed to do in a different state—must prove competency. Legal authority is required before a provider can undertake an expanded scope of practice, but it is difficult to demonstrate that competency when the performance is prohibited. Legislators, most of whom are not clinicians, have great difficulty weighing the conflicting arguments about the safety or risks related to changes in scope of practice for providers. Therefore, dental and medical practice acts are very difficult to amend even though they should be updated regularly to ensure that the public benefits from advances in science, education, and the health care system.

Physicians and dentists see medical and dental practice acts as crucial to their control over their profession. They fight any "encroachments" by other providers seeking amendments to recognize their training or ability to perform new functions. Their objections to changes in the law may not consider objectively the clinical competency of other providers or the quality of care they could provide but rather seem to derive from an interest in retaining hegemony over the profession and an understandable desire to control their ability to operate profitable businesses in the face of uncertain economies and reimbursements.[19] The viability of health care providers' businesses is and should remain a concern for policymakers; but it should be balanced against the state's responsibility to ensure access to care for citizens and to promote competition and consumer choice. These considerations are major factors in the regulation of almost all other services and sectors of the economy (eg, transportation, utilities, and telecommunications) and should be no different for medicine and dentistry.

Given the challenges in regulating health providers, change can be slow. Although the integration of dental hygienists into dental practice is a given today, it was not always so. The first state to recognize hygienists was Connecticut in 1907, followed by Massachusetts and New York in 1915 and 1916, respectively. By 1948, only two thirds of the states licensed hygienists, and some limited their practice to schools and clinics because of opposition from organized dentistry. Many dentists in private practice who performed dental cleanings themselves "looked upon this new intruder as a competitor."[18] Now, most dentists employ dental hygienists. A sizable portion of visits to the dentists, and of private practice income, stems from services hygienists provide.

In practical terms, legislatures enact dental practice acts, and state boards of dentistry or dental examiners implement them by writing and enforcing rules and regulations. The fact that this process occurs in each state, rather than at the federal level, leads to a confusing patchwork of laws governing the profession. These laws bear little relationship to the actual clinical competency of the providers they govern or the needs of patients, neither of which vary by jurisdiction, or to the most efficient use of health care resources. Instead, the great differences between what a specific type of provider can do in each state reflects the relative political and financial power of different provider groups, not their education, training, or competency. For example, in Washington State, dental assistants who meet certain requirements in experience and training can apply sealants and fluorides under general supervision in school-based programs,[20] but in eight states registered dental hygienists (who typically have more training than dental assistants) cannot apply sealants without a dentist present.[21] Variation across states in teeth, or patients, or even provider education, does not account for those differences. According to workforce experts at the University of California, "Because legal scopes of practice can facilitate or hinder patients from seeing a particular type of health provider, the regulations have direct impacts on access to and cost of care. Quality of care may also be affected **Fig. 3**."[22]

An example that highlights an opportunity for state policymakers to improve access is the requirement in some states for supervision of hygienists when applying sealants. Sealants are clear plastic coatings applied to the chewing surfaces of molars that keep cavity-causing bacteria from invading. Ninety percent of cavities occur in molars, so a population-based strategy of applying sealants in second

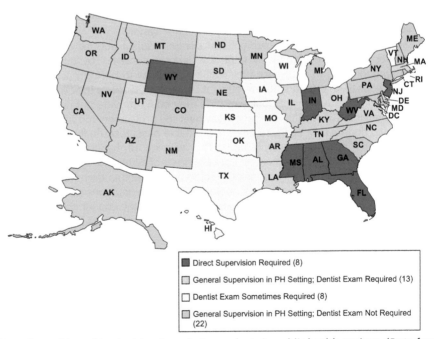

Fig. 3. Supervision of hygienists when placing sealants in public health settings. (*Data from* American Dental Hygienists' Association. Sealant application—settings and supervision by state. September 2008. Available at: http://www.adha.org/governmental_affairs/downloads/sealant.pdf. Accessed December 10, 2008.)

and third grade (when a child's first permanent molars come in) can deliver signifi-cant preventive benefits for many years afterward. Most sealant programs target chil-dren in at-risk schools and communities, particularly children receiving free or reduced-cost lunch programs, those on Medicaid, and racial and ethnic minorities, who are less likely to have regular access to oral health care. Children in racial and ethnic minorities are three times more likely to have untreated decay and are only one third as likely to receive sealants.[23]

Dental hygienists are widely recognized as the appropriate providers to apply seal-ants to children's teeth. In many states, however, organized dentistry has insisted that children be seen by a dentist before a hygienist applies sealants. The requirement that dentists screen a child first and be present while the sealants are applied is scientifi-cally unnecessary and economically impractical. A committee of the ADA issued new guidelines in March, 2008 indicating that sealants are protective against the progres-sion of decay, even if a molar has "incipient decay." (Detection of "incipient decay" had been the most frequently cited reason for requiring a dentists' diagnosis before sealant placement.[24]) Requiring dentists to examine a child raises the cost of sealant programs, makes the programs more difficult to administer (because dentists willing to participate are in short supply), and limits the number of children that can be pro-tected from future decay.

Policymakers have a number of levers at their disposal to affect the regulation of the profession and improve access. Governors appoint members to the state board of dentistry and thus can influence decisions by varying the background and expe-rience of appointees. State legislatures can influence a state board by changing the number and types of members the board should include, such as such as hygien-ists, public health dentists, and members of the public. Both appointments and membership structure can affect board decisions. In addition, workforce experts cite an "inherent conflict of allowing one professional board to govern members of a different profession" as a reason for establishing a different regulatory structure for each profession.[22] (Thus nurses are self-regulated rather than governed by state boards of medicine.) State policymakers can establish separate committees of a state board to provide advice or to oversee the practice of dental hygiene, can spell out what power those committees have, and can assure the committees' recommendations to the full board are considered seriously. At least three states have established a separate regulatory structure for hygienists. Since the 1980s, the State of Washington has had a dental hygiene advisory committee that functions independently of the dental commission. New Mexico has had a dental hygienists' committee since 1994, and Iowa has had one since 1999. These committees make recommendations to the Board of Dental Examiners that must be followed unless some reasonable objection is made.[22]

States also set requirements for licensure and certification that govern the move-ment of providers between states and countries. State dental practice acts set the requirements for licensure of providers in a state, but state boards have latitude in in-terpreting the law. Because there is a great uniformity in dental education in the United States, 46 states allow licensure by credential or reciprocity, so that a dentist with a valid license who has been in practice for a set period (usually 5 years) in another state can get a license without sitting for the state examination (only four states do not: Delaware, Florida, Hawaii, and Nevada).[25] The movement of dentists between countries, however, is made difficult or impossible by licensing laws in most states that require all dentists to have graduated from an American or Canadian dental school accredited by the ADA Council on Dental Accreditation.[26] A few states, however, have programs that draw foreign dental graduates into underserved areas and allow them to practice for 2 years, after which they can pursue a regular license. In Maryland, for instance, the board of dentistry issues licenses to pediatric dentists that are limited to graduates of a United States–based residency program who practice in a sponsoring hospital, clinic, or dental school.[27]

A few states have changed their legal and regulatory framework to foster innovation, improve consistency, and make scientifically sound recommendations to legislatures. California has established a legal authority for its health department to operate workforce pilot projects.[28] Under this program, schools, clinics, hospitals, or government entities can apply to develop a new type of provider or to propose a new scope of practice or supervision level for existing providers. This program was used to develop and test Registered Dental Hygienists in Alternative Practice, and the authority was made permanent by the legislature in 1997. It currently is being used to develop a Community Oral Health Professional, an innovative dental auxiliary designed to assist patients who have special needs; hygienists with a slightly expanded scope of practice will work in collaborative practice with a dentist, using teledentistry communication technology to provide consultations.

Further, to reduce the difficulty with interstate movement and consumer and regulatory confusion, the Pew Commission favored uniform standards to measure providers' knowledge and skills and recommended that states use consistent regulatory terminology coupled with reciprocal licensure by endorsement. The Physician Payment Review Commission endorsed model practice acts for practitioners. Three national associations have called for standardized terminology.[29] Montana adopted a Uniform Licensing Act in 1995.

Another key element of dental practice acts is a little-known set of provisions that govern who can own a dental practice or employ a dentist. Few state legislators are familiar with these laws, which are called "bans on the corporate practice of dentistry." Their modification is a seldom-exercised policy lever that has potential to improve access to care. The ADA believes these laws are necessary to prevent "interference with the professional judgment of a dentist,"[30] but they also have been used to keep out managed care, to stifle alternative delivery system models, to limit the expansion of the safety net, and to preserve dentistry as a cottage industry.[31] They also strictly limit dentists' choices in how and where they can practice. Fully 26 states define the ownership of a dental practice as an element of practicing dentistry, and five more prohibit anyone but a dentist from operating a dental practice.[32] Exceptions are narrow. For instance, many states have altered the law so that widows of dentists can operate the practice while seeking a buyer. Other exceptions have been made to allow community health centers or charity clinics to hire a dentist, but even these exceptions can be controversial in some states among dentists who believe that clinics are unfair competition. It is important for policymakers to take a fresh look at these laws and to work closely with their state dental society, state health officials, coalitions, safety net hospitals and clinics, and community groups to examine the potential for common-sense safety net exceptions, as well as exceptions for new models of service delivery. For example, access to care could be increased for vulnerable people if a group of nursing homes could employ a dentist to serve its residents or a rural hospital could open a dental clinic and employ a dentist to staff it. Dentists would have more choices for employment if they could belong to a group practice that included pediatricians, nurses, pediatric dentists, hygienists, and orthodontists who wanted to provide "one-stop shopping" for children and their families. Currently, most dental practice laws prohibit all these "corporate" options, although none of them poses a threat to public health or safety.

PUBLIC HEALTH

The third critical function that states perform in regard to oral health is the maintenance of a public health infrastructure to monitor the oral health status of citizens and to organize public health responses to identified needs. Public health responses are interventions intended to prevent disease in the population as a whole, not just for people in a public program. Although these programs have the greatest potential for improving oral health of all policy areas, they often are given short shrift in funding battles and policy debates. States monitor oral health status and deliver population-based preventive care through fluoridation and school-based or school-linked sealant programs. The state health department coordinates those responses, usually through a state dental director who provides leadership and internal support for the state's efforts.

The most effective public oral health program, bar none, is community water fluoridation, which the Centers for Disease Control and Prevention (CDC) has identified as one of 10 great public health achievements of the twentieth century. Adjusting fluoride levels (because it occurs naturally in water) is a safe, low-cost way to reduce decay rates by up to 60%, but only 69% of Americans on public water systems have optimal levels of fluoride in their water, a percentage that is below the Healthy People 2010 goal of 75%.[33] Some states, such as Illinois, have instituted state mandates for water fluoridation,[34] and some, such as Kentucky, have achieved almost universal fluoridation through regulation. In most states, the decision to fluoridate is made by individual cities and towns through ballot initiatives or referenda. These ballot measures often fail because of misperceptions about fluoride or lack of funding. Opponents of fluoridation spread unfounded beliefs and instill fear about adverse health consequences from exposure to fluoride, even though the safety of water fluoridation has been well documented by more than half a century of scientific study. Further, a recent CDC report suggested that more than $1.5 billion dollars could be saved annually, and the oral health of high-risk communities could be improved significantly, if the remaining public water supplies were fluoridated.[35,36] Louisiana and Texas also have performed state-specific estimates of the averted costs in Medicaid from community water fluoridation.[37,38] In a "local control" situation, state policymakers can promote water fluoridation by providing grants, matching funds, or short-term loans to localities for the initial purchase of equipment and by serving as credible champions in public debates surrounding fluoridation referenda.

The other major dental public health strategy that states have adopted is school-based and school-linked sealant programs. State oral health programs often have to cobble together limited funding for these programs from federal, state, and philanthropic sources, limiting the reach of sealant programs. As **Fig. 4** shows, 22 states reported having less than $1 million in combined funding from all federal and state sources – including Medicaid, the CDC, the Maternal and Child Health Block Grant, and state appropriations. In fact, in 2007, only three fourths of states reported having any state-organized sealant program,[39] and only six states were able to assure that at least 50% of third-grade children had received at least one sealant.[40] Policymakers can mobilize their state's resources to harness the preventive power of sealants by ensuring that the state dental director has adequate support to guide development of county/local programs, dedicating state funds to bulk purchasing sealant materials, financially supporting local sealant programs, streamlining the process for these programs to bill Medicaid and SCHIP for eligible patients, and adopting practice laws that maximize dental hygienists' ability to reach at-risk children in schools without overly burdensome requirements for the presence or prescription of a dentist.

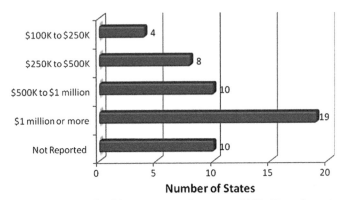

Fig. 4. Funding for state oral health programs, all sources, 2007. (*Data from* Association of State and Territorial Dental Directors. Summary report: synopses of state dental public health programs—data for FY 2006–2007. New Bern, NC: Association of State and Territorial Dental Directors; 2008. p. 14.)

A state dental director is a valuable resource for policymakers who are seeking to advance an oral health agenda. The director is a dental public health professional (often holding a dental or dental hygiene degree, as well as a master's degree in public health) who provides leadership for the state's fluoridation and sealant programs, coordinates local efforts, and keeps initiatives moving. The CDC has funded 16 states to bolster their dental directors' ability to perform three critical functions: (1) to develop an oral health plan that specifies goals and responsibilities among state and community actors; (2) to build an oral health coalition that includes representation from stakeholders such as professional organizations, safety net providers, families, employers, and others to meet those goals; and (3) to perform surveillance of sealant and other programs to assess progress toward the state's oral health goals.[41] Forty-six states reported having a dental director in 2007, but staffing beyond that position is lean. Almost half of states reported having three or fewer full-time employees dedicated to oral health, and four states had a less than-full-time dental director.[39] To support smart decision making, state policymakers should ensure that there is sufficient public health infrastructure and relevant data to know the extent of the burden of unmet dental disease and to determine whether the state's interventions to combat that disease are working.

EDUCATION AND TRAINING OF THE HEALTH CARE WORKFORCE

The fourth key state function is the education and training of health care providers. Although this function attracts less attention than provider regulation, it is enormously important and commands significant resources. The public operates dental schools; in 2000, there were 35 schools of dentistry at public universities, 14 dental schools at private universities, and 5 that were public/private. Likewise, many of the 280 dental hygiene programs in the United States are housed in state and community colleges and university dental schools. The public commits funds to dental education: in 2000, about one third of dental school funding ($500 million) came from public sources (although state support has been dwindling).[42] The public has a legitimate interest in having a dental workforce that is trained to provide care to people who need it most, but the skills and practice habits that dental students acquire often prepare them to treat only highly compliant, relatively noncomplex, adolescents and adults. This situation leads to practicing dentists who have little familiarity with or comfort in caring for the oral health needs of groups such as very young children or people who have disabilities. Indeed, the ADA's Commission on Dental Accreditation requires that "Graduates [of accredited dental schools] must be competent in assessing the *treatment needs* of patients with special needs" (emphasis added) but not that graduates be competent in the special techniques required to provide care to those patients.[43] Likewise, the education of dentists is poorly integrated with the education of medical providers, a situation that contributes to poor coordination between practicing doctors and dentists. Many state public health and Medicaid programs are trying to change the situation by attaching incentive payments to training for general dentists to treat children under age 3 years (eg, Washington State's "Access to Baby and Child Dentistry" program, which has been operating in counties across the state since the 1990s, provides enhanced Medicaid payments to general dentists who receive training on how to manage very young children in the dental office),[44] for dentists to care for people who have developmental disabilities (eg, New Mexico allows dentists who complete in-person and online training in care-management techniques for people who have developmental disabilities to receive an enhanced per-visit fee through a "Special Needs Code"),[45] and for physicians to provide limited preventive oral health services (eg, North Carolina's "Into the Mouths of Babes" project, which works in tandem with the state Medicaid program and was the first in the nation to train pediatricians and family practice physicians to provide basic oral health assessments, anticipatory guidance, and fluoride varnish applications).[46] Currently, more than half the states reimburse physicians for some oral health services.[47]

Increased or redesigned state support, which is important in funding clinic space, maintaining equipment, subsidizing tuition, and recruiting faculty, could be used to shape the dental school curriculum better, to encourage or require admissions of qualified students from underserved groups or geographic areas, and to establish community-based rotations for dental students. Such a redesigned curriculum could emphasize ways to incorporate Medicaid into a practice's payor mix, help build bridges between dentistry and other health professions, and convey messages about dentists' social responsibilities as health care providers and not just as business owners.[47] There is significant interest across the country in the model pursued by the new Arizona School of Dentistry and Oral Health at A.T. Still University, a private school. Its admission criteria include not just academic merit but also "demonstrated community service through volunteerism or service-oriented employment."[48,49] Although it is a rather new school, a much higher proportion of its graduates enter dental public health and accept Medicaid when they graduate than do the graduates of traditional model dental schools.

One reason that many new dentists focus on the "business" aspect of dentistry is the high debt burden that they carry when they graduate. In 2002, graduating students had an average debt burden of $107,500. Only 12% of students graduate without debt.[50] Lower levels of debt—achieved either through keeping tuition rates reasonable or offering more financial aid—make it easier for dentists to consider a public health career or to maintain a private practice that accepts Medicaid and other low-income patients. Reasonable tuition and more financial aid also open dental education to more students from disadvantaged backgrounds. Loan repayment programs are one strategy that states use to give new dentists incentives to practice in rural and underserved areas for a set period of time.[51] In 2005, about half of the states reported having formal loan repayment programs, either specifically for dentists or for providers including dentists.[52,53] Loan repayment programs gained popularity in the 1990s as a cheaper and more effective alternative to scholarship programs.

States have long funded dental and other health care professional education because of the hope that at least a portion of the graduates would stay in the state to practice and improve residents' access to care. In fact, more graduates of publicly funded dental schools than graduates of private schools tend to stay in the state where they were trained.[51] Some rural states purchase seats for students from underserved areas, in exchange for their agreement to return to the area to practice. The 18 states without a dental school often belong to or operate interstate compacts, paying a subsidy to reserve a set number of slots for residents of their states to attend and pay in state tuition. A well-known example is the Western Interstate Commission on Higher Education, in which 15 states purchase slots for their residents in a variety of professional training programs.[42] Maine also has an agreement to purchase slots for its residents outside the country, in a Canadian dental school.

SUMMARY

Space does not permit full discussion of the other state functions mentioned in the introduction, but policy in those other areas contributes substantially to access to dental care as well. State policymakers should not ignore the functions of regulating insurance, cost containment, informing the public about dental health and the functioning of the health system, and monitoring the system. Historically, organized dentistry has exerted a great deal of control over many aspects of the profession and has resisted many policy changes pushed by advocates or policymakers to expand access to care for underserved groups. The policy framework for dental care set out by states is intended to do many things: to provide a financial base for care for low-income citizens; to deliver care directly; to establish rules for credentialing and licensing an adequate supply of competent providers; to ensure the health of the public through population-based initiatives; and to educate (and, it is hoped, to retain) health care providers. Actions by legislators and executive branch officials to regulate dentistry and influence dental practice are an essential function of governance that is needed to ensure access to care and public safety and to establish a level playing field; these regulations are not unfair or unnecessary interference, as dental groups sometimes suggest. This article has outlined the basic structure of public policy in access to dental care and has highlighted the many opportunities for policy change that can expand access to dental care for those who lack it. As discussed here, decision makers in the state legislative and executive branches have a broader array of tools than many realize to build a dental system that delivers the health care that citizens need.

REFERENCES

1. McDonough JE. Introduction to state health policy: workshop for new legislators. Powerpoint presentation at the Agency for Healthcare Research and Quality, May 15, 2005.
2. Monthly Medicaid enrollment for children and monthly SCHIP enrollment. Available at: http://www.statehealthfacts.org. Accessed December 1, 2008.
3. Snyder A. SCHIP dental benefits. Portland (ME): National Academy for State Health Policy; 2007.
4. U.S. Congress House. Children's Health Insurance Program Reauthorization Act of 2007, Title V, Section 501, Dental Benefits. 110th Congress. H.R. 3963. Available at: http://frwebgate.access.gpo.gov/cgi-bin/getdoc.cgi?dbname=110_cong_bills &docid=f:h3963enr.txt.pdf. Accessed December 1, 2008.

5. Perkins J. National Health Law Program: docket of Medicaid cases to improve dental access. Available at: http://www.healthlaw.org/library/item.157322; 2007. Accessed December 10, 2008.
6. Manski RJ, Brown E. MEPS Chartbook No. 17. Dental use, expenses, dental coverage, and changes: 1996 and 2004. Rockville (MD): Agency for Healthcare Research and Quality; 2007. p. 13.
7. New York State Department of Health. Oral health care in pregnancy and early childhood. In: Kumar J, Samuelson R, editors. Oral health care during pregnancy and early childhood practice guidelines. Albany (NY): New York State Department of Health; 2006. p. 14–5.
8. Milgrom P, Ludwig S, Shirtcliff RM, et al. Providing a dental home for pregnant women: a community program to address dental care access—a brief communication. J Public Health Dent 2008;68:170–3.
9. McGinn-Shapiro M. Medicaid coverage of adult dental services. Portland (ME): National Academy for State Health Policy; 2008.
10. Snyder A, Gehshan S. State health reform: how do dental benefits fit in? Options for policy makers. Portland (ME): National Academy for State Health Policy; 2008.
11. Social Security Act §1902(a)(30)(A). Available at: http://www.ssa.gov/OP_Home/ssact/title19/1902.htm.
12. Gehshan S, Snyder A, Paradise J. Filling an urgent need: improving children's access to dental care in medicaid and SCHIP. Washington, DC: Kaiser Commission on Medicaid and Uninsured; 2008.
13. Borchgrevink A, Snyder A, Gehshan S. The effects of Medicaid reimbursement rates on access to dental care. Portland (ME): National Academy for State Health Policy; 2008.
14. CMS Medicaid Statistical Information System. Available at: http://www.cms.hhs.gov/MedicaidDataSourcesGenInfo/02_MSISData.asp. Accessed October, 2007.
15. Snyder A. Increasing access to dental care in Medicaid: targeted programs for four populations. Washington, DC: National Academy for State Health Policy and Pew Charitable Trusts; 2009.
16. Cantrell C. Physicians' role in children's oral health. Portland (ME): National Academy for State Health Policy; 2008.
17. Bailit H, Beazoglou T, Drodzdowski M. Financial feasibility of a model school-based program in different states. Public Health Rep 2008;123(6):761–7.
18. Bremner MDK. The story of dentistry from the dawn of civilization to the present. Brooklyn (NY): Dental Items of Interest Publishing House; 1946. p. 125, 301, 302.
19. Safriet BJ. Closing the gap between can and may in health-care providers' scopes of practice: a primer for policymakers. Yale J Regul 2002;19:301, 316.
20. Dental Assisting National Board. State-specific dental assisting information. Available at: http://danb.org/PDFs/Charts/Washington.pdf. Accessed November 29, 2008.
21. American Dental Hygienists' Association. Dental hygiene practice act overview, permitted functions and supervision levels by state. Available at: http://adha.org/governmental_affairs/downloads/fiftyone.pdf. Accessed November 29, 2008.
22. Dower C, Christian S, O'Neil E. Promising scope of practice models for the health professions. University of California, San Francisco Center for the Health Professions. San Francisco (CA): University of California; 2007. p. 1.
23. Gehshan S, Wyatt M. Improving oral health care for young children. Portland (ME): National Academy for State Health Policy; 2007.

24. Beauchamp J, Caufield P, Crall JJ, et al. Evidence-based clinical recommendations for the use of pit-and-fissure sealants. J Am Dent Assoc 2008;139: 257–68.

25. American Dental Association, Department of State Government Affairs. License recognition: dentists. Available at: http://ada.org/prof/prac/licensure/licensure_recognition.pdf. Accessed November 29, 2008.

26. Summary of state educational requirements for international dentists. Available at: http://creativesmileinstitute.com/Documents/licensure_state_requirements_intl.pdf. Accessed December 11, 2008.

27. Maryland State Board of Dental Examiners. Forms and applications. Available at: http://dhmh.md.gov/dental/forms_original.htm. Accessed December 10, 2008.

28. California Office of Statewide Health Planning and Development, Healthcare Workforce Development Division. Health workforce pilot projects program: frequently asked questions. Available at: http://www.oshpd.ca.gov/HWDD/HWPP_faqs.html. Accessed December 8, 2008

29. Sage WM, Aiken LH. Regulating interdisciplinary practice. In: Jost TS, editor. Regulation of the healthcare professions. Chicago (IL); Health Administration Press: p. 71–1.

30. American Dental Association. Available at: http://ada.org/prof/advocacy/issues/ownership_practices.pdf. Accessed November 23, 2008.

31. Gehshan S, Straw T. Access to oral health services for low income people: policy barriers and opportunities for intervention for the Robert Wood Johnson Foundation. Washington, DC; National Conference of State Legislatures; October, 2002.

32. American Dental Association, Department of State Government Affairs. Number 22, ownership interference, October 16, 2007. Available at: http://ada.org/prof/advocacy/issues/ownership_practices.pdf. Accessed November 29, 2008.

33. Centers for Disease Control and Prevention. Water fluoridation statistics for 2006. Available at: http://www.cdc.gov/fluoridation/statistics/2006stats.htm. Accessed December 31, 2008.

34. IFLOSS Coalition. Illinois oral health plan II. Springfield (IL): IFLOSS Coalition; 2007. p. 7. Available at: http://www.ifloss.org/OralHealth/plan2.html. Accessed December 31, 2008.

35. Chadwick A, Lamia T, Zaro-Moore J. Building capacity to fluoridate—literature review. Centers for Disease Control and Prevention. Available at: http://www.cdc.gov/fluoridation/pdf/fluoride_campaign_lit_review.doc. Accessed December 31, 2008.

36. Centers for Disease Control and Prevention. Preventing dental caries with community programs. Available at: http://www.cdc.gov/Oralhealth/factsheets/dental_caries.htm. Accessed April 13, 2009.

37. National Conference of State Legislatures. State health lawmakers' digest: water fluoridation March 2003; vol. 3, No. 2. Available at: http://www.ncsl.org/programs/health/forum/shld/32.pdf. Accessed December 31, 2008.

38. Texas Department of Health. Water fluoridation reduces cost of dental care. Disease Prevention News 2002;62:4. Available at: http://www.dshs.state.tx.us/idcu/health/dpn/issues/dpn62n04.pdf. Accessed December 12, 2008.

39. Association of State and Territorial Dental Directors. Summary report: synopses of state dental public health programs—data for FY 2006–2007. New Bern (NC): Association of State and Territorial Dental Directors; 2008. p. 14.

40. National Oral Health Surveillance System. Available at: http://www.cdc.gov/nohss. Accessed November 15, 2008.

41. Centers for Disease Control and Prevention. CDC-funded states: cooperative agreements. Available at: http://www.cdc.gov/oralhealth/state_programs/cooperative_agreements/index.htm. Accessed December 31, 2008.

42. Byck GR, Kaste LM, Cooksey JA, et al. Dental student enrollment and graduation: a report by state, census division, and region. J Dent Educ 2006;70(10): 1023–37.

43. Commission on Dental Accreditation. Accreditation standards for dental education programs. Chicago: American Dental Association; 2008. Available at: http://www.ada.org/prof/ed/accred/commission/news/proposed_predoc.pdf. Accessed November 15, 2008.

44. Access to Baby and Child Dentistry program. Available at: http://www.abcd-dental.org. Accessed December 10, 2008.

45. Association of State and Territorial Dental Directors Best Practice Approaches for State and Community Oral Health Programs. Practice #34005 – The New Mexico special needs dental procedure code. Available at: http://www.astdd.org/bestpractices/pdf/DES34005NMspecialneedsdentalcode.pdf.

46. Into the Mouths of Babes project. Available at: http://www.communityhealth.dhhs.state.nc.us/dental/Into_the_Mouths_of_Babes.htm.

47. Maternal and Child Oral Health Resource Center. State medicaid reimbursement policies for oral health services provided by medical staff. Available at: http://www.mchoralhealth.org/feedback/reimbursementchart6_08.pdf. Accessed November 23, 2008

48. Nash D. A larger sense of purpose: dentistry and society. J Am Coll Dent 2007; 74(2):27–33.

49. Davis E, et al. Serving the public good: challenges of dental education in the twenty-first century. J Dent Educ 2007;71(8):1009–19.

50. Arizona School of Dentistry and Oral Health. Doctor of Dental Medicine Admission Guidelines. Available at: http://www.atsu.edu/asdoh/programs/dental_medicine/admission_requirements.htm. Accessed December 31, 2008.

51. Neumann LM. Trends in dental and allied dental education. J Am Dent Assoc 2004;135:1253–9.

52. Lin HL, Rowland ML, Fields HW. In-state graduate retention for US dental schools. J Dent Educ 2006;70(12):1320–7.

53. National Conference of State Legislatures Forum for State Health Policy Leadership. In: Goodwin K, editor. State experiences with dental loan repayment programs. Washington, DC: National Conference of State Legislatures; 2005.

Innovations to Improve Oral Health Care Access

Gary A. Colangelo, DDS, MGA*

KEYWORDS

• Oral • Health • Care • Access • Innovation

Concern about access to oral health care has been expressed by the dental profession since its organizing years in the nineteenth century. Concern by patients or their advocates, non-dental health care professionals, and policy makers is articulated most often after the realization that uncontrolled oral diseases have negative effects for both individuals and society. Each individual or organization addressing access to oral health care has its own motivations, perspectives, experiences, and tools, and these assets often lead to innovations that improve access. Effective innovations often are the result of collaborations between dentists, advocacy groups, and policy makers, but innovations also can result from changes in public policy or judicial decisions that are not related to the issues of oral health care access. In the twenty-first century the process of collaboration, development of health care policy, initiatives for care delivery, and legislative changes continues to be the wellspring of innovation to improve access.

This article highlights past and contemporary innovations and initiatives that have improved access or have the potential to improve access. These innovations are grouped into six categories: the dental profession; public health; community-based care delivery; oral health care funding, dental education; and evidence-based dentistry.

THE DENTAL PROFESSION

Innovation to improve access to oral health care began with the founding of the dental profession in the nineteenth century. Current innovations by the American Dental Association are discussed elsewhere in this issue, but the dental profession has a rich history in improving access through the marketing of professional services. Edgar Randolph ("Painless") Parker (1872–1952) promoted his practice empire using blatant advertising that was characterized as unethical and fraudulent by the dental profession. Parker defended his advertising by saying, "I have spent more time fighting for better teeth for more people than any other man."[1] Although Parker was

---

Baltimore College of Dental Surgery, Dental School, University of Maryland, 650 West Baltimore Street, Baltimore, MD, USA
* Corresponding author. 39 Kenmare Way, Rehoboth Beach, DE 19971-1071.
E-mail address: garycolangelo2@comcast.net

Dent Clin N Am 53 (2009) 591–608
doi:10.1016/j.cden.2009.03.002
0011-8532/09/$ – see front matter © 2009 Elsevier Inc. All rights reserved.

shunned by the dental profession, his innovative advertising techniques became standard practice in the twentieth century. In 1931 the American Dental Association, with the financial support of manufacturers of oral health products, embarked on a $500,000 advertising campaign to promote oral health to the more than 36 million Americans who did not take care of their teeth.[2] The dental profession continued to forbid the use of advertising by individual dentists until 1977, when the Supreme Court ruled in *Bates-O'Steen v. State Bar of Arizona* that the legal profession's restrictions on advertising were in restraint of trade. The Federal Trade Commission applied this decision to all learned professions and in 1979 settled out of court with the American Dental Association, which no longer could restrict truthful advertising by dentists.[3] Since the Federal Trade Commission settlement, advertising has become a standard dental business practice that, along with the advertising of oral health products, improves access to care by increasing awareness of oral health, reducing costs through increased competition, and increasing consumer knowledge of the availability of service and the importance of disease prevention.[1] Dentists and dental service organizations continue to innovate in advertising through brand development, electronic and printed media, Web sites, e-mail communications, direct mail, and billboards. Although advertising may increase awareness of the importance of oral health, it is not known which form of dental advertising is most effective in improving awareness or what specific effects advertising has on access to oral health care.

The dental profession is regulated by state law through dental boards that typically are composed of dentists, dental hygienists, and consumer representatives. Because workforce qualifications and scope of practice are controlled by state boards, an opportunity to improve access to oral health care exists in permitting alternative models of care delivery by expanding the scope of practice of dental hygienists, physicians, and other health care professionals. In six states (Connecticut, Iowa, New Mexico, North Carolina, South Carolina, and Washington) where dental practice laws or regulations were changed to allow dental hygienists or physicians an expanded role in providing preventive services, however, there was no immediate effect on the delivery of preventive health care. Impediments to establishing a new workforce model can include provider acceptance, lack of funding, and facility costs. Improved access through permitted alternative models of care remains elusive.[4]

Mobile dental care is an innovative alternative for patients who cannot access conventional office-based care. The State of South Carolina regulates mobile and portable dental operations by requiring the registration of these facilities to prevent perceived fraudulent operations. Dental Access Mobile Clinics, LLC successfully applies an entrepreneurial model to deliver comprehensive care to children at their schools in six South Carolina counties. In 2001, 14,700 visits of 5000 children were recorded.[5] Other attempts to deliver mobile dental care may not be successful because of the reliance on low and inconsistent Medicaid dental funding rather than a mixed funding stream of self-pay, private insurance, and Medicaid. Dental Access Mobile Clinics, LLC also may be successful because it is a dentist-developed enterprise.

It is projected that in 2010 there will be 180,875 professionally active dentists in the United States, most of whom were trained in United States dental schools.[6] The projected number of professionally active foreign-trained dentists is not known. Information about the success rate of foreign-trained graduates in qualifying examinations could provide insight on foreign-trained graduates who practice, but privacy concerns limit this indicator.[7] From 1993 to 2002 the number of foreign-trained dentists admitted to United States dental schools decreased from 930 to 441.[8] Because the most common path to dental licensure for foreign-trained dentists is completion of a United States dental degree, the licensing of foreign graduates seems to be declining. This decline may affect dental manpower and thus access to oral health care. In contrast, nearly 25% of United States physicians are foreign trained, and many of these physicians practice in the inner city, in small communities, and in poor rural areas.[9] Indeed, without professionally active foreign-trained physicians in the United States, the lack of medical care access would be catastrophic. The lack of dentists willing to treat the underserved could be improved if the number of foreign-trained dentists practicing in the United States was comparable to the medical professions.

PUBLIC HEALTH INTERVENTIONS

The concept of public health, as it is known today, did not exist in this country in the eighteenth and nineteenth centuries, and dealing with outbreaks of disease was stymied by a lack of knowledge of disease causation.[10] Oral disease was treated on an individual basis with no population-based disease control. It was not until the 1860s that the federal government began to consider the importance of access to oral health care. In the context of military preparedness, Secretary of War Jefferson Davis, serving under President Pierce, advocated for a dental corps, and as President of the Confederacy Davis instituted a dental program, which the Union Army lacked.[11] An Atlanta dentist, James Baxter Bean, established the first military hospital program to treat maxillofacial trauma using interdental splints. Confederate Surgeon General Moore promoted this technique by having Bean establish a ward at a hospital in Richmond that provided maxillofacial trauma care and also elevated the status of the dental profession by recognizing the importance of dentistry in the treatment of trauma.[11]

After the Civil War, The Quarantine Act of 1878 conferred national quarantine authority on the Marine Hospital Service, which evolved into the Public Health and Marine Hospital Service in 1902. The growth of biologic knowledge and sanitary reform in the late nineteenth century coupled with political influence of the Progressive Movement provided the impetus for rapid expansion of the Service and its renaming by Congress as the Public Health Service with broad national authority over disease control and sanitation. The importance of dentistry in public health was demonstrated by Frederick McKay and H. Trendley Dean, who promoted the importance of optimal fluoride in the water supply. Dean was one of the first dentists commissioned in the Public Health Service and became the first dental research scientist of the new National Institute of Health in 1931.[10]

The innovations of fluoridated water to prevent dental caries, immunization, and the establishment of potable water supplies were collectively the greatest disease prevention initiatives in the history of man. In 2006, 69.2% of the United States population received optimally fluoridated water, although these percentages vary by state.[12] It would not be considered acceptable to have only 69.2% of the United States population immunized against contagious diseases or to have access to potable water, so continued innovations in public policy are needed to establish optimal dietary fluoride levels for all Americans. Current best practice for fluoride prevention therapy includes twice-daily use of a fluoridated dentifrice for children in optimally fluoridated communities and, in fluoride-deficient communities, the additional use of office-applied topical fluoride gel, foam, or varnish.[13] For children without access to fluoridated water or regular oral health care, school-based dental care is an important means of providing oral screening and prevention intervention, including topical fluoride applications. One study, however, determined that children who were susceptible to decay did not benefit appreciably more from any of these preventive measures than did children in general.[14] Other methods of accessing the benefits of fluoride in non-fluoridated communities include school water fluoridation and the use of dietary supplements, fluoride varnish or gel, and fluoride rinses. Communal water fluoridation remains the most cost-effective means to prevent decay at an annual cost of $0.72 (1999 dollars) per capita, whereas fluoride mouth rinses cost $3.29 per capita.[15] Innovation and change in public health policy are needed to improve access to water fluoridation and to meet the Healthy People 2010 objective that 75% of the United States population using public water sources receive fluoridated water. Between 1992 and 2002 five additional states joined the 22 states that already had achieved the Healthy People objective of 75%.[16] Recently, Louisiana enacted Act 761, mandating that community water systems with at least 5000 hookups work with the state to find grants and state funds to implement fluoridation. The Louisiana Dental Association estimates that nearly 2 million citizens will be affected by the new law.[17]

In the United States more than 30,000 new cases and 8000 deaths occur annually from oral and pharyngeal cancers. Public health preventive innovations have focused on tobacco use and alcohol consumption, two factors implicated in these cancers. Oral Health America's National Spit Tobacco Education Program was founded in 1994 as an effort to educate the American public about the dangers of smokeless or spit tobacco, to prevent young people from using spit tobacco, and to help users quit. The program enlists professional baseball personalities to advocate for spit tobacco cessation for both the American public and professional athletes.[18] Recently, many state health departments have conducted oral cancer awareness campaigns aimed at both the general public and non-dental health care providers. The Nevada State Health Division partnered with the University of Nevada School of Medicine Office of Continuing Education, the Northeastern Area Health Education Center, and the Northern Nevada Dental Society to provide all-day continuing education courses on the prevention and detection of oral cancer. The Health Division also maintains an educational oral cancer Web site.[19] There have been no large-scale intervention initiatives for preventing oral cancer by targeting alcohol abuse, but most communities have programs that stress responsible drinking by adults and discourage drinking by young people. These programs are sponsored by local health departments, law enforcement agencies, and alcohol producers and vendors.

There are few initiatives promoting access to early detection of oral and pharyngeal cancers. These conditions are diagnosed most often by dental professionals, but many Americans do not see dentists regularly. All primary care providers should include oral cancer detection in their examinations, but one study found that fewer than 24% of family physicians provided an oral cancer examination to patients 40 years of age and over.[20] In Illinois, a cancer-control partnership was convened, supported by the Illinois Department of Public Health, with representatives from public, private, professional, and voluntary agencies and policymakers in Illinois concerned about cancer. The partnership was charged with providing leadership and a forum for identifying and implementing Illinois' cancer-control priorities. The inclusion of oral cancer into a state comprehensive cancer-control plan capitalizes on resources not normally available to a state oral health program; as a result, Illinois has been able to educate stakeholders on the impact of oral cancer, to build capacity for oral cancer prevention and control, and to obtain funds through the National Institutes of Health to leverage funds from the tobacco master settlement agreement for activities supporting oral cancer prevention.[21]

COMMUNITY-BASED INNOVATIONS

The concept of community-based care began with innovations in primary care delivery in Great Britain in the 1930s[22] and was defined and embodied in the United States by the Institute of Medicine in 1983.[23] Community-based oral health care can replicate or be part of the model of community-based primary care, which has one or more of the following characteristics: provision of population-based care using an assessment of needs; community participation; a focus on health and prevention rather than illness; providing continuous and comprehensive care; sponsorship by religious, secular, or government organizations; integration of social service programs; outreach activities; and demonstration of cultural competency.

The delivery of community-based oral health care is aimed primarily at the dentally underserved. The 1996 Medical Expenditures Panel Survey estimates that 43% of the United States population 2 years of age and older had at least one dental visit during the survey year.[24] Data from the National Health Survey states that in 1997 65.1% of the United States population 2 years of age and older reported having visited a dentist in the preceding year.[25] Even though estimates of overall access to oral health care, as measured by annual dental visits, vary by study, it is well documented that use of and access to professional services also varies by gender, race/ethnicity, and socioeconomic standing and that these differences lead to substantial disparities in care.[26] Americans who belong to populations with a disproportionate lack of access to professional services are or can be served by the delivery of community-based care.

There are five federal resources supporting community-based programs, each offering opportunities for innovation in financing, organizational structure, or outreach to improve access.

Dental Health Professions Shortage Areas (D-HPSAs) are areas identified as having a shortage of dental providers (a population to practitioner ratio of less than 3000:1) and may be urban or rural areas, population groups, or medical or other public facilities. Currently 47 million people live in 3951 identified Health Professions Shortage Areas (HPSAs).[27] The HPSA designation calls attention to areas where access to professional health care services may be inadequate and makes community-based programs eligible for resources such as the assignment of a public health dentist.

The National Health Service Corps (NHSC) is dedicated to improving the health of underserved Americans by supporting communities in need (as identified by D-HPSAs), recruiting and retaining health professionals, developing and preparing sites, and seeking innovative solutions. The NHSC offers programs for both students and clinicians, including scholarships, loan repayment programs, and rotations in Community Health Centers.[28] In 2000, approximately 2526 clinicians, including 306 dental care providers, delivered care to more than 4.6 million people through these programs. Only about 6% of the dental need was being met in the approved 1198 D-HPSAs with a population of 25.9 million persons. It is estimated that an additional 4873 dental care providers are needed to meet the current demand.[29]

Area Health Education Centers are academic and community partnerships that train health care providers in sites and programs that are responsive to state and local needs with the intent of improving the supply, distribution, diversity, and quality of the health care workforce. In a typical year, 37,000 health professions students (17,000 medical students and 20,000 in other health professions, including dental students) are placed in community-based sites.[30]

Federally Qualified Health Centers (FQHCs) are the backbone of community health centers in the United States, with one in three providing dental care.[31] Federal support for entities that later would be called health centers began in 1962 with passage of the Migrant Health Act. Two years later, the Economic Opportunity Act of 1964 provided federal funds for two "neighborhood health centers," which were launched in 1965 by Jack Geiger and Count Gibson, physicians at Tufts University in Boston. In 1991, FQHC's were authorized as part of Medicare when Congress amended §1861(aa) of the Social Security Act. FQHCs were intended to be "safety net" providers for public housing centers, outpatient Indian Health Service facilities, and programs serving migrants and the homeless, but their mission has changed since their founding. They now bring primary health care to the underserved, underinsured, and non-insured people in urban and rural communities through more than 1000 health centers that operate 6000 service delivery sites in every state, the District of Columbia, Puerto Rico, the U.S. Virgin Islands, and the Pacific Basin. FQHCs qualify for enhanced reimbursement from Medicare and Medicaid, as well as other benefits. FQHCs must serve an underserved area or population, offer a sliding fee scale, provide comprehensive services, have an ongoing quality assurance program, and have a governing board of directors.[32] In 2002, the Health Centers Program sought to increase significantly the access to primary health care services through FQHC's. As a result of this initiative, FQHCs provided care for more than 15 million patients in 2006, an increase of more than 4.7 million over 2001. Nearly 2.6 million patients received dental services in 2006, an increase of more than 80% over 1.4 million in 2001.[33]

Medicare Direct Graduate Medical Education (DGME) payment compensates teaching hospitals for some of the costs related directly to the graduate training of physicians, dentists, and other professionals. Medicare does not pay the costs of the clinical portion of medical education of students that occurs in teaching hospitals. In fiscal year 1997, DGME payments for residents were about $2 billion.[34] Academic health centers, teaching hospitals, and community hospitals that receive DGME payments may be located in underserved regions and provide additional manpower through the education program for care or may participate in community-based dental care programs through resident placement. Community-based oral health care programs also can rely on DGME facilities for specialty care referrals.

Examples of Innovative Community-based Dental Programs

Chase Brexton Health Services in Baltimore, Maryland evolved from a single urban location serving only the gay community into a multifaceted health center offering a continuum of care to a diverse, medically underserved community. The program now has two suburban and one rural locations and has incorporated oral health services in two of the community-based programs. The dental population has grown from 743 in 2002 to more than 5000 in 2007 and offers a sliding fee schedule as well as accepting commercial insurance and Medicaid. In the current dental patient population, 57% of the patients are uninsured, 79% are over 21 years of age, 51% are African American, and 16% identify themselves as gay.[35]

"Into the Mouths of Babes" is a collaborative effort of six partners: the North Carolina Academy of Family Physicians, the North Carolina Pediatric Society, the North Carolina Division of Medical Assistance, the North Carolina Oral Health Section, the University of North Carolina School of Dentistry, and the University of North Carolina School of Public Health. Grant funding has been provided by the Centers for Disease Control, the Center for Medicare and Medicaid Services, the Health Resources and Services Administration, and, most recently, the State Oral Health Collaborative Systems. The objective of the "Into the Mouths of Babes" program is to train medical providers to deliver preventive oral health services to high-risk children from the time of tooth eruption until the third birthday, including oral screening, parent/caregiver education, and fluoride varnish application. Since year 2000, medical and dental services have increased 30-fold with participation by 425 practices and local health departments, training of more than 3000 providers, and more than 100,000 visits per year. Services now are provided in every county in the state; formerly one third of the counties did not have these services. Because of dentist referrals, there is a significant increase in the use of restorative care with improved dental health.[36]

Community Dental Care in Texas has provided dental care and education about the prevention of oral disease to low-income families for more than 4 decades by working with local school districts and county health agencies to provide dental services through seven strategically located Community Dental Centers. Since 1982, the population of Community Dental Care's service area has increased by more than 1 million people. The organization now operates 11 Community Dental Centers and is the largest nonprofit provider of dental care to low-income individuals in Texas. Community Dental Care has partnerships with Baylor College of Dentistry and five Dallas County clinics and has conveniently co-located dental programs with community primary health care centers. In 1997, Community Dental Care and Baylor's College of Dentistry entered into a program to incorporate undergraduate students into the Community Dental Care staff, and in 1998, graduate pediatric residents were added. A staff of 70 dentists, dental assistants, and hygienists provides care and dental health education to children, adults, and senior citizens. The patient base includes the homeless, patients who have HIV/AIDS, low-income expectant mothers, and persons who have physical or mental disorders.[37]

The Choptank Community Health System is an FQHC that received more than $3 million in Health Resources Services Administration funding in 2007. This amount is less than 30% of the annual operating budget, which exceeds $10 million. Federal funding supports services to the uninsured and provides additional enabling services for all patients. The Choptank Community Health System offers services to all in need and maintains appropriate services for a diverse community through seven primary care facilities and programs for migrant health, school-based wellness, and pharmacy assistance. A dental program started in 2000 with BlueCross BlueShield and federal block grant funding, expanded to a second primary care facility in 2005, and linked to school-based programs by providing dental screenings and preventive care. In 2005, the Choptank Community Health System partnered with a regional hospital system and Area Health Education Center to create a hospital-based pediatric dental surgery program.[38]

The Ohio State University Geriatric Dentistry Program, Appalachian Outreach Project provides dental service in Appalachian Ohio, which has high unemployment, high poverty rates, substandard housing, and poor access to medical care, including dental services. Supervised senior-year dental students provide community-based basic dental services using mobile dental equipment; patients needing more extensive dental care are referred to the Ohio State University Geriatric Dental Clinic in Columbus. More than 700 older adults had been served through December 2004. The clinic is set up in senior centers, senior housing units, or nutrition sights.[39]

FirstHealth of the Carolinas attempts to meet the health care and dental needs of residents of the mid-Carolinas. In a dental needs assessment, oral health care was cited as the primary unmet need for low-income children in the region, but only 10% of dentists participated in publicly assisted programs. FirstHealth developed an integrated model of dental service delivery by creating an oral health task force to identify strategies to address the lack of access to oral health care. With support from the W. K. Kellogg Foundation and local philanthropies, including the Duke Endowment and the Kate B. Reynolds Charitable Trust, FirstHealth opened a community-based dental care center in three counties. Two of the three dental care centers use existing medical centers, and the third operates in a newly constructed facility. These dental care centers provide comprehensive dental care for more than 7000 children, or nearly 60% of the targeted underserved population.[40]

The Community DentCare delivery system provides oral health services to Northern Manhattan residents across the entire age spectrum, from children in the Head Start program to the elderly. A network of community-based health centers, school-based health centers, neighborhood practices, a mobile dental van, the Columbia University School of Dental and Oral Surgery, and the Harlem Hospital Dental Service are used to deliver care to residents regardless of their ability to pay for services. The Network recorded 50,000 patient visits and provided 7000 school children with preventive dental services in 2003. The DentCare model's success comes from its focus on providing services, building a strong foundation of community-based support, and developing a sustainable funding stream that relies on patient revenue rather than soft-money grant funding.[41]

In 2005, the Health Resources Services Administration initiated the Oral Health Disparities Collaborative pilot study to investigate whether a planned-care model could be applied to manage oral disease within a group of four community health centers. The aim of the collaborative was to develop comprehensive changes in the primary oral health care system that would lead to major improvements in process and outcome measures for perinatal oral health and early childhood caries prevention and treatment. A core principal of the model was to change oral health care from emergency care to outreach, prevention, and proactive management. The four centers have 18 full-time dentists and 360 medical providers and have instituted a physician-training program to screen pregnant women and children from birth to 5 years of age for obvious oral health problems and to provide some initial oral health counseling. Medical staff has access to the dental schedule and provides follow-up counseling to assure that dental treatment and preventive care has been received. Between December 2005 and June 2006, the percentage of pregnant women receiving dental care nearly tripled, and the percentage of very young children in care increased eightfold.[42]

The Head Start Dental Home Initiative is a collaboration of the American Academy of Pediatric Dentistry and the Office of Head Start, which awarded a 5-year, $10 million contract to the American Academy of Pediatric Dentistry to help establish dental homes for approximately 1 million children across America. The objectives of the collaborative are to provide quality dental homes for children, to train teams of dentists and Head Start personnel in optimal oral health care practices, and to assist Head Start programs in obtaining comprehensive services to meet the full range of Head Start children's oral health needs.[43]

INNOVATIONS IN FUNDING
Medicaid

Medicaid is a state and federal partnership to provide health services for designated populations and is the primary source of health care funding for low-income people. The provision of dental services for the adult population is optional but is required for most Medicaid-eligible individuals under the age of 21 years, as specified in the Early and Periodic Screening, Diagnostic and Treatment benefit. This benefit is a mandatory comprehensive child health program focusing on prevention and early diagnosis, including oral health care. The State Children's Health Insurance Program (SCHIP), similar to Medicaid, is financed jointly by the federal and state governments and is administered by the states. Within broad federal guidelines, each state determines the design of its SCHIP program, eligibility groups, benefit packages, payment levels for coverage, and administrative and operating procedures.[44] Medicaid covers about 29 million poor children, and SCHIP covers an additional 6 million low-income children.[45] In total, 25% of all children and about half of the low-income children are covered through these public programs. Medicaid and SCHIP provide a significant amount of resources to support community-based programs in addition to paying claims to participating dentists in the private sector.

Medicaid and SCHIP improve access to oral health care, but there are conflicting conclusions when survey data are compared with state encounter data summaries. The "Summary Health Statistics for US Children: National Health Interview Survey, 2006" states that 37% of uninsured children had no dental contact for more than 2 years (including those who never had a contact), compared with 17% of children with Medicaid and 13% of children with private health insurance.[46] Medicaid encounter data, however, show a less robust access picture: only 20% of children and adolescents under age 19 years at or below 200% of the federal poverty level received any preventive dental service in 1996.[47] Current Centers for Medicare and Medicaid Service Form-416 data for fiscal year 2006 show that one in three individuals under age 21 years received a dental service during the year. This figure is an increase of 10% from the 2003 data and of 22% from the 2000 data.[48] A National Medical Expenditure Panel survey shows that 35.1% of children under age 21 years covered by public dental care programs had a dental visit in 2006, compared with 58.0% of those who who had private dental coverage.[49] Regardless of how Medicaid dental access is quantified, it is clear that there is need for improvement in access for Medicaid- and SCHIP-eligible children.

Researchers analyzed a year's worth of Medicaid dental claims for children in Alabama (1999) and Georgia (1997), before these states undertook efforts to increase dentist participation in Medicaid, to determine which Medicaid-enrolled children were more likely to receive dental care and what dental services were used most frequently. Researchers found that only 22% of Medicaid-eligible children in Alabama and 39% of comparable children in Georgia received dental care during the study period. In both Alabama and Georgia, nearly one third of the children enrolled in Medicaid who received medical care also received dental care. In contrast, children who did not receive medical care were much less likely to receive dental care (3% in Alabama and 23% in Georgia). The Alabama Medicaid program implemented a dental initiative in October 2000 to recruit and retain dental providers and educate families enrolled in Medicaid about the importance of preventive dental care. Under the initiative, dentists typically were reimbursed at 100% of regular BlueCross BlueShield rates. The Georgia Medicaid program implemented the "Take Five" program in October 2000 to encourage dental providers to serve at least five children enrolled in Medicaid per year. Medicaid reimbursement fees for the 56 most-used dental services were increased significantly.[50] This study demonstrates that improved dental access can be achieved with better medical access by Medicaid recipients and shows ways that states are innovating to further improve access.

The Healthy People 2010 program has set a target of 56% for the proportion of children and adults who use the oral health care system each year.[51] If this goal is applied to Medicaid and SCHIP dental programs, there is a clear need for further innovation to improve access to Medicaid oral health care services for children. In the monograph series "Innovations in Dental Medicaid,"[52] the American Dental Association (ADA) identified three areas of concern that discourage dentist participation and limit access to care: inadequate reimbursement, burdensome program administration, and ineffective outreach and care coordination services. The ADA suggests reimbursements should approach the 75th percentile of charges, meaning that dentists should be paid 25% higher than usual and customary reimbursements. To conserve limited resources, however, the level of reimbursement can be the lowest possible to maintain an adequate network of dentists for access, which typically is 25% to 40% less than average charges. A recent study showed that although increases in provider payments were necessary for the success of the states' reform efforts, they were not sufficient to produce substantial gains in either dentist participation or patients' access to care. The study concludes that, in addition to raising reimbursement rates, Medicaid agencies must revamp their administrative procedures and build partnerships with dental societies.[53]

Commercial dental plans are very innovative in setting reimbursement rates high enough to maintain a network for plan members while keeping premium costs competitive. In the Michigan Healthy Kids Dental program, the prevailing reimbursement schedule of a commercial carrier was used to increase access by 31.4% overall and by 39% for children who were enrolled continuously for 12 months, when compared with the previous year under Medicaid. The increase in dentists' participation and in their locations cut the distance traveled by patients for appointments in half. Costs were 2.5 times higher because of the increased access, because more children received care that shifted to more comprehensive care.[54]

Burdensome program administration can be corrected by employing the efficient benefit management systems used by commercial dental insurance. Administrative efficiencies also can be gained by eliminating pre-certification requirements, by the use of advanced claim process platforms that use standard dental codes, electronic claims processing, and other electronic data transfer systems, and by online provider credentialing with streamlined provider enrollment.

The final innovation highlighted in the ADA dental Medicaid monographs is outreach, which is a systematic attempt to provide services beyond conventional limits for a particular segment of a community. Outreach includes education and engagement of the members of the community for ongoing assistance and service coordination to achieve access to oral health care service.[55] Many Medicaid and SCHIP enrollees encounter significant barriers to accessing dental care that often cannot be addressed by the patient's family or community: transportation, availability of a parent or guardian to accompany a minor, distrust of the dental care delivery system, language and cultural differences, and lack of understanding of the importance of good oral health. Innovative outreach programs, as described in the article by Doris and colleagues elsewhere in this issue, attempt to address these barriers.

Examples of Dental Professional Foundations

The California Dental Association Foundation is the philanthropic affiliate of the California Dental Association. Its mission is to improve the oral health of Californians by supporting dental health professionals and to meet community needs. The purpose of the California Dental Association Foundation is to promote the concept that oral health and general health are inseparable and to provide grants to community-based organizations and individuals to reduce disparities in access to oral health care. Grants have been provided to support migrant oral health care, care for low-income children, a mobile clinic serving geriatric and other underserved populations, and programs to integrate preventive services into community-based primary care sites.[56]

The Children's Dental Care Foundation is an affiliate of Cincinnati Children's Hospital Medical Center and was incorporated in 1955 to provide care for underserved children with dental care needs and special medical conditions. The Foundation was one of the nation's first centers providing dental care for handicapped children and postgraduate training in pediatric dentistry. The Foundation annually provides funding for more than 30 children who live throughout the Greater Cincinnati area and who need significant dental care but otherwise could not afford it. Financial assistance is available for a variety of dental needs for well children and those who have medical, mental, and physical challenges. The Children's Dental Care Foundation funds research and training to support the pediatric dental residents at Cincinnati Children's and the dental professionals who are serving the children with the most serious oral health needs in the community.[57]

The National Foundation of Dentistry for the Handicapped operates the Donated Dental Services (DDS) program in which more than 13,000 dentists and 3000 dental laboratories provide comprehensive dental care for disabled, elderly, or medically compromised individuals who cannot afford necessary treatment and do not receive public assistance. Medicare has no dental benefits, and Medicaid primarily provides dental care to children and pregnant mothers. DDS serves disabled and/or low-income adults who have dental needs. At least one DDS coordinator in each state screens applicants and refers eligible patients to volunteer dentists. Dental care is pro bono, and laboratory costs are donated or discounted. In fiscal year 2007, volunteers provided $16.4 million in dental services for 6258 people.[58]

Private Foundations and Public Agency Partnerships

The Rhode Island Oral Health Access Project is a partnership between the Rhode Island Department of Human Services, The Rhode Island Foundation, and Rhode Island KIDS COUNT program and is funded by the Robert Wood Johnson Foundation. The purpose of the Project is to increase access to dental services for children and families covered by Medicaid and for underserved citizens. In 2004, 14 new grants totaling $737,308 were made to increase the number of dental professionals, to support community-based health organizations providing oral health services, and to expand school-based dental examinations and treatment.[59]

The Health Foundation of Greater Cincinnati provided $190,400 to establish Bellevue Dental Services to provide dental services for low-income and uninsured patients in northern Kentucky. Four dental operatories were equipped for the Bellevue Health Center, and staff were hired, including a full-time dentist, a dental hygienist, and support staff. The clinic opened on December 15, 2005, and achieved two times the projected patient load in the first year of operation. It now employs an additional full-time dentist. From January 1 through December 31, 2006, 2957 patients were seen in 7598 visits. A total of $910,000 in patient revenue was generated.[60]

The W.K. Kellogg Foundation funded the Community Voices New Mexico initiative through the University of New Mexico Health Sciences Center. In 1999, there was a chronic shortage of dentists in both rural and urban New Mexico. A majority of New Mexicans, especially rural residents, could not get the oral health care they needed. Activities to improve access include increasing the number of oral health providers, enhancing the skills of dentists and providers already in place within communities in need, expanding the number of practitioners providing service for uninsured community members by increasing the reimbursements received from Medicaid, creating interdisciplinary health care teams in which primary care physicians can work together with dental hygienists, and creating and encouraging more comprehensive oral health policy. In underserved areas the number of patient visits grew from 580 in 1999 to 9000 in 2000, with estimates of more than 15,000 patient visits in 2001.[61]

The Quantum Foundation provided $175,000 to the Palm Beach County, Florida Health Department to expand the School-Based Dental Sealant Project, which began in 1997 at eight elementary schools. The program was expanded to 13 elementary schools in 2001. It provided 1122 dental screenings to second graders and placed sealants on 2590 first molars. Each of the children screened received a form to take home to parents advising the parents of the status of the child's oral health.[62]

Innovations in Dental Insurance

The business of dental insurance plans is to provide access to oral health services for plan subscribers by reducing costs through discounting reimbursements from the usual charges paid to dentists. The number of participating dentists and their locations directly affect plan members' ability to access care. Dental plans must balance the premiums charged to participate in the plan with covered services and their limitations and the reimbursements paid to dentists. To remain competitive and cost effective, dental plans must attract enough dentists willing to accept discounted reimbursements. The amount of discount dentists will accept varies by geographic location and dental specialty, but other variables in addition to the discount level affect a dentist's willingness to participate. Actuarial analysis of plan allowances and network dentist participation indicates that the way dentists are recruited to participate, the use of provider-specific targeted allowances, and the volume of dentists already participating in a specified area are factors that seem to affect participation rates.[63] Dentists may participate in dental plans out of fear they will not have adequate patients or income or with the hope that plan participation somehow will give the dentist a positive credential. Conversely, dentists in certain regions may collectively not participate in dental plans, and some have been charged with conspiracy in this practice.[64] Dental plan administrators innovate to maintain an adequate network while controlling care costs by recruiting dentists who already participate with a competitive plan, negotiating allowances, offering reimbursement guarantees to dentists in underserved areas, offering "value added" benefits such as discounted supplies, laboratory services, and education programs, and employing provider representatives to train dental offices in optimizing the use of dental benefits and improving administrative efficiencies.

DENTAL EDUCATION

In addition to developing professional skills in future dentists, dental schools are responding to issues regarding access to oral health care with initiatives to increase minority enrollment in dental school, to conduct clinical programs in dentally underserved areas, to provide didactic programs in public health, health services delivery, and population-based care, to increase awareness of oral health care access and social justice issues, and to advocate for programs that address disparities on health care.[65] The most effective way to reduce disparities in health care is to increase the representation of minority of students, because minority dentists tend to return to their communities, which can be underserved.[66]

The American Dental Education Association and the Association of American Medical Colleges created the Summer Medical and Dental Education Program to enroll students from disadvantaged backgrounds to spend 6 weeks at an academic campus gaining clinical experience, academic training, learning skills, and career-planning experiences.[67] African American dentists in Texas practice in lower socio-economic, predominantly African American, areas,[68] but the number of Kentucky dental students recruited from the Appalachian region of Kentucky and returning to their home area declined in the last 10 years of a 30-year survey of graduates, possibly because of the rising cost of dental education and increased student debt.[69] The Robert Wood Johnson Foundation program, "Pipeline Profession & Practice: Community-Based Dental Education," demonstrated that 15 dental schools potentially could improve access to care through their educational programs by enhancing recruitment of students of color or from disadvantaged backgrounds. First-year enrollment of minority students nearly doubled, from 6.5% to 12%, over 5 years. In addition, time spent in community clinics doubled from 2 to 10 weeks. A second round of funding will allow additional dental schools to put strategies in place to increase the enrollment of minorities.[70]

The American Dental Education Association reported on three allied dental work-force models that could expand dental personnel, particularly for underserved areas. The models are the advanced dental hygiene practitioner, the community dental health coordinator, and the dental health aide therapist.[71] Specialty training programs leading to licensure of foreign-trained dentists is another innovation in manpower development. The Pediatric Dentistry Fellowship Program of the University of Maryland Dental School provides additional training to pediatric dentists by placing them in urban and rural community-based health care clinics throughout Maryland to provide comprehensive clinical dental care to underserved children, including Head Start children. This program is the only one in which graduates of dental schools outside the United States and Canadian are eligible for full dental licensure in Maryland after completing the fellowship.[72]

EVIDENCE-BASED DENTISTRY

Allocating health care resources toward effective disease prevention and therapeutic interventions can improve access to oral health care by redirecting resources from ineffective care to expand coverage for more people. Evidence-based dentistry is "an approach to oral health care that requires the judicious integration of systematic assessments of clinically relevant scientific evidence, relating to the patient's oral and medical condition and history, with the dentist's clinical expertise and the patient's treatment needs and preferences."[73] Because many oral health care interventions lack rigorous longitudinal, randomized, controlled clinical trials,[74] the strength of the scientific evidence is assessed using a hierarchy of criteria that includes study methodology, analytic strength, and validity. In this way all evidence of efficacy can be considered, even though the validity of any conclusion may be reduced.

Because the use of evidence-based dentistry is a new approach to oral health care efficacy, the potential to improve health outcomes and improve access is not known. Three examples can demonstrate this potential.

First, there is insufficient evidence for the beneficial or harmful effects of changing recall intervals between dental check-ups.[75] The efficacy of the traditional 6-month interval is in doubt. Perhaps a risk-based recall interval, as proposed by the American Academy of Pediatric Dentistry,[76] would be more valid for prevention and early intervention of oral diseases. Saved resources could be redirected to expand population coverage. Considering that diagnostic and preventive dental services consume 30% of the resources of a typical commercial insurance plan,[77] a savings of a few percentage points from the national cost of personal dental services ($96.9 billion in 2007)[78] could provide considerable resources to improve access.

Second, the use of composite restorations for posterior teeth is an example of a new application of an existing technology that had inadequate evidence of efficacy when it was introduced. Indeed, accumulating evidence shows that posterior composite restorations are not as effective as amalgam for restoring posterior teeth.[79,80] Many dentists use posterior composite restorations, however, because of their esthetic qualities and as a reaction to unfounded public concern about amalgam. The additional costs of placing posterior composites, of the replacement of failed restoration, and of additional care resulting from restoration failure have not been determined.

Third, new technologies with unproven benefits may be increasing the cost of oral health care. Localized antimicrobial therapy used as an adjunct to periodontal root planning to treat periodontal inflammation has questionable clinical efficacy.[81] If localized antimicrobial therapy proves to be only marginally effective for treating periodontal disease, the resources applied to this treatment could be redirected to improve access.

SUMMARY

Improving access to oral health care requires an understanding of the social, cultural, political, financial, and manpower factors that influence access. Armed with this knowledge, individuals and organizations desiring to improve access can innovate to change public policy, garner resources, create clinical programs, and expand public health interventions as demonstrated by the examples in this article. Although access to oral health care is a complex and vexing issue, solutions can be found by those who understand the issues, create collaborations, and are persistent in implementing their innovations.

REFERENCES

1. Christen AG, Pronych PM. Painless parker: a dental renegade's fight to make advertising "ethical." Baltimore (MD): National Museum of Dentistry; 1995. p. 451–48.
2. Advertising dentists. Time Magazine; November 2, 1931. Available at: http://www.time.com/time/magazine/article/0,00.html,9168,753095. Accessed September 12, 2008.
3. Schiedermayer DL. The process of de-professionalization: getting down to business in dentistry; the effect of advertising on a profession. J Am Coll Dent 1988; 55(1):10–6.
4. Nolan L, Kamoie B, Jennel H, et al. The effects of state dental practice laws allowing alternative models of preventive oral health care delivery to low-income children. Washington, DC: Center for Health Services Research and Policy; 2003. School of Public Health and Health Services, the George Washington University Medical Center.
5. Hamilton J. Mobile dentistry: entrepreneurial boom spurs debate. AGD Impact 2007;35(12):38–40.
6. Total number of professionally active dentists, 2004–2025 (projected), American Dental Education Association Trends in Dental Education. Available at: http://www5.adea.org/tde/3_1_1_3.htm. Accessed September 14, 2008.
7. Sweis LE, Guay AH. Foreign-trained dentists licensed in the United States: exploring their origins. J Am Dent Assoc 2007;138(2):219–24.
8. American Dental Association Survey Center Survey of predoctoral dental education institutions and various surveys on predoctoral education [unpublished survey data]. Available at: http://jada.ada.org/content/vol138/issue2/images/large/219tbl5.jpeg. Accessed September 14, 2008.
9. Mcguire P. A coming shortage of foreign-trained doctors? Am Col Physicians 2001. Available at: http://www.acponline.org/clinical_information/journals_publications/acp_internisi/sep01/imgs.htm. Accessed September 15, 2008.
10. Mullan F. Plague and politics. New York: Basic Books; 1989. p. 14–31, 112–4.

11. Cunningham HH. Doctors in gray: the confederate medical service. Baton Rouge (LA): Louisiana State University Press; 1993. p. 243, 244–56.
12. Populations receiving optimally fluoridated public drinking water: United States, 1992–2006. MMWR 2008;57(27):737–74 CDC Surveillance Summaries (Atlanta GA). Available at: http://www.cdc.gov/mmwr/preview/mmwrhtml/mm5727a1.htm. Accessed August 15, 2008.
13. Adair SM. Evidence-based use of fluoride in contemporary pediatric dental practice. Pediatr Dent 2006;28(2):133–42 [discussion: 192–8].
14. Klein SP, Bohannan HM, Bell RM, et al. The cost and effectiveness of school-based preventive dental care. Am J Public Health 1985;75(4):382–91.
15. American Dental Association Survey Center. Key dental facts. Chicago (IL): American Dental Association; 2004. p. 17.
16. Progress toward healthy people 2010 targets; midcourse review Healthy People 2010 oral health. Available at: http://www.healthypeople.gov/data/midcourse/html/focusareas/FA21ProgressHP.htm. Accessed October 20, 2008.
17. Crozier S. Louisiana law clears path for fluoridation. ADA News 2008;39(14):1,14.
18. Smokeless does not mean harmless. National Spit Tobacco Education Program. Available at: http://www.nstep.org/index.htm. Accessed September 17, 2008.
19. Nevada State Health Division. Prevention and detection of oral cancer website. Available at: http://health.nv.gov/index.php?option=com_content&task=view&id=342&Itemid=539. Accessed September 17, 2008.
20. Canto MT, Horowitz AM, Drury TF, et al. Maryland family physicians' knowledge, opinions and practices about oral cancer. Oral Oncol 2002;38(5):416–24.
21. Association of State and Territorial Dental Directors. Dental public health activities & practices. Available at: http://www.astdd.org/bestpractices/pdf/DES16003ILcancerplan.pdf. Accessed September 18, 2008.
22. Pickles WN. Epidemiology in country practice. Baltimore (MD): Williams and Wilkins; 1939.
23. Community oriented primary care: new directions for health services delivery. Washington, DC: Institute of Medicine; 1983. Board on Health Care Services.
24. Medical Expenditure Panel Survey 1996. Analysis by center for cost and financing studies. Rockville (MD): Agency for Healthcare Research and Quality; 2000.
25. National Center for Health Statistics. Prevalence of selected chronic conditions: United States, 1990–92. Series 10: data from the national health survey no. 194. Hyattsville (MD): U.S. Department of Health and Human Services, Centers for Disease Control and Prevention; DHHS Pub. no. PH-S97-1522, 1997.
26. Utilization of professional care: what do we know about the relationship of oral health and use of dental services? Table 4.3; Percentage of persons 25 years of age and older with a dental visit within the previous year, by selected patient characteristics, selected years. Available at: http://www2.nidcr.nih.gov/sgr/sgrohweb/tables/table43.htm. Accessed August 20, 2008.
27. Health Resources and Services Administration National Health Service Corps. Available at: http://nhsc.bhpr.hrsa.gov/about/. Accessed October 21, 2008.
28. US Department of Health and Human Services. Oral health in America: a report of the surgeon general. Rockville (MD): U.S. Department of Health and Human Services, National Institute of Dental and Craniofacial Research, National Institutes of Health, 2000. p. 237
29. Shortage designation: HPSAs, MUAs & MUPs; US Department of Health and Human Services, Health Resources and Services Administration. Available at: http://bhpr.hrsa.gov/shortage/. Accessed August 25, 2008.

30. Area Health Education Centers; US Department of Health and Human Services, Health Resources and Services Administration, Bureau of Health Professions. Available at: http://bhpr.hrsa.gov/ahec. Accessed August 25, 2008.

31. Federally Qualified Health Centers (FQHC); US Department of Health and Human Services, Centers for Medicare and Medicaid Services. Available at: http://www.cms.hhs.gov/center/fqhc.asp. Accessed August 25, 2008.

32. Health Resources and Services Administration. Opportunities to use medicaid in support of access to health care services; Oral health services. Available at: http://www.hrsa.gov/medicaidprimer/oral_part3only.htm. Accessed September 18, 2008.

33. Health Resources and Services Administration primary health care. The Health Center Program. Available at: http://bphc.hrsa.gov. Accessed September 10, 2008.

34. Centers for Medicare and Medicaid Direct Graduate Medical Education (DGME). Available at: http://www.cms.hhs.gov/AcuteInpatientPPS/06_dgme.asp. Accessed September 26, 2008.

35. Woodward B. Engaging consumers and providers: education to improve access to dental services. In: developing comprehensive oral health policy symposium: challenges and opportunities for state health policy makers. Baltimore (MD): The Hilltop Institute; 2008.

36. NC Oral Health Section. Into the mouths of babes. Available at: http://www.communityhealth.dhhs.state.nc.us/dental/Into_the_Mouths_of_Babes.htm. Accessed September 8, 2008.

37. Community dental care. Available at: http://www.communitydentalcare.org/who.html#services. Accessed September 8, 2008.

38. Choptank Community Health System annual report 2007. Available at: http://www.medbankmd.org/Choptankhealth.htm. Accessed September 26, 2008.

39. The Ohio State University Geriatric Dentistry Program Appalachian Outreach Project. Area Agency on Aging District 7 (Ohio). Available at: http://www.aaa7.org/appdentistry2.htm. Accessed September 18, 2008.

40. First Health of the Carolinas. Available at: http://www.firsthealth.org. Accessed September 18, 2008.

41. WK Kellogg Foundation Lessons from three innovative models; case study in community dental care. Available at: http://www.wkkf.org/oralhealth/InteriorPage.aspx?PageID=38&LanguageID=0. Accessed September 18, 2008.

42. Institute for Health Improvement. Better oral health for mothers and children. Available at: http://www.ihi.org/IHI/Topics/ChronicConditions/AllConditions/ImprovementStories/FSBetterOralHealthforMothersandChildren.htm. Accessed September 19, 2008.

43. The Head Start Dental Home Initiative partnering to provide dental homes and optimal oral health for Head Start children throughout the U.S. Available at: http://www.aapd.org/members/headstart/files/January2008HS.pdf. Accessed September 19, 2008.

44. Center for Medicare and Medicaid and SCHIP. Available at: http://www.cms.hhs.gov/home/medicaid.asp. Accessed September 26, 2008.

45. Dental coverage and care for low-income children: the role of Medicaid and SCHIP. The Kaiser Commission on Medicaid and uninsured. Available at: http://www.kff.org/medicaid/upload/7681-02.pdf. Accessed August 26, 2008.

46. Summary health statistics for US children: National Health Interview Survey, 2006. Vital Health Stat 2007;10(234):6–7.

47. U.S. Department of Health and Human Services, Office of Inspector General; Children's dental services under Medicaid: access and utilization. Washington, DC 1996. Pub. No. OEI-09-93-00240. Available at: http://www.oig.hhs.gov/oei/reports/oei-09-93-00240.pdf. Accessed September 15, 2008.
48. Hearings before the House Oversight and Government Reform Subcommittee on Domestic Policy. 110th Cong., 1st Sess. (2008) (testimony of Dennis G. Smith, Director, Center for Medicaid & State Operations Centers for Medicare & Medicaid Services on issues with pediatric dental services in the Medicaid program).
49. Manski RJ, Brown E. Dental coverage of children and young adults under age 21, United States, 1996 and 2006. Medical Expenditure Panel Survey Agency for Healthcare Research and Quality Statistical Brief #221. September 2008. Available at: http://www.meps.ahrq.gov/mepsweb/data_stats/Pub_ProdResults_Details.jsp?pt=Chartbook&opt=2&id=827. Accessed November 15, 2008.
50. Children's dental care access in Medicaid, the role of medical care use and dentist participation. Agency for Healthcare Research and Quality. Available at: http://www.ahrq.gov/chiri/chirident.htm. Accessed September 18, 2008.
51. Health People 2010 oral health. Available at: http://www.healthypeople.gov/document/html/volume2/21oral.htm. Accessed September 26, 2008.
52. Innovations in dental medicaid. Chicago: American Dental Association; March 2004.
53. National Academy for State Health Policy. Increasing access to dental care in Medicaid: does raising provider rates work? Available at: http://www.chcf.org/topics/medi-cal/index.cfm?itemID=133606. Accessed September 19, 2008.
54. Eklund SA, Pittman JL, Clark SJ. Michigan Medicaid's Healthy Kids dental program: an assessment of the first 12 months. J Am Dent Assoc 2003; 134(11):1509–15.
55. Outreach. Available at: http://en.wikipedia.org/wiki/Outreach. Accessed September 26, 2008.
56. California Dental Foundation. Available at: http://www.cdafoundation.org/impact/cda_foundation_grant_program_recipients. Accessed September 3, 2008.
57. Children's Dental Care Foundation. Available at: http://www.cincinnatichildrens.org/svc/alpha/c/dental/default.htm. Accessed September 4, 2008.
58. Volunteer dental opportunities. National Foundation of Dentistry for the Handicapped. Available at: http://nfdh.org/joomla_nfdh/content/view/16/37. Accessed September 5, 2008.
59. Rhode Island Oral Health Access Project. Oral health access grant program technical assistance grants. Available at: http://www.rikidscount.org/matriarch/documents/Dental%20RFP%281%29.pdf. Accessed September 6, 2008.
60. The Health Foundation of Greater Cincinnati HealthPoint Family Care. Available at: http://www.healthfoundation.org/grants/organizations/healthpoint.html. Accessed September 6, 2008.
61. Community Voices New Mexico Program. Improving oral health of underserved residents. Available at: http://www.wkkf.org/default.aspx?tabid=102&CID=7&CatID=7&ItemID=70187&NID=20&LanguageID=0. Accessed September 6, 2008.
62. Quantum Foundation $175,000 to expand school-based dental sealant program. Available at: http://www.quantumfoundation.org/public/news/index.cfm?fuseaction=one_news&content_id=22. Accessed September 6, 2008.
63. Woodley RA, Groffman A. Measuring the value of your dental network through competitive intelligence. Presented at the Dental Benefits Summit. Orlando (FL), February 25–26, 2008.

64. United States of America before the Federal Trade Commission; Puerto Rico Association of Endodontist Corp.; Docket C-4166; Decision and Order. August 24, 2006.

65. Graham BS. Educating dental students about oral health care access disparities. J Dent Educ 2006;70(11):1208–11.

66. Smedley BD, Stith AY, Colburn L, et al. The right thing to do, the smart thing to do; enhancing diversity in the health professions. Institute of Medicine. Washington, DC: National Academy Press; 2001. p. 57–90.

67. Summer medical and dental education program. Available at: http://www.smdep.org/. Accessed September 26, 2008.

68. Solomon ES, Williams CR, Sinford JC. Practice location characteristics of black dentists in Texas. J Dent Educ 2001;65(6):571–5.

69. Osborne PB, Haubenreich JE. Underserved region recruitment and return to practice: a thirty-year analysis. J Dent Educ 2003;67(5):505–8.

70. Pipeline profession, practice. Community based dental education. Available at: http://www.dentalpipeline.org. Accessed September 26, 2008.

71. McKinnon M, Luke G, Bresch J, et al. Emerging allied dental workforce models: considerations for academic dental institutions. J Dent Educ 2007;71(11): 1476–91.

72. Pediatric Dentistry Fellowship Program. Baltimore College of Dental Surgery, Dental School, University of Maryland. Available at: http://www.dental.umaryland.edu/dentaldepts/pediatric/fellowship.html. Accessed September 6, 2008.

73. American Dental Association glossary of terms. Available at: http://www.ada.org/prof/resources/ebd/glossary.asp#ebd. Accessed August 13, 2008.

74. Hayden WJ. Dental health services research utilizing comprehensive clinical databases and information technology. J Dent Educ 1997;61(1):47–55.

75. Beirne PV, Clarkson JE, Worthington HV. Recall intervals for oral health in primary care patients. The Cochrane Collaboration. Available at: www.cochrane.org/reviews/en/ab004346.html. Accessed August 13, 2008.

76. Guideline on periodicity of examination, preventive dental services, anticipatory guidance/counseling, and oral treatment for infants, children, and adolescents. American Academy of Pediatric Dentistry 2008-09 Definitions, Oral Health Policies, and Clinical Guidelines 2008;29(7):102–8.

77. Del Aguila MA, Anderson M, et al. Patterns of oral care in a Washington state dental service population. J Am Dent Assoc 2002;133(3):343–51.

78. National Health Expenditure Data. Centers for Medicare and Medicaid Services. Available at: http://www.cms.hhs.gov/NationalHealthExpendData/03_NationalHealthAccountsProjected.asp#TopOfPage. Accessed September 15, 2008.

79. Hickel R, Manhart J, García-Godoy F. Clinical results and new developments of direct posterior restorations. Am J Dent 2000;13(Spec No):41D–54D.

80. Bernardo M, Luis H, Martin MD, et al. Survival and reasons for failure of amalgam versus composite posterior restorations placed in a randomized clinical trial. J Evid Based Dent Pract 2008;8(2):83–4.

81. Arthur JB, Kathleen N, Lohr LL, et al. Effectiveness of antimicrobial adjuncts to scaling and root-planing therapy for periodontitis. Agency for Healthcare Research and Quality. Available at: http://www.ncbi.nlm.nih.gov/books/bv.fcgi?rid=hstat1a.chapter.7321. Accessed September 26, 2008.

Index

Note: Page numbers of article titles are in **boldface** type.

A

Advanced Dental Health Practitioner (ADHP), 563, 564
Age, as barrier to oral health care, 525
Alcohol consumption, and tobacco use, oral and pharyngeal cancers and, 592
American Dental Association (ADA), advertising by dentists and, 590
   American Indian/Alaska Native Oral Health Assess Summit, 531
   National Oral Health Literacy Advisory Committee (NOHLAC), 531
   recommendations for improvement of oral health of underserved, 527, 529
American Dental Education Association (ADEA), 564, 600, 601
American Dental Hygienists Association (ADHA), 562, 563
Association of American Medical Colleges, 600

B

Bon Secours Health System, Inc., 427

C

Cancer(s), oral, 406
   and pharyngeal, tobacco use and alcohol consumption and, 592
   prevention and detection of, 592
CARES model, 549
   community outreach programs of, 553
   education and, 553
   for improving patient retention and access to care, as social work in dentistry, **549–558**
   growth of, 550–551
   origins of, 550
   research and, 554–557
      demographic information of, 555–557
   services provided by, 552–553
   transportation and, 552–553
   use in financial problems, 552
   use in mental health problems, 553
Caries, 401–404
   clinical risk assessment of, 514, 515–516
   decline in, fluoride exposure and, 436
   incidence of, 402, 403
   primary prevention of, 402–403
   secondary prevention of, 403
   tertiary prevention of, 403–404
Centers for Disease Control and Prevention (CDC), 532

Dent Clin N Am 53 (2009) 609–615
doi:10.1016/S0011-8532(09)00046-9
0011-8532/09/$ – see front matter © 2009 Elsevier Inc. All rights reserved.

dental.theclinics.com

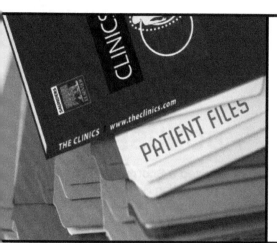
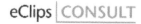
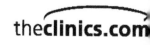

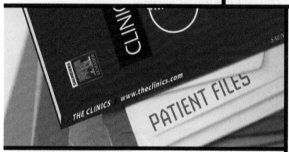

Moving?

Make sure your subscription moves with you!

To notify us of your new address, find your **Clinics Account Number** (located on your mailing label above your name), and contact customer service at:

E-mail: elspcs@elsevier.com

800-654-2452 (subscribers in the U.S. & Canada)
314-453-7041 (subscribers outside of the U.S. & Canada)

Fax number: 314-523-5170

Elsevier Periodicals Customer Service
11830 Westline Industrial Drive
St. Louis, MO 63146

*To ensure uninterrupted delivery of your subscription, please notify us at least 4 weeks in advance of move.

ELSEVIER

Printed and bound by CPI Group (UK) Ltd, Croydon, CR0 4YY

03/10/2024

01040463-0003